The Brain and Behavior

An Introduction to Behavioral Neuroanatomy

Second Edition

This new edition of *The Brain and Behavior* builds on the success of the previous edition and retains the core aim of providing an accessible introduction to behavioral neuroanatomy. Human behavior is a direct reflection of the anatomy of the central nervous system, and it is the goal of the behavioral neuroscientist to uncover the neuroanatomical basis of behavior. Recent developments in neuroimaging technologies have led to significant advances on this front.

The text is presented in a highly structured and organized format to help the reader distinguish between issues of anatomical, behavioral, and physiological relevance. Simplified and clear diagrams are provided throughout the chapters to illustrate key points. Case examples are explored to set the neuroanatomy in the context of clinical experience.

The book is written for behavioral clinicians, trainees, residents, and students, and will also be of interest to psychiatrists, psychologists, neurologists, and neuroscientists seeking an accessible overview of behavioral neuroanatomy.

David L. Clark is Associate Professor in the School of Biomedical Sciences at The Ohio State University.

Nashaat N. Boutros is Professor of Psychiatry and Neurology, Department of Psychiatry and Behavioral Neurosciences, Wayne State University School of Medicine.

Mario F. Mendez is Director of the Neurobehavior Unit for the Veterans Affairs Greater Los Angeles Healthcare System.

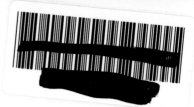

The **Brain**
and **Behavior**

An Introduction to Behavioral Neuroanatomy

David L. Clark

The Ohio State University

Nashaat N. Boutros

Wayne State University School of Medicine

Mario F. Mendez

David Geffen School of Medicine at UCLA

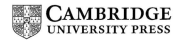

CAMBRIDGE
UNIVERSITY PRESS

CAMBRIDGE UNIVERSITY PRESS

Cambridge, New York, Melbourne, Madrid, Cape Town, Singapore, São Paulo

CAMBRIDGE UNIVERSITY PRESS

The Edinburgh Building, Cambridge CB2 2RU, UK

Published in the United States of America by Cambridge University Press, New York

www.cambridge.org
Information on this title: www.cambridge.org/9780521840503

© D. L. Clark, N. N. Boutros & M. F. Mendez 2005

First published 2005

Printed in the United Kingdom at the University Press, Cambridge

A catalog record for this publication is available from the British Library

ISBN-13 978-0-521-84050-7 hardback
ISBN-10 0-521-84050-3 hardback
ISBN-13 978-0-521-54984-4 paperback
ISBN-10 0-521-54984-1 paperback

To our wives,
Jane (D.L.C.), Sylvia (N.N.B.), and Mary (M.F.M.)
And to our children,
Jennifer, Julie and Amy (D.L.C.)
Tammer and Alexandria (N.N.B.)
Paul and Mark (M.F.M.)

Contents

Preface

The last ten years has witnessed an explosion in the understanding of the neurochemical and neurophysiological processes that underlie behavior. Our understanding of the pathophysiology of many psychiatric disorders has increased as well. Clinicians are now faced with the overwhelming challenge of the need to keep up with the flood of basic neuroscientific knowledge that appears monthly in scientific journals, as well as the need to assimilate it with an ever-increasing number of reports in the clinical journals that identify structural and biochemical abnormalities associated with clinical disorders. The gap that has always existed between the basic science of neuroanatomy and clinical behavioral science seems to be widening at an increasing rate.

Although the current level of knowledge of behavior and psychopathology does not necessitate a detailed understanding of all neuroanatomy, a basic level of some neuroanatomical knowledge is necessary. Familiarity with those brain regions that are heavily implicated in both normal and abnormal behavior will help the clinician assimilate new knowledge as the field evolves. As the clinician becomes more aware of the structure and function of the behaviorally sensitive regions of the brain, the concept that brain abnormalities can produce the symptomatology that is seen in the clinic becomes progressively more understandable.

Currently available neuroanatomy books are written with the neurologist in mind. Emphasis is placed on the neuroanatomy that is examined during a standard neurological exam. Areas that are known to be heavily involved in behavior such as the nucleus accumbens and the nucleus locus ceruleus receive only passing mention. We wrote this volume with the behavioral clinician in mind. It is meant to be an introduction rather than a comprehensive neuroanatomy text. We hope to be able to convey the immense complexity of the neuronal circuitry that subserves our cognitive and emotional lives. At the same time we hope to present the reader with a simplified view of the complexity of the neuroanatomy that underlies certain behaviors.

We will have accomplished our mission if we can convince the reader that the brain is an organ worthy of being the seat for the immensely complex function of behavior. Each chapter includes a list of suggested texts, as well as selected references for those who find the topic interesting and would like further details.

In preparing this volume many sources were utilized (textbooks and published articles). We encountered some discrepancies, particularly in the description of anatomical regions subserving behavior. We either elected to exclude that particular detail or chose the version compatible with the excellent and highly recommended *Principles of Neural Science*, by Kandel, Schwartz and Jessell, and its companion text, *Neuroanatomy: Text and Atlas*, by John Martin. One goal of our book is to provide a summary view of each topic. Every effort has been made to make that view as accurate as possible. Many details have been omitted because of the summary nature of the text. We hope the accuracy of the text has not been distorted by the process of summarization. Please contact us if you find errors in the material or in its interpretation (clark.32@osu.edu, nboutros@med.wayne.edu, mmendez@ucla.edu).

In order to facilitate reading this book, anatomical details appear in regular type, while behavioral implications are in bold type. Physiological implications are in small type. Cross chapter references are provided to help the reader link the related parts of the different chapters. Simplified diagrams are provided throughout the text. Selected material from clinical experience (N.N.B. and M.F.M.) is included to help relate the dry science of neuroanatomy to our everyday clinical encounters. Other clinical material is referenced. It is not the purpose of this book to present a complete picture of what is currently known about behavioral/anatomical relationships. This is the domain of clinical neuropsychiatry, for which many excellent textbooks are now available. Much ongoing research is aimed at defining the neuroanatomical bases of the various psychopathological states. A complete discussion of this research is beyond the scope of this introductory volume. Selected references regarding this fascinating research are included and may be used as starting points for readers who would like to obtain a more complete understanding of one specific area.

Two introductory chapters covering an overall view of the brain are included. Neuroanatomy has its own language. Such language tends to make reading neuroanatomy literature even more difficult. Chapter 1 includes definitions of the more commonly used neuroanatomy terms. Chapter 2 reviews some critical gross brain structures.

Many of the central nervous system (CNS) regions that are thought not to be central to behavior are mentioned only in passing in the two introductory chapters. It should be noted that as knowledge about brain and behavior increases such areas may attain more central positions. A chapter on histology includes an introduction to synaptic structure and to neurotransmission.

The book targets brain areas that are known to be heavily involved in behavior. Each chapter begins with a brief introduction. The majority of each chapter consists of anatomy and behavioral considerations. In some chapters further behavioral considerations are included before the select bibliography and references. We have allowed ourselves to speculate on the possible function of some of the CNS circuits for the purpose of stimulating the reader's interest. The speculative nature of such statements are clearly stated.

We suggest that the reader reads through the entire book at least once to develop an overview of the brain. Be sure to examine the orientation and terminology displayed in Figure 1.1. The reader can then return to individual chapters to develop a further understanding of a particular region.

REFERENCES

Kandel, E. R., Schwartz, J. H., and Jessell, T. M. 2000. *Principles of Neural Science.* New York: Appleton and Lange.

Martin, J. 1996. *Neuroanatomy: Text and Atlas.* New York: Appleton and Lange.

1 Introduction

Human behavior is a direct reflection of the anatomy and physiology of the central nervous system (CNS). The goal of the behavioral neuroscientist is to uncover the neuroanatomical substrates of behavior. Complex mental processes are represented in the brain by their elementary components. Elaborate mental functions consist of subfunctions and are constructed from both serial and parallel interconnections of several brain regions. An introduction to the nervous system covers general terminology and the ventricular system.

Major subdivisions

The nervous system is divided anatomically into the central nervous system (CNS) and the peripheral nervous system (PNS).
- The CNS is made up of the brain and spinal cord.
- The PNS consists of the cranial nerves and spinal nerves.

Physiologically, the nervous system can be divided into somatic and visceral (autonomic) divisions.
- The somatic nervous system deals with the contraction of striated muscle and the sensations of the skin (pain, touch, temperature), the innervation of muscles and joint capsules (proprioception), and the reception of sensations remote to the body by way of special senses. The somatic nervous system senses and controls our interaction with the environment external to the body.
- The autonomic nervous system controls the tone of the smooth muscles and the secretions of glands. It senses and controls the condition of the internal environment.

Common terms

The neuraxis is the long axis of the brain and spinal cord (Figure 1.1). A cross section (transverse section) is a section taken at right angles to the neuraxis. The neuraxis in the human runs as an imaginary straight line through the center of the spinal cord and brainstem (Figure 1.1). At the level of the junction of the midbrain and diencephalon, however, the neuraxis changes orientation and extends from the occipital pole to the

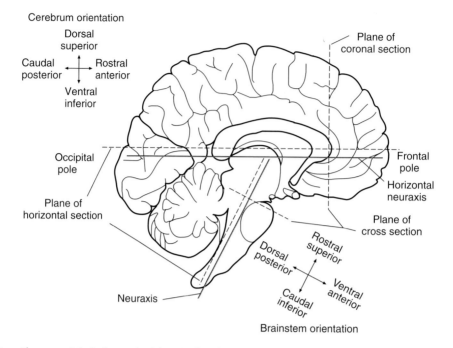

Figure 1.1.   The neuraxis is the long axis of the spinal cord and brain. The neuraxis of the human brain changes at the junction of the midbrain and diencephalon. Caudal to this junction, orientation is as shown in the *lower right* (brainstem orientation). Rostral to this junction, orientation is as shown in the *upper left* (cerebrum orientation).

frontal pole (Figure 1.1). The neuraxis located above the midbrain is the neuraxis of the cerebrum and is sometimes called the *horizontal neuraxis*. A cross section taken perpendicular to the horizontal neuraxis is called a *coronal (frontal) section*.

With regard to the neuraxis of the spinal cord and brainstem:

- *Dorsal* (posterior) means toward the back.
- *Ventral* (anterior) means toward the abdomen.
- *Rostral* means toward the nose.
- *Caudal* means toward the tail.
- The *sagittal (midsagittal) plane* is the vertical plane that passes through the neuraxis. Figure 1.1 is cut in the sagittal plane.
- The *parasagittal plane* is parallel to the sagittal plane but to one side or the other of the midline.
- A *horizontal section* is a cut of tissue taken parallel to the neuraxis (see Figure 9.1).
- A *cross section (transverse section)* is a cut taken perpendicular to the neuraxis (see Figures 10.1–10.4).

With regard to the neuraxis of the cerebrum (horizontal neuraxis):

- *Dorsal (superior)* means toward the top (crown) of the skull.
- *Ventral (inferior)* means toward the base of the skull.
- *Rostral (anterior)* means toward the nose.

- *Caudal (posterior)* means toward the occipital bone of the skull.
- The *sagittal (midsagittal) plane* is the vertical plane that passes through the neuraxis.
- The *parasagittal plane* is parallel to the sagittal plane but to one side or the other of the midline.
- A *horizontal section* is a cut of tissue taken parallel to the horizon.
- A *coronal section (transverse section)* is a cut taken perpendicular to the neuraxis.

Other terms that relate to the CNS:

- *Afferent* means to or toward and is sometimes used to mean sensory.
- *Efferent* means away from and is sometimes used to mean motor.
- *Ipsilateral* refers to the same side; *contralateral* refers to the opposite side.

The CNS differentiates embryologically as a series of subdivisions called encephalons. Each encephalon can be identified in the adult brain. In many regions of the brain, the embryological terminology is applied to adult brain subdivisions:

- The prosencephalon is the most rostral of the embryonic subdivisions and consists of the telencephalon and diencephalon. The cerebrum of the adult corresponds with the prosencephalon.
    - The telencephalon consists of the two cerebral hemispheres. These include the superficial gray matter of the cerebral cortex, the white matter beneath it, and the corpus striatum of the basal ganglia.
    - The diencephalon is made up of the thalamus, the hypothalamus below it, and the epithalamus located above it (pineal and habenula; see Figure 13.5).
- The brainstem lies caudal to the prosencephalon. It consists of the following:
    - The mesencephalon (midbrain).
    - The rhombencephalon, which is made up of the following:
        - The metencephalon, which contains the pons and cerebellum.
        - The myelencephalon (medulla oblongata).

The ventricular system

The central canal of the embryo differentiates into the ventricular system of the adult brain. The ventricular cavities are filled with cerebrospinal fluid (CSF), which is produced by vascular tufts called *choroid plexes*. The ventricular cavity of the telencephalon is represented by the lateral ventricles (Figure 1.2). The lateral ventricles are the first and second ventricles. They connect to the third ventricle of the diencephalon by the interventricular foramina (of Monro). Continuing caudally, the cerebral aqueduct of the midbrain opens into the fourth ventricle. The fourth ventricle occupies the space dorsal to the pons and medulla and ventral to the cerebellum. Cerebrospinal fluid flows from the fourth ventricle to the subarachnoid space through the median aperture (of Magendie) and the lateral apertures (of Luschka). Most of the CSF is produced by the choroid plexus of the lateral ventricles, although tufts of choroid plexus are found in the third and fourth ventricles as well. The fluid circulates through the subarachnoid space and is resorbed

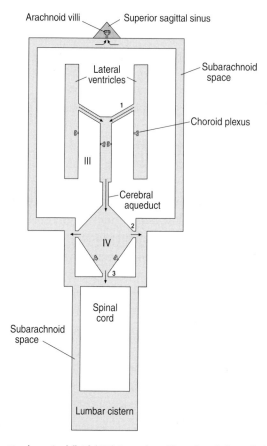

Figure 1.2.   Cerebrospinal fluid (CSF) is produced by tufts of choroid plexus found in all four ventricles. CSF exits the lateral ventricles through the interventricular foramina (of Monro) (1). CSF exits the ventricular system through the lateral apertures (of Luschka) (2) and the median (aperture of Magendie) (3). CSF is reabsorbed into the blood by way of the arachnoid villi that project into the superior sagittal sinus.

into the venous system by way of the arachnoid villi (granulations) that project into the superior sagittal sinus.

The lateral as well as the third ventricles have been noted to be enlarged in a number of psychiatric disorders, particularly schizophrenia (Daniel *et al.,* 1991; Elkis *et al.,* 1995). Enlargement of the ventricles usually reflects atrophy of surrounding brain tissue. The term hydrocephalus is used to describe abnormal enlargement of the ventricles. In the condition known as normal pressure hydrocephalus, the ventricles enlarge in the absence of brain atrophy or obvious obstruction to the flow of the CSF. Normal pressure hydrocephalus is classically characterized by the clinical triad of progressive dementia, ataxia, and incontinence (Friedland, 1989). Dementia accompanied by gait ataxia strongly suggests normal pressure hydrocephalus (Meier *et al.,* 2004). However, symptoms may range from apathy and anhedonia to aggressive or obsessive-compulsive behavior or both (Abbruzzese *et al.,* 1994).

Clinical vignette

A 61-year-old male reported that his work performance was slipping. He was forgetting names and dates more than usual. Because of recent losses in his family, he assumed he was depressed. He saw a psychiatrist (wife had a history of depression), who prescribed an antidepressant. Soon after this he had an episode of urinary incontinence. A neurology consultation was obtained and revealed the presence of gait problems. A computed tomographic scan showed enlarged ventricles without enlarged sulci (which would have indicated generalized brain atrophy). The diagnosis of normal pressure hydrocephalus was made. Progressive improvement of the patient's clinical condition was seen following the installation of a ventricular shunt.

REFERENCES

Abbruzzese, M., Scarone, S., and Colombo, C. 1994. Obsessive-compulsive symptomatology in normal pressure hydrocephalus: a case report. *J. Psychiatr. Neurosci.* **19**:378–380.

Daniel, D. G., Goldberg., T. E., Gibbons, R. D., and Weinberger, D. R. 1991. Lack of a bimodal distribution of ventricular size in schizophrenia: a Gaussian mixture analysis of 1056 cases and controls. *Biol. Psychiatry* **30**:886–903.

Elkis, H., Friedman, L., Wise, A., and Meltzer, H. Y. 1995. Meta-analyses of studies of ventricular enlargement and cortical sulcal prominence in mood disorders. *Arch. Gen. Psychiatry* **52**:735–746.

Friedland, R. P. 1989. Normal-pressure hydrocephalus and the saga of the treatable dementias. *J. Am. Med. Assoc.* **262**:2577–2593.

Meier, U., Konig, A., and Miethke, C. 2004. Predictors of outcome in patients with normal-pressure hydrocephalus. *Eur. J. Neurol.* **51**(2):59–67.

2 Gross anatomy of the brain

The brain is that portion of the central nervous system (CNS) that lies within the skull. Three major subdivisions are recognized: the brainstem, the cerebellum, and the cerebrum. The cerebrum includes both the cerebral hemispheres and the diencephalon.

Brainstem

The brainstem is the rostral continuation of the spinal cord. The foramen magnum, the hole at the base of the skull, marks the junction of the spinal cord and brainstem. The brainstem consists of three subdivisions: the medulla, the pons, and the midbrain (Figure 2.1).

Medulla

The caudal limit of the medulla lies at the foramen magnum. The central canal of the spinal cord expands in the region of the medulla to form the fourth ventricle (IV in Figure 1.2). Cranial nerves associated with the medulla are the hypoglossal, spinal accessory, vagus, and the glossopharyngeal.

Pons

The pons lies above (rostral to) the medulla (see Figure 2.1). The bulk of the medulla is continuous with the pontine tegmentum. The tegmentum consists of nuclei and tracts that lie between the basilar pons and the floor of the fourth ventricle (IV in Figure 1.2; see Figure 10.2). The basilar pons consists of tracts along with nuclei that are associated with the cerebellum. The fourth ventricle narrows at the rostral end of the pons to connect with the cerebral aqueduct of the midbrain (see Figures 1.2, 10.2–10.4). Cranial nerves associated with the pons are the statoacoustic (previously known as the auditory), facial, abducens, and trigeminal.

Midbrain

The dorsal surface of the midbrain is marked by four hillocks, the corpora quadrigemina (tectum). The caudal pair form the inferior colliculi (see Figure 10.3; auditory system); the cranial pair, the superior colliculi (see Figure 10.4; visual system). The ventricular cavity of the midbrain is the cerebral aqueduct. Most nuclei and tracts found in the midbrain lie

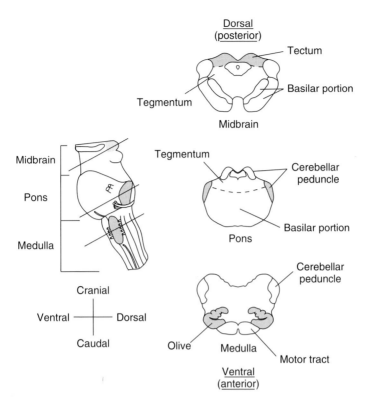

Figure 2.1.   The brainstem consists of the medulla, the pons, and the midbrain. A lateral view of the brainstem (*left*) is marked to indicate the level from which each of the cross sections (*right*) is taken. See Chapter 10 for significant structures found in each cross section. *Cranial* refers to the top of the head, and *caudal* refers to the spinal cord.

ventral to the cerebral aqueduct and together make up the midbrain tegmentum (see Figure 2.1). The basilar midbrain contains the crus cerebri ("motor pathway" in Figures 10.3 and 10.4) and the substantia nigra, one of the basal ganglia. Cranial nerves associated with the midbrain are the trochlear and oculomotor.

Ischemia (particularly transient ischemia) of the midbrain tectum can result in visual hallucinations (peduncular hallucinosis). Auditory hallucinations have also been reported with lesions of the tegmentum of the pons and lower midbrain (Cascino and Adams, 1986). The sounds have the character of noise: buzzing and clanging. To one patient, the sounds reportedly had a musical character like chiming bells.

Clinical vignette
A 71-year-old retired man had no prior history of psychiatric or neurological problems. While at home with his two sons, daughter and wife, he suddenly experienced weakness in all four extremities and started seeing policemen entering the front door of his house. He became irritable and fearful that the police would take him away. He was brought to the emergency room (ER). A neurological examination was normal, and the hallucinations ceased. The patient was released with follow-up at the psychiatry clinic. Three days later he was brought to the ER completely comatose due to a brainstem stroke. In retrospect, the patient's attack was found to be a brainstem transient ischemic attack (TIA), which caused him to experience peduncular hallucinosis.

Cerebellum

The cerebellum arises embryologically from the dorsal pons. In the mature brain the cerebellum overlies the pons and medulla (Figure 2.2) and is connected with them by the three paired cerebellar peduncles (see Figures 10.1 and 10.2). The cerebellum is separated from the pons and medulla by the cavity of the fourth ventricle. Like the cerebrum, it displays a highly convoluted surface. The cortex of the cerebellum is gray and a layer of white matter lies deep to it.

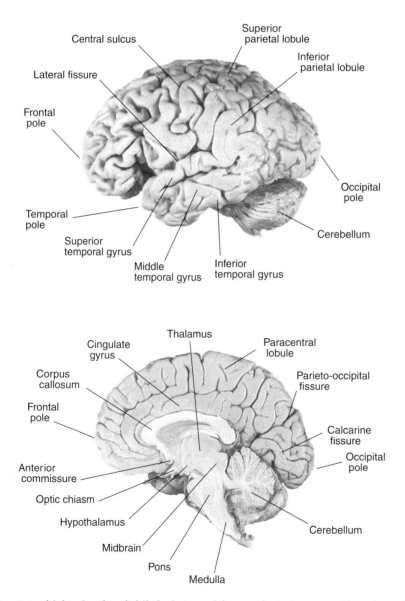

Figure 2.2.   Lateral (*above*) and medial (*below*) views of the gross brain. Compare with Brodmann's areas, Figure 2.3.

Traditionally the cerebellum is thought to be involved in the control and integration of motor functions that subserve coordination, balance, and gait. Accumulating evidence suggests that the cerebellum also plays a role in affective and higher cognitive functions (Berntson and Torello, 1980; Fiez, 1996; Katsetos *et al.*, 1997, an authoritative review). The progressive expansion of the cerebellum and the proliferation and specialization of its connections to the prefrontal cortex in the human may contribute to the enhancement of mental and language skills. Activation of cerebellar nuclear structures has been demonstrated during cognitive processing (Kim *et al.*, 1994). Accumulated evidence suggests that the older cerebellar regions (the medial structures: flocculonodular lobe, vermis, and fastigial and globose nuclei) are associated with limbic functions. The lateral cerebellar lobes (including the dentate and emboliform nuclei) may be more involved with cognitive functions such as strategic planning, learning, memory, and language (see Schmahmann, 1991, for a complete review).

Structural abnormalities of the cerebellar vermis including a loss of tissue volume in chronic schizophrenia have been demonstrated (Jacobsen *et al.*, 1997; Okugawa *et al.*, 2003). The patients evaluated include those with no history of alcoholism or repeated electroconvulsive treatments (Heath *et al.*, 1979). An increase in vermis volume and white matter volume was reported in male schizophrenic patients that correlated with positive symptoms, thought disorder and impaired verbal memory (Levitt *et al.*, 1999). The loss of cerebellar volume is progressive throughout adolescence (Keller *et al.*, 2003) and duration of illness (Velakoulis *et al.*, 2002). Schizophrenic patients prone to auditory hallucinations compared with controls showed bilateral attenuation of activation of the cerebellum, greater on the right, during the perception of auditory verbal imagery (Shergill *et al.*, 2000). Left greater than right cerebellar hemisphere volume suggests a correlation with left greater than right cerebral cortex anomalies (Shenton *et al.*, 2001). It is hypothesized that a cortical–cerebellar–thalamus–cortical–circuit (CCTCC) functions to provide smooth coordination of cognitive as well as motor function (Schmahmann, 1996). A model has been proposed suggesting that abnormalities in connectivity of the CCTCC may be responsible for the "cognitive dysmetria" seen in schizophrenia (Andreasen *et al.*, 1998, 1999).

An increase in blood flow in the cerebellar vermis has been seen in depression (see Figure 6.8; Dolan *et al.*, 1992). The anterior cerebellar vermis has been reported to be significantly smaller using magnetic resonance imaging (Shah *et al.*, 1992) and functionally abnormal based on oculomotor tasks (Sweeney *et al.*, 1998) in patients with major depression. Cerebellar atrophy has been reported in patients with manic symptoms, depression, hyperactivity, and hypersexuality (Lauterbach, 1996, 2001).

Lotspeich and Ciaranello (1993) reviewed studies of autistic subjects in which abnormalities were reported in the cerebellar cortex and the cerebellar nuclei that were consistent with delayed development. A significant correlation between slowed attentional orientation to visual cues and cerebellar hypoplasia was reported in autistic children (Harris *et al.*, 1999). Impairments in procedural learning may also be related to the cerebellar deficit (Mostofsky *et al.*, 2000). The posterior inferior vermis was significantly smaller in males (Mostofsky *et al.*, 1998) and females (Castellanos *et al.*, 2001) with attention-deficit/hyperactivity disorder.

Cerebrum

The diencephalic portion of the cerebrum consists of the thalamus (see Chapter 9), the hypothalamus, and the epithalamus (see Chapter 8). The thalamus is an integrative center through which most sensory information must pass in order to reach the cerebral cortex (i.e., the level of consciousness). The hypothalamus serves as an integrative center for control of the body's internal environment by way of the autonomic nervous system (see Figure 8.1). The pituitary gland (hypophysis) extends ventrally from the base of the hypothalamus. The epithalamus consists of the habenula and pineal gland. The ventricular cavity of the diencephalon is the third ventricle (III in Figure 1.2). The optic nerve is associated with the diencephalon (dotted lines, Figure 8.4).

The cerebral hemisphere includes the cerebral cortex and underlying white matter, as well as a number of nuclei that lie deep to the white matter. Traditionally, these nuclei are referred to as the *basal ganglia* (see Chapter 7). One of these forebrain nuclei, the amygdala (see Figure 11.1), is now included as part of the limbic system (see Chapters 11–13).

The surface of the cortex is marked by ridges (gyri) and grooves (sulci). Several of the sulci are quite deep, earning them the status of fissure. The most prominent fissure is the longitudinal cerebral fissure (sagittal or interhemispheric fissure), which is located in the midline and separates the two hemispheres. Each of the hemispheres is divided into four separate lobes: frontal, parietal, occipital, and temporal.

The frontal lobe lies rostral to the central sulcus and dorsal to the lateral fissure (see Figures 2.2 and 2.3). An imaginary line drawn from the parieto-occipital sulcus to the preoccipital notch separates the occipital lobe from the rest of the brain (see Figure 5.1). A second imaginary line, perpendicular to the first and continuing rostrally with the lateral fissure, divides the parietal lobe above from the temporal lobe below. Spreading the lips of the lateral fissure reveals the smaller insular region deep to the surface of the cortex.

The limbic system (limbic lobe) is made up of contributions from several areas. The parahippocampal gyrus and uncus can be seen on the ventromedial aspect of the temporal lobe (see Figure 5.2). The hippocampus and amygdaloid nucleus lie deep to the ventral surface of the medial temporal lobe (see Figure 11.1), and the cingulate gyrus lies along the deep medial aspect of the cortex (see Figure 12.1). These structures are joined together by fiber bundles and form a crescent or limbus (see Figure 13.1).

The basal ganglia represent an important motor control center.
- The neostriatum is made up of the caudate nucleus and putamen (see Figure 7.1).
- The paleostriatum is also known as the globus pallidus.
- Two additional nuclei that are included as basal ganglia are the subthalamic nucleus (subthalamus) and the substantia nigra.

The internal capsule is made up of fibers that interconnect the cerebral cortex with other subdivisions of the brain and spinal cord. The anterior and posterior commissures as well as the massive corpus callosum interconnect the left side with the right side of the cerebrum.

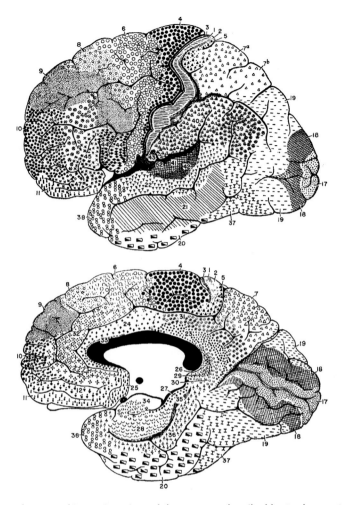

Figure 2.3.   The cytoarchitectonic regions of the cortex as described by Brodmann. Compare with the surface of the brain, Figure 2.2.

Vasculature

Two major systems supply blood to the brain (Figure 2.4). The vertebral arteries represent the posterior supply and course along the ventral surface of the spinal cord, pass through the foramen magnum then merge medially as the basilar artery on the ventral aspect of the medulla. The basilar artery splits at its rostral terminus to form the paired posterior cerebral arteries.

The internal carotid system represents the anterior supply and arises at the carotid bifurcation. Major branches of the internal carotid include the anterior cerebral and the middle cerebral arteries. The vertebral–basilar and internal carotid systems join at the base of the brain to form the cerebral arterial circle (of Willis).

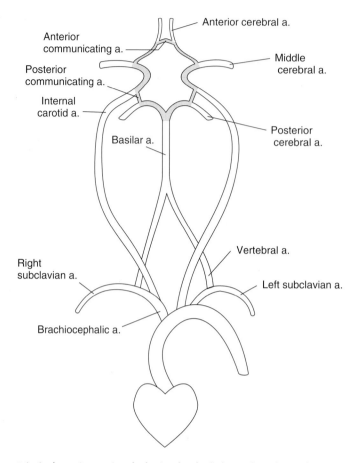

Figure 2.4.   Principal arteries serving the brain. The shaded vessels make up the cerebral arterial circle (of Willis).

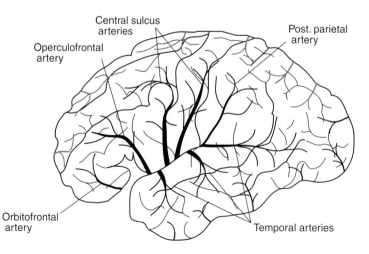

Figure 2.5.   The stippled area represents the cortex served by the middle cerebral artery. The vessels emerging from the longitudinal cerebral fissure represent the area served by the anterior cerebral artery (after Waddington, 1974; compare with Figure 2.6).

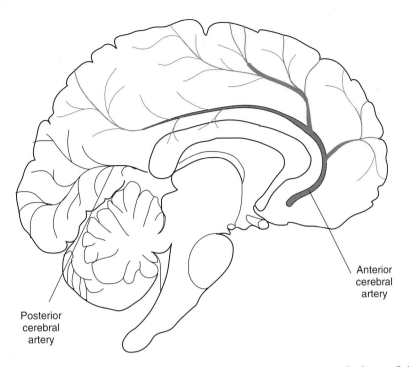

Anterior
cerebral
artery

Posterior
cerebral
artery

Figure 2.6.   The distribution of the anterior cerebral artery (right) and the posterior cerebral artery (left) on the medial aspect of the brain.

The cerebral cortex is served by the three major cerebral arteries (Figures 2.5 and 2.6).

- The anterior cerebral artery supplies the medial aspect of the frontal and parietal cortices, with terminal branches extending a short distance out of the sagittal fissure onto the lateral surface of the brain.
- The posterior cerebral artery serves the medial and most of the lateral aspect of the occipital lobe, as well as portions of the ventral aspect of the temporal lobe.
- The large middle cerebral artery serves the remainder of the cortex, including the majority of the lateral aspect of the frontal, parietal, and temporal cortices.

The blood–brain barrier is a physiological concept based on the observation that many substances including many drugs, which may be in high concentrations in the blood, are not simultaneously found in the brain tissue. The location of the barrier coincides with the endothelial cells of the capillaries found in the brain. These endothelial cells, unlike those found in capillaries elsewhere in the body, are joined together by tight junctions. These tight junctions are recognized as the anatomical basis of the blood–brain barrier.

Blood flow to the brain was reported to be reduced in elderly patients diagnosed with major depressive disorder when compared with age-matched control subjects. Overall blood flow was reduced by 12%. The distribution of the effect was uneven, and there were brain regions in which the reduction was even greater (Sackeim *et al.*, 1990).

Electroencephalogram

The electroencephalogram (EEG) uses large recording electrodes placed on the scalp (Figure 2.7). The activity seen on the EEG represents the summated activity of large ensembles of neurons. More specifically, it is a reflection of the extracellular current flow associated with the summed activity of many individual neurons. Most EEG activity reflects activity in the cortex, but some (e.g., sleep spindles) shows activity in various subcortical structures. The record generated reflects spontaneous voltage fluctuations. Abnormalities in the brain can produce pathological synchronization of neural elements that can be seen, for example, as spike discharges representing seizure activity. The detection of seizure activity is one of the most valuable assets of the EEG.

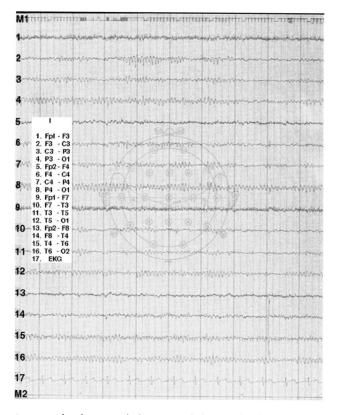

Figure 2.7.   An example of a normal electroencephalogram (EEG). Metal sensors (electrodes) placed on various scalp locations are used to record the electrical activity of the brain. The actual brain electrical signal is amplified 10 000 times before it can be recorded for visual inspection. The various electrodes are electronically connected to form montages. The particular montage used for the example shown is listed on the left of the figure. Note that the rhythmic sinusoidal alpha activity is most developed on the occipital regions (electrodes 4, 8, 12, and 16).

Meninges

The brain and spinal cord are surrounded by three meninges: the dura mater, the arachnoid, and the pia mater. Blood vessels as well as cranial and spinal nerves all pierce the meninges. The pia mater is intimate to the surface of the brain and spinal cord and envelops the blood vessels that course along its surface. The dura mater is a thick, heavy membrane that forms the internal periosteum of the skull. The dura is made up of two layers, and these layers separate at several locations to form venous sinuses such as the superior sagittal sinus (see Figure 1.2). The epidural space and the subdural space are only potential spaces. The arachnoid lies between the pia mater and the dura mater and forms a very thin layer along the inner surface of the dura mater. The subarachnoid space is filled with cerebrospinal fluid.

REFERENCES

Andreasen, N. C., Paradiso, S., and O'Leary, D. S. 1998. "Cognitive dysmetria" as an integrative theory of schizophrenia: a dysfunction in cortical–subcortical–cerebellar circuitry? *Schizophr. Bull.* **24**:203–218.

Andreasen, N. C., Nopoulos, P., O'Leary, D. S., Miller, D. D., Wassink, T., and Falum, M. 1999. Defining the phenotype of schizophrenia: cognitive dysmetria and its neural mechanisms. *Biol. Psychiatry.* **46**(7):908–920.

Berntson, G., and Torello, M. W. 1980. Attenuation of septal hyperemotionality by cerebellar fastigial lesions in the rat. *Physiol. Behav.* **24**:547–551.

Cascino, G. D., and Adams, R. D. 1986. Brainstem auditory hallucinosis. *Neurology* **36**:1042–1047.

Castellanos, F., Xavier, M. D., Giedd, J. N., Berquin, P. C., Walter, J. M., Sharp, W., Tran, T., Vaituzis, A. C., Blumenthal, J. D., Nelson, J., Bastain, T. M., Zijdenbos, A., Evans, A., and Rapoport, J. L. 2001. Quantitative brain magnetic resonance imaging in girls with attention-deficit/hyperactivity disorder. *Arch. Gen. Psychiatr.* **58**(3):289–295.

Dolan, R. J., Bench, C. J., Brown, R. G., Scott, L. C., Friston, K. J., and Frackowiak, R. S. J. 1992. Regional cerebral blood flow abnormalities in depressed patients with cognitive impairment. *J. Neurol. Neurosurg. Psychiatry* **55**:768–773.

Fiez, J. A. 1996. Cerebellar contributions to cognition. *Neuron* **16**:13.

Harris, N. S., Courchesne, E., Townsend, J., Carper, R. A., and Lord, C. 1999. Neuroanatomic contributions to slowed orienting of attention in children with autism. *Brain Res. Cogn. Brain Res.* **8**(1):61–71.

Heath, R. G., Franklin, D. E., and Shraberg, D. 1979. Gross pathology of the cerebellum in patients diagnosed and treated as functional psychiatric disorders. *J. Nerv. Ment. Dis.* **167**:585–592.

Jacobsen, L. K., Giedd, J. N., Berquin, P. C., Krain, A. L., Hamburger, S. D., Kumra, S., and Rapoport, J. L. 1997. Quantitative morphology of the cerebellum and fourth ventricle in childhood-onset schizophrenia. *Am. J. Psychiatry* **154**:1663–1669.

Katsetos, C. D., Hyde, T. M., and Herman, M. M. 1997. Neuropathology of the cerebellum in schizophrenia – an update: 1996 and future directions. *Biol. Psychiatry* **42**:213–224.

Keller, A., Castellanos, X., Vaituzis, C., Jeffries, N. O., Giedd, J. N., and Rapoport, J. 2003. Progressive loss of cerebellar volume in childhood-onset schizophrenia. *Am. J. Psychiatry* **160**:128–133.

Kim, S. -G., Ugurbil, K., and Strick, P. L. 1994. Activation of cerebellar output nucleus during cognitive processing. *Science* **265**:949.

Lauterbach, E. C. 1996. Bipolar disorders, dystonia, and compulsion after dysfunction of the cerebellum, dentatorubrothalamic tract, and substantia nigra. *Biol. Psychiatry* **40**:726–730.

Lauterbach, E. C. 2001. Cerebellar-subcortical circuits and mania in cerebellar disease. *J. Neuropsychiatry Clin. Neurosci.* **13**(1):112.

Levitt, J. J., McCarley, R. W., Nestor, P. G., Petrescu, C., Donnino, R., Hirayasu, Y., Kikinis, R., Jolesz, F. A., and Shenton, M. E. 1999. Quantitative volumetric MRI study of the cerebellum and vermis in schizophrenia: clinical and cognitive correlates. *Am. J. Psychiatry* **156**:1105–1107.

Lotspeich, L. J., and Ciaranello, R. D. 1993. The neurobiology and genetics of infantile autism. *Int. Rev. Neurobiol.* **35**:87–129.

Mostofsky, S. H., Reiss, A. L., Lockhart, P., and Denckla, M. B. 1998. Evaluation of cerebellar size in attention-deficit hyperactivity disorder. *J. Child Neurol.* **13**(9):434–439.

Mostofsky, S. H., Goldberg, M. C., Landa, R. J., and Denckla, M. B. 2000. Evidence for a deficit in procedural learning in children and adolescents with autism: implications for cerebellar contribution. *J. Int. Neuropsychol. Soc.* **6**(7):752–759.

Okugawa, G., Sedvall, G. C., and Agartz, I. 2003. Smaller cerebellar vermis but not hemisphere volumes in patients with chronic schizophrenia. *Am. J. Psychiatry* **160**(9):1614–1617.

Sackeim, H. A., Prohovnik, I., Moeller, J. R., Brown, R. P., Apter, S., Prudic, J., Devanand, D. P., and Mukerjee, S. 1990. Regional cerebral blood flow in mood disorders. I. Comparison of major depressives and normal controls at rest. *Arch. Gen. Psychiatry* **47**:60–70.

Schmahmann, J. D. 1991. An emerging concept. The cerebellar contribution to higher function. *Arch. Neurol.* **48**:1178–1187.

— 1996. From movement to thought: anatomic substrates of the cerebellar contribution to cognitive processing. *Hum. Brain Map.* **4**:174–198.

Shah, S. A., Doraiswamy, P. M., Husain, M. M., Escalona, P. R., Na, C., Figiel, G. S., Patterson, L. J., Ellinwood, E. H. Jr., McDonald, W. M., Boyko, O. B., Nemeroff, C. B., and Krishnan, K. R. R. 1992. Posterior fossa abnormalities in major depression: a controlled magnetic resonance imaging study. *Acta Psychiatr. Scand.* **85**:474–479.

Shenton, M. E., Dickey, C. C., Frumin, M., and McCarley, R. W. 2001. A review of MRI findings in schizophrenia. *Schizophr. Res.* **49**:1–52.

Shergill, S. S., Bullmore, E., Simmons, A., Murray, R., and McGuire, P. 2000. Functional anatomy of auditory verbal imagery in schizophrenic patients with auditory hallucinations. *Am. J. Psychiatry* **157**:1691–1693.

Sweeney, J. A., Strojwas, M. H., Mann, J. J., and Thase, M. E. 1998. Prefrontal and cerebellar abnormalities in major depression: evidence from oculomotor studies. *Biol. Psychiatry* **43**:584–594.

Velakoulis, D., Wood, S. J., Smith, D. J., Soulsby, B., Brewer, W., Leeton, L., Desmond, P., Suckling, J., Bullmore, E. T., McGuire, P. K., and Pantelis, C. 2002. Increased duration of illness is associated with reduced volume in right medial temporal/anterior cingulate grey matter in patients with chronic schizophrenia. *Schizophr. Res.* **57**:43–49.

Waddington, M. M. 1974. *Atlas of Cerebral Angiography with Anatomic Correction.* Boston, Mass.: Little, Brown.

3 Histology

The brain weighs between 1100 and 2000 g. It contains an estimated 100 billion neurons. The average neuron has up to 10 000 synapses. Almost one-third of this immensely complex system is dedicated to the function of behavior.

Anatomy and behavioral considerations

Two types of cells make up the nervous system: neurons and neuroglial cells. Neurons are specialized to conduct bioelectrical messages, whereas the glial cells play a supportive role.

The neuron

The neuron is the structural and functional unit of the nervous system. It is made up of four distinctive regions: the soma (nerve cell body), the dendrites, the axon, and the synapse (Figures 3.1 and 3.4). The soma is the metabolic center of the cell and contains the cell nucleus. The nucleus is centrally located in the soma, and the cytoplasm immediately surrounding the nucleus is called the *perikaryon*. The cytoplasm of the axon is called the *axoplasm*.

Most neurons have several dendrites. Each neuron has a single axon (Figure 3.2). The axon arises from a specialized region of the cell body called the *axon hillock* (see Figure 3.1), which is specialized to facilitate the propagation of the all-or-none action potential.

Nissl substance (rough endoplasmic reticulum) and Golgi apparatus are restricted to the perikaryon and to the base of the dendrites. They synthesize proteins for use throughout the neuron. Three classes of proteins are produced. One of these classes produced in the perikaryon includes the neurotransmitters. Substances to be used in the axon for growth, for membrane repair, and for neurotransmitters must be packaged into vesicles and transported along the axon to the presynaptic axon terminal. Therefore, the axon and its synaptic terminal are dependent on the cell body for their normal function and survival.

Axon

The axon is typically depicted as being many times longer than the dendrites and, in fact, may extend up to a meter from the cell body. Microtubules and neurofilaments (microfilaments) are found in the cytoplasm of axons. Microtubules measure approximately

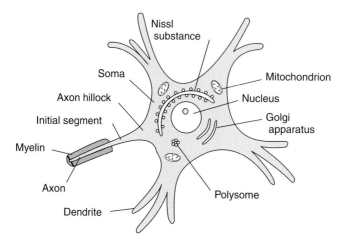

Figure 3.1.   Major components of a typical neuron cell body. The cytoskeleton and lysosomes have been omitted.

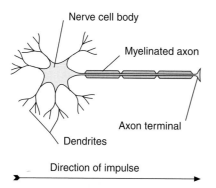

Figure 3.2.   Signals pass from the dendrite to the cell body to the axon of the neuron.

20–25 nm in diameter (nanometer = 1 billionth of a meter = 10 μm), are hollow cylinders, and are made of the protein tubulin. Microtubules are involved in the transport of macromolecules throughout the axon. Neurofilaments are approximately 10 nm in diameter and provide skeletal support for the neuron.

Substances produced in the soma must be transported along the axon in order to reach the cell membrane of the axon as well as the axon terminal (Figure 3.3). Substances are normally thought of as being transported from the soma to the axon terminal. However, transport from the axon terminal back to the soma also occurs.

- Anterograde (orthograde) axon transport carries substances from the soma to the axon terminal. Anterograde transport may be fast (3–4 cm/day) or slow (1–4 mm/day). Fast axon transport moves synaptic vesicles or their precursors via motor molecules along the external surface of microtubules. Organelles, vesicles, and membrane glycoproteins are carried by fast axon transport. Slow axon transport reflects the movement of the

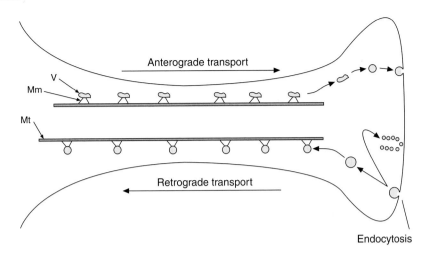

Figure 3.3.   Microtubules are important in fast axon transport. Motor molecules (Mm) attach the vesicles (V) to the microtubules (Mt). Vesicles and mitochondria move at rates of up to 4 cm per day. Microtubules do not extend the entire length of the axon. Vesicles can transfer across overlapping microtubules. Anterograde and retrograde transport can take place at the same time over a single microtubule.

entire axoplasm of the axon. Neurofilaments and components of microtubules are two elements that move by slow axon transport.

- Retrograde axon transport carries substances back from the axon terminal to the nerve cell body. Microtubules are involved in retrograde axon transport, and the speed of transport is about half that of fast anterograde transport. Metabolic by-products and information about the condition of the axon terminal are sent back to the cell body by retrograde transport. Viruses (e.g., herpes, rabies, polio) as well as toxic substances taken up by the nerve terminal may be transported back to the cell body by this same mechanism.

The axon cell membrane is electrically excitable. When at rest, a difference in electrical potential of about 65 mV is maintained across the cell membrane. This electrical potential represents the unequal distribution of ions across the membrane. The difference in ion distribution is maintained by an ion pump. When triggered by events at the axon hillock, pores in the cell membrane open, ions stream across the membrane in the direction opposite to that maintained by the pump, and the axon membrane depolarizes. A wave of electrical depolarization (excitation) is produced that moves from the region of the axon hillock toward the presynaptic axon terminal. This wave of electrical depolarization is called the *action potential*. The axon is covered by an insulating sheath, myelin. The myelin is not continuous along the entire length of the axon but is regularly separated by gaps called *nodes (of Ranvier)*. The axon cell membrane is exposed at the nodes to the extracellular space, and it is at the nodes that the action potential regenerates as it passes down the axon.

Dendrites

Dendrites are extensions of the cell body and expand the receptive surface of the cell. They branch repeatedly and, beginning a short distance from the cell body, are covered by cytoplasmic extensions called *gemmules* or *dendritic spines*. The spines increase the receptive surface area of the dendrites.

Neuron cell membrane

There are four specialized regions of the neuron cell membrane:

- The *receptive region* is represented by the dendrites and, to a lesser extent, the neuron cell body. When the dendrite membrane is depolarized, a wave of negativity passes down the dendrite toward the cell body and the axon hillock. As the wave continues, the amplitude of its voltage decreases because of the resistance inherent in the cell membrane.
- The *trigger region* is represented by the axon hillock. If the wave of negativity from the dendrite is of sufficient magnitude when it arrives at the axon hillock, an all-or-none action potential is produced.
- The *conductance region* of the neuron cell membrane is represented by the axon. Where the axon is myelinated, there are no sodium ion channels and the electrical signal must pass through the cytoplasm to the next node of Ranvier. The neuron cell membrane at the node contains many ion channels where the action potential is renewed.
- The *output region* of the neuron is represented by the axon terminal.

Synapse

The synapse is the junctional complex between the presynaptic axon terminal and the postsynaptic tissue (Figure 3.4). Within the central nervous system (CNS), the postsynaptic tissue is usually another neuron. There are two types of synapses: the electrical synapse and the chemical synapse. Electrical synapses provide for electrotonic coupling between neurons and are found at gap junctions between neurons. They permit bidirectional passage of ions directly from one cell to another. Electrical synapses are found in situations in which rapid stereotyped behavior is needed and are uncommon in the human nervous system.

Electrotonic coupling is found between axons of the neurons of the locus ceruleus (see Chapter 10). It is proposed that these junctions help synchronize the discharge of a small grouping of closely related locus ceruleus neurons to optimize the regulation of tonic and phasic activity of the locus ceruleus (G. Aston-Jones, personal communication, 1998).

A gap (synaptic cleft) exists between the axon terminal and the postsynaptic neuron of a chemical synapse. The chemical synapse can be identified by the large number of synaptic vesicles clustered in the axon terminal on the presynaptic side of the synaptic cleft (Figure 3.4). Each synaptic vesicle is filled with several thousand molecules of a chemical neurotransmitter. The arrival at the axon terminal of the action potential triggers an influx of calcium ions across the axon membrane into the axon terminal (2, in Figure 3.4). The influx of calcium ions causes synaptic vesicles located near the presynaptic membrane to fuse with

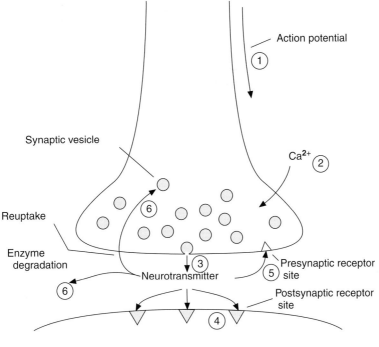

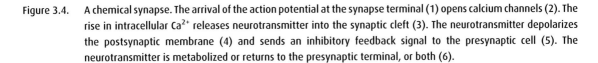

Figure 3.4.   A chemical synapse. The arrival of the action potential at the synapse terminal (1) opens calcium channels (2). The rise in intracellular Ca^{2+} releases neurotransmitter into the synaptic cleft (3). The neurotransmitter depolarizes the postsynaptic membrane (4) and sends an inhibitory feedback signal to the presynaptic cell (5). The neurotransmitter is metabolized or returns to the presynaptic terminal, or both (6).

the membrane and to release neurotransmitter into the synaptic gap (exocytosis; 3, in Figure 3.4).

Chemical transmission consists of two steps. The first is the *transmitting* step, in which the neurotransmitter is released by the presynaptic cell. The second is the *receptive* step, in which the neurotransmitter is bound to the postsynaptic cell. Chemical receptor sites located in the membrane of the postsynaptic cell respond to the presence of a neurotransmitter. In the case of an excitatory neurotransmitter, ion channels in the postsynaptic cell membrane open and the postsynaptic cell membrane depolarizes. Neurotransmitters are potent and typically only two molecules of a neurotransmitter are required to open one postsynaptic ion channel. The response seen in the postsynaptic cell is dependent on the properties of the receptor rather than on the neurotransmitter; that is, the same neurotransmitter may excite one neuron and inhibit another.

Receptors and receptor mechanisms

Ion channels exist in the membrane of the neuron. There are several kinds of ion channels, and they may be found in different concentrations in different regions of the cell. Some ion channels are sensitive to voltage (voltage-gated channels) and open in response to the

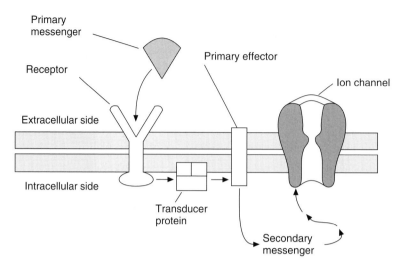

Figure 3.5.   The opening of an indirect ion channel is a multistep process. The receptor, primary effector, and ion channel span the cell membrane. The primary messenger is the neurotransmitter. The receptor activates a transducer protein, which excites primary effector enzymes to produce a secondary messenger. Secondary messengers may act directly on the ion channel or may involve several steps.

depolarization of the cell membrane, such as the calcium channel found in abundance at the axon terminal of many neurons. Some channels are sensitive to neurotransmitters or other chemical substances or both, and are described as *ligand-gated channels*. Ligand-gated channels may have receptor sites located directly on the ion channel itself (direct gating). Other ligand-gated channels may have receptor sites located at some distance from the ion channel (indirect gating; Figure 3.5). Receptor sites located directly on the ion channel are associated with a fast response (milliseconds). Receptor sites located some distance from the ion channel are associated with a slower response (up to minutes). Fast receptors include those that are sensitive to glutamate, glycine, and gamma-aminobutyric acid (GABA). Slow receptors include those in the CNS that are sensitive to norepinephrine and serotonin.

The configuration of the receptor determines the neuron's response to a particular neurotransmitter. For example, there are at least four types of glutamate receptor, and some of these receptors have subtypes. An ion channel that is controlled by one type of glutamate receptor is permeable to both Na^+ and K^+ but not to Ca^{2+}, whereas another ion channel controlled by a second type of glutamate receptor is permeable to all three ions. A third type of glutamate receptor has a docking site for Mg^{2+}, the presence of which modifies the neuron's response to glutamate. **The glutamate receptor sensitive to *N*-methyl-ᴅ-aspartate (NMDA) is believed to be involved in schizophrenia. Phencyclidine, an NMDA receptor antagonist, produces effects in normal persons that resemble schizophrenia (Tamminga, 1999).**

The fast receptor consists of an ion channel that spans the neuron cell membrane. The neurotransmitter receptor site is located on the extracellular surface of the wall of the ion channel. Some ion channels have a binding site for a regulator molecule, such as an anesthetic, or Mg^{2+} as described for the glutamate receptor.

The slow receptor has a different configuration. It spans the neuron cell membrane just as the ion channel does, but it cannot open to allow the passage of ions (Figure 3.5). The slow receptor is linked by a protein to the ion channel that the receptor controls. The linking protein is called a *G-protein* (guanine nucleotide-binding protein), and the receptors are called *G-protein-linked receptors*. G-protein receptors include alpha- and beta-adrenergic, serotonin, dopamine, and muscarinic acetylcholine (ACh) receptors as well as receptors for neuropeptides. The G-protein is loosely associated with the inner layer of the neuron cell membrane and consists of three subunits. The subunits vary with the receptor with which they are affiliated. They also vary with the effector enzyme with which they communicate and vary as to whether they excite or inhibit the effector enzyme.

When activated by a receptor, the α subunit of the G-protein binds with a second messenger. Four different second messengers are recognized (cyclic adenosine monophosphate, inositol polyphosphate, diacylglycerol, and arachidonic acid). The second-messenger molecule may directly open (or close) an ion channel but more often initiates a cascade of enzymatic activity within the neuronal cytoplasm. More than one second-messenger system may exist within a neuron, and cross-talk can occur during the operation of two or more second-messenger systems. Amplification of the signal can occur with second messengers. More than one G-protein is activated by a single receptor, and second messengers can diffuse to affect a distant part of the neuron. Second-messenger systems also can induce the synthesis of new proteins by altering gene expression, thus altering the long-term function of the neuron, including cell growth. Second-messenger systems: (1) operate relatively slowly, (2) can interact with other transmitter systems within the neuron, and (3) operate at some distance from the receptor site. The resulting action, which is relatively slow, is often described as one that modulates neuron activity.

Synapses located on dendrites tend to be excitatory. Both excitatory and inhibitory synapses are found on the nerve cell body. Synapses found on axon terminals tend to be inhibitory in function.

Neurotransmitter removal

Timely removal of neurotransmitters from the synaptic cleft prepares the synapse for continued usage. All neurotransmitters are passively removed to some degree by diffusion into the adjacent extracellular space. Acetylcholine at the neuromuscular junction is removed by enzymatic degradation. Active reuptake of the transmitter substance into the presynaptic nerve terminal is the most common inactivation mechanism. Uptake mechanisms have been described for norepinephrine, dopamine, serotonin, glutamate, GABA, and glycine.

Many drugs take advantage of neurotransmitter removal mechanisms. Monoamine oxidase inhibitors block the degradation of amine transmitters and are used for treating depression. Cocaine blocks the reuptake of monoamines (norepinephrine, dopamine, serotonin). Tricyclic antidepressants block the reuptake of epinephrine and serotonin.

Selective serotonin reuptake inhibitor drugs (SSRI) selectively block the reuptake of serotonin.

Neurotransmitters

In order to qualify as a neurotransmitter, a chemical must be recognized to be synthesized in the neuron, to be present in the presynaptic terminal, and to depolarize the postsynaptic membrane, and finally must be removed from the synaptic cleft.

There are three classes of neurotransmitters: amino acids, monoamines, and neuropeptides. Amino acid and monoamine neurotransmitters as a group are called *small-molecule neurotransmitters*. Small-molecule neurotransmitter precursors are synthesized in the soma. Following synthesis, they are transported to the axon terminal by way of rapid anterograde axon transport. The small-molecule neurotransmitters are assembled in the axon terminal from the precursors and stored in synaptic vesicles. Neuropeptide neurotransmitters are less well understood. They are short-chain amino acids and are supplied to the axon terminal in final form. They are also stored in vesicles in the synaptic terminal.

Examples of amino acid neurotransmitters include glutamate, aspartate, glycine, and GABA. Monoaminergic neurotransmitters include ACh, dopamine, epinephrine, norepinephrine, and serotonin. Neuropeptides include the opioids and substance P.

All axon terminals of the same neuron contain the same neurotransmitters. However, there may be more than one transmitter found in a single neuron. When two or more neurotransmitters coexist within a single neuron, one is usually a small-molecule transmitter, whereas the second (or more) is usually a peptide.

The enzymes that assemble small-molecule neurotransmitters are found throughout the cytoplasm of the cell. Therefore, the production of much of these transmitter substances takes place in the axon terminal. On the other hand, the neuropeptides are produced only in the cell body.

Amino acid neurotransmitters

Glycine, aspartate, and glutamate are amino acids and are recognized neurotransmitters. More than half the neurons in the CNS express receptors for amino acid transmitters. Glycine is found in spinal cord neurons, where it acts as an inhibitory neurotransmitter. Glutamate is believed to be excitatory and is important in learning as well as in sensitization to drugs such as amphetamine (Wolf, 1998). Glutamate is sometimes found in inhibitory cells, but it does not function as a transmitter in those cells. Two forms of glutamate are recognized: a neurotransmitter and a metabolite. Glutamic acid decarboxylase is an enzyme that synthesizes GABA from glutamate. GABA is also an amino acid. It is widely distributed in the CNS and is an inhibitory neurotransmitter. Quantitative estimates of glutamate levels in the brain have been made using magnetic resonance spectroscopy and appear to remain constant from 0 to 39 years with a slight decrease approaching 60 years (Pouwels *et al.*, 1999; Schubert *et al.*, 2004).

Evidence indicates a decreased production or release, or both, of glutamate in the brains of schizophrenic patients, especially in the hippocampus, parahippocampal gyrus, and dorsolateral prefrontal cortex. This is accompanied by an increase in glutamate receptors and in receptor sensitivity (Tsai *et al.*, 1995). Agents that enhance the activity of the glutamate NMDA receptor improve symptoms in schizophrenia (Goff, 2000). These results along with reports of alterations in dopamine in schizophrenia have produced the "glutamate hypothesis of schizophrenia." This hypothesis describes a balance between dopamine and glutamate in the cortex. These two neurotransmitters normally produce a balanced signal in the basal ganglia (striatum) that results in an optimal feedback from the basal ganglia and thalamus to the cortex. An increase in dopamine or a decrease in glutamate would upset this balance and could result in psychosis (Tamminga, 1998; Carlsson *et al.*, 1999).

Glutamate and aspartate are excitatory, and most neurons in the CNS contain receptors to one or the other. Normally, only small quantities of these excitatory amino acids appear in the synapse at any one time. If extraneuronal concentrations of these excitatory amino acids exceed the ability of uptake mechanisms to remove them, the affected neurons will die. This process of neuron cell death is referred to as *excitotoxicity* and is an important mechanism of neuron loss following hypoxia or ischemia. It appears that the influx of calcium into the neuron plays a major role in excitotoxicity.

Excitotoxicity has been implicated in schizophrenia. Coyle and Puttfarcken (1993) suggest that glutamate-stimulated intracellular oxidation in CNS neurons gradually produces neurotoxic damage and finally cell death. Olney and Farber (1995) propose that ACh overactivation secondary to reduced glutamatergic transmission can result in cell damage or death.

Glutamate may be involved in both the establishment and maintenance of addictive behavior. A greater number of glutamate receptors is established in sensitive regions as cocaine addiction is established. It is proposed that increased levels of glutamate in the amygdala may mediate the craving experienced by cocaine addicts (Kalivas *et al.*, 1998).

Monoaminergic neurotransmitters

Acetylcholine

The components of acetylcholine (ACh) can be synthesized in the axon terminal. Only the storage vesicle and choline acetyltransferase must be transported from the soma. Acetylcholine is in a class by itself. It is synthesized by choline acetyltransferase (CAT) from acetyl coenzyme A (CoA) and choline. Choline cannot be synthesized by the nervous system. It must be derived from the diet. Acetylcholine has been described as the neurotransmitter of the peripheral nervous system. It is the transmitter for all preganglionic autonomic neurons and for the postganglionic parasympathetic neurons. It is also the neurotransmitter of the axons serving all skeletal muscles. The enzyme acetylcholinesterase hydrolyzes ACh and is concentrated in the pre- and postsynaptic membranes. Acetylcholinesterase is an efficient enzyme, and ACh does not spread beyond the synaptic cleft.

Acetylcholine released by interneurons in the amygdala facilitates consolidation of long-term memory of emotionally arousing experiences (McGaugh *et al.*, 1996). ACh is also found within the cerebral cortex and is the neurotransmitter of the neurons that make up the nucleus basalis (of Meynert). Axons that arise from the nucleus basalis have widespread distribution to the cortex.

Degeneration of the nucleus basalis is a finding in Alzheimer's disease. Both human and animal research on aging have demonstrated a decline in the enzyme choline acetyltransferase in all cortical regions and particularly in the temporal lobe (Struble *et al.*, 1986). This deficiency is believed to contribute to the cognitive decline as well as the decrease in insight and judgment seen with aging. Altered cholinergic function in schizophrenia has been proposed (Tandon, 1999).

Biogenic amines (catecholamines)

The class of biogenic amine transmitters includes the catecholamines [dopamine (DA) and norepinephrine (NE)] and serotonin (5-hydroxytryptamine). All three catecholamine neurotransmitters are derived from the amino acid tyrosine.

Dopamine

There are four major dopamine systems in the brain:

- One extends from the hypothalamic nuclei to the median eminence, where dopamine inhibits the release of prolactin from the pituitary gland (see Chapter 8).
- The second system extends from the substantia nigra to the striatum (nigrostriatal system) and is associated with motor activity of the basal ganglia (see Chapter 7).
- The third arises from cells located in the ventral tegmental area of the ventral striatum (see Figure 10.3) and extends to the nucleus accumbens (mesolimbic system).
- The fourth arises from cells in the ventral tegmental area and projects to limbic system structures and to the prefrontal cortex (mesocortical system).

Dopamine suppresses the spontaneous activity of cortical neurons to new input (Thierry *et al.*, 1992) and at the same time is important in tonic activation that precedes motor action (Tucker and Williamson, 1989). It is hypothesized that dopaminergic input to the prefrontal cortex functions to lock out new information and at the same time heightens the individual's ability to respond to the task at hand (Pliszka *et al.*, 1996). Novelty-seeking behavior may be dopamine dependent (Menza *et al.*, 1993). It has been suggested that the higher the level of dopamine or the more responsive the brain is to dopamine, the more likely a person is to be sensitive to incentives and rewards. Activation of the dopamine system facilitates the pursuit of goals or rewards such as food, sex, money, or education (Depue, 1996).

An estrous female elicits the release of dopamine in three systems in the male rat. Dopamine in the nigrostriatal tract primes the male for the motor component of copulation. Dopamine in the mesolimbic system increases sensitivity to stimuli of motivational significance. Dopamine in the medial preoptic area increases responsiveness to sexual stimuli (Hull *et al.*, 1998).

Dopamine plays an important role in the reward mechanisms, and cocaine increases extracellular levels of dopamine. Prolonged use of cocaine may dysregulate brain dopaminergic systems and can result in persistent hypodopaminergia. The downregulation of dopaminergic pathways due to long-term cocaine abuse may underlie anhedonia and relapse in cocaine addicts (Majewska, 1996).

Table 3.1. *The areas of greatest concentration of the five different subtypes of dopamine receptors. More modest numbers of dopamine receptors are found in other regions of the brain (Levant, 1996: Goldman-Rakic and Selemon, 1997).*

	D_1	D_5	D_2	D_3	D_4
Frontal cortex	X	X			X
Caudate/putamen	X	X	X		
Amygdala					X
Nuc. accumbens	X		X	X	
Ventral pallidum	X		X	X	
Hippocampus		X			
Hypothalamus		X			
Substantia nigra			X		
Brainstem					X

Permanent changes are seen in anterior cingulate cortex pyramidal cell dendrites in rabbits exposed prenatally to cocaine (Levitt *et al.*, 1997; see Chapter 12*)*.

The dopamine theory of schizophrenia proposes an excess of dopaminergic stimulation and is based on two observations (Snyder *et al.*, 1974). First, there is a high correlation between the effective dose of traditional neuroleptics and the degree to which they block D_2 dopamine receptors. Second, the paranoid psychosis that is often seen in amphetamine and cocaine addicts can be clinically indistinguishable from paranoid schizophrenia and appears to be due to dopamine activation (Manschreck *et al.*, 1988). A dopamine/glutamate theory of schizophrenia has been proposed (Carlsson and Carlsson, 1990; Carlsson *et al.*, 1999).

Dopamine receptors are found in high concentrations in limbic regions of the cerebral cortex. Since the mid 1970s, it has been thought that two dopamine receptor subtypes exist, D_1 and D_2 (Table 3.1). In the past few years, three additional subtypes have been recognized. D_3 and D_4 show pharmacological similarities to the D_2 receptor subtype. Some authors group D_2, D_3, and D_4 into the D_2-like family (Levant, 1996). A fifth receptor subtype has also been recognized, D_5, which is similar to the D_1 receptor. D_1 and D_5 are sometimes referred to as the D_1-like "family" of dopamine receptors (Nestler, 1997). Type D_1 receptors are particularly prominent in the prefrontal cortex (Goldman-Rakic *et al.*, 1990). D_5 receptors are found predominantly in the hippocampus and thalamus (Meader-Woodruff *et al.*, 1992). Type D_2 receptors are concentrated in the striatum and limbic structures and may play a role in the reward deficiency syndrome (Blum *et al.*, 1996). D_3 receptors are found in the nucleus accumbens and in very low levels in the caudate nucleus and putamen (Landwehrmeyer *et al.*, 1993).

Neuroleptics block the D_2 receptor. Blockade of the receptors in limbic areas such as the nucleus accumbens and prefrontal cortex accounts for the antipsychotic effects. Blockade of the receptors in the caudate nucleus and putamen results in the extrapyramidal side-effects. Clozapine has a high affinity for the D_4 receptor, suggesting that blockade of the D_4 receptor may be related to the efficacy of neuroleptics (Seeman, 1992; Sawa and Snyder, 2002).

Reduced cortical dopamine function has been reported in schizophrenia and in Parkinson's disease (Brozoski *et al.*, 1979). Raising dopamine levels in these same groups improves performance on tests that examine working memory (Daniel *et al.*, 1991; Lange *et al.*, 1992). Low dopamine levels may be associated with dysfunctional eating patterns (Ericsson *et al.*, 1997).

Evidence suggests that the D_1 receptor located in the dorsolateral prefrontal cortex may be particularly important in working memory and that an optimal level of dopamine is critical in facilitating working memory. Novelty-seeking behavior in humans and exploratory activity in animals are analogous (Cloninger, 1987) and may be related to the level of dopamine. Patients with Parkinson's disease have reduced levels of dopamine and exhibit personality characteristics consistent with reduced novelty seeking that can be described as compulsive, industrious, rigidly moral, stoic, serious, and quiet (Menza *et al.*, 1993).

In the cortex, D_1 receptors are concentrated in the dorsolateral prefrontal cortex. These D_1 receptors are found predominantly on the dendritic spines of pyramidal neurons, which places them in a position to directly affect corticothalamic, corticostriatal, and corticocortical projections. D_5 receptors are also associated with pyramidal neurons but are localized to the shafts of the dendrites. It is not surprising to find that a hyperactive dopaminergic (DA) system can result in increased motor activity, whereas a hypoactive DA system can result in decreased motoric activity (hypokinesia or akinesia) and a tendency to physical weariness. D_2 receptors appear to be on GABA-containing interneurons and on some pyramidal neurons (Goldman-Rakic and Selemon, 1997).

Clinically effective antipsychotic drugs are antagonists of D_2 receptors. For this reason, high levels of D_2 receptors or excessive dopamine-mediated neurotransmission was thought to underlie schizophrenia (Nestler, 1997). Comparison of drug-free schizophrenic patients with a control group showed no difference in the density of D_2 receptors in the striatum. However, a significant reduction in D_1 receptor density was seen in the prefrontal cortex of schizophrenics that related to the severity of negative symptoms and cognitive defects. These findings suggest that a dysfunction in the D_1 receptor system in the prefrontal cortex may contribute to the negative symptoms and cognitive dysfunction seen in schizophrenia (Okubo *et al.*, 1997).

Dopamine is found in high concentrations in the retina, where it functions as a neurotransmitter and neuromodulator in conjunction with color vision. Patients recently withdrawn from cocaine show abnormalities in the electroretinogram accompanied by a significant loss of blue–yellow color vision (Desai *et al.*, 1997). Abnormalities in retinal dopaminergic transmission in patients with seasonal affective disorder also have been suggested (Partonen, 1996).

Norepinephrine and epinephrine

Norepinephrine (NE) is produced by cells that make up the locus ceruleus of the brainstem. Axons of these neurons extend to many regions of the brain and spinal cord. NE input to the right superior parietal lobe is greater than to the left. The right superior parietal lobe is part of the posterior attentional system (Posner and Petersen, 1990).

Norepinephrine released in the cortex inhibits the spontaneous activity of cortical neurons. At the same time these neurons become more sensitive to specific sensory inputs indicating that NE functions to increase the signal-to-noise ratio for sensory signals (Segal and Bloom, 1976).

Norepinephrine is associated with arousal, vigilance, and reward dependency (Cloninger, 1987; Menza *et al.*, 1993). NE hyperactivity can lead to insomnia, weight loss, irritability, agitation, and a reduction in the pain threshold. Peripheral NE hyperactivity results in symptoms of anxiety (i.e., tachycardia, muscular cramps, and increased blood pressure). A decrease in NE activity is associated with some forms of depression, and an increase of NE is linked with mania (Schildkraut, 1965). Abnormal regulation of NE levels in the central nervous system is implicated in attention-deficit hyperactivity disorder (Pliszka *et al.*, 1996).

Epinephrine released by the adrenal medulla activates the vagus nerve (see Chapter 11). In this same circuitry, NE released in the amygdala is important in modulating consolidation of long-term memory of emotionally arousing experiences (McGaugh *et al.*, 1996).

Serotonin

Serotonin (5-hydroxytryptamine, or 5-HT) is classified as an indolamine and is synthesized from tryptophan. Two enzymes, tryptophan hydroxylase and 5-hydroxytryptophan decarboxylase, are required to synthesize serotonin from tryptophan. Plasma tryptophan is provided by the daily diet, and a reduction in dietary tryptophan can dramatically reduce the levels of brain serotonin (Cooper *et al.*,1991). Serotonin is found throughout the body but does not cross the blood–brain barrier. Within the brain, serotonergic neurons are found in the raphe nuclei of the brainstem, and their axons range widely throughout the brain and spinal cord.

Serotonin is regarded as a modulatory neurotransmitter with inhibitory effects in the areas of mood, arousal, cognition, and feeding behavior (Trestman et al., 1995). Serotonin neurons that are normally active fall silent during rapid eye movement (REM) sleep. With decreased serotonergic activity, sleep becomes fragmented and disrupted. It is hypothesized that abnormalities in serotonin function in the prefrontal cortex may be a primary factor in impulsive aggressive and violent behavior (Davidson et al., 2000). Evidence indicates that expression of the serotonin transported gene can regulate fear and anxiety-related behavior through its effect on the amygdala (Hariri *et al.*, 2002).

Selective serotonin reuptake inhibitors (SSRIs) slow the reuptake of serotonin, making it more available to the postsynaptic cell and prolonging its effect in the synaptic cleft. Low serotonin levels can trigger high carbohydrate consumption and are associated with binge eating and with carbohydrate preference in obese women (Bjorntorp, 1995; Brewerton, 1995). In contrast, high levels of serotonin are associated with harm avoidance, anorexia nervosa, and with compulsive behavior (Cloninger, 1987; Menza *et al.*, 1993; Brewerton, 1995; Jarry and Vaccarino, 1996).

Low levels of serotonin turnover are associated with alcoholism, social isolation, and impaired social function, depression and similar behaviors in nonhuman primates (Heinz *et al.*, 1998; Bremner *et al.*, 2003). Serotonin may also be altered in panic disorder (Gorman *et al.*, 1989; Knott *et al.*, 1994), in schizophrenia (Gurevich and Joyce, 1997), in aggressive behavior (Unis *et al.*, 1997), and in borderline personality disorder (Martial *et al.*, 1997). It has been hypothesized that obsessive-compulsive disorder (OCD) may involve brain regions that are modulated by normally functioning serotonin neurons. Drugs that affect serotonin output improve symptoms of OCD by action on the involved brain regions (Baumgarten and Grozdanovic, 1998; Delgado and Moreno, 1998).

A significant decline in the number of serotonin receptors in some parts of the brain has been reported with age. This decline may predispose the elderly to major depression (Meltzer *et al.*, 1998).

Neuroactive peptide neurotransmitters

More than 50 short peptides have been described as being neuroactive. Some of these are particularly important since they have relatively long-lasting effects. Since these effects make them different from neurotransmitters, which by definition are short acting, this class of long-lasting peptides is referred to as "neuromodulators. " There are five families of neuroactive peptides. The families of opioids, neurohypophyseal peptides, and tachykinins are better known. The opioids consist of the opiocortins, enkephalins, dynorphin, and FMRFamide. Neurohypophyseal peptides include vasopressin, oxytocin, and the neurophysins. Substance P is a tachykinin.

Among the neuropeptides, substance P and the enkephalins have been linked to the control of pain. Substance P is prevalent in the prefrontal cortex and is being examined for its role in depression (Holden, 2003). Neuropeptide Y is a potent stimulator of food intake in rats (White *et al.*, 1994). Gamma-melanocyte-stimulating hormone, adrenocorticotropin, and beta-endorphin regulate responses to stress. A neuropeptide may coexist with a small molecule transmitter within the same neuron.

Some obese individuals, particularly those who binge eat, have elevated beta-endorphin levels. Increased levels of beta-endorphin are also associated with bingeing in bulimia nervosa (Hubner, 1993; Ericsson *et al.*, 1997).

Neuroglia

Myelin

There are four neuroglial cells. Two of these produce myelin. Myelin consists of multiple wrappings of the cell membrane of the myelin-producing cell around segments of axons. Myelin insulates the axon from the extracellular environment. As the myelin-producing cell wraps around a segment of an axon, the cytoplasm is squeezed out from between the layers of cell membrane of the myelin-producing cell. The cell membrane is a lipoprotein sheath and contains large amounts of lipid. The multiple wrappings produce a white, glistening appearance in the fresh state, accounting for the white matter of the brain and spinal cord. Myelin from one myelin-producing cell extends for only up to approximately a 1-cm segment along an axon. The segment of myelin does not overlap significantly with the next myelin segment. The discontinuity between myelin sheaths is called the *node (of Ranvier)*. The myelin-covered length is called the *internode* and insulates the axon. The insulating effect of myelin is minimal at the node, and depolarization of the axon membrane occurs at the node. Because the internodal distance is insulated, the action potential hops (saltates) along the axon from one node to the next.

The oligodendroglial cell produces myelin in the CNS. The neurilemmal cell (of Schwann) produces myelin in the peripheral nervous system (PNS). After injury, neurilemmal cells (of

Schwann) support the regeneration of PNS axons. However, within the CNS, axonal regrowth is insignificant following injury. The oligodendrocyte does not appear to provide the same support for regenerating CNS axons as does the neurilemmal cell for PNS axons.

Astrocytes

Astrocytes are found only within the CNS and are of several types. In general, astrocytes provide structural and physiological support to CNS neurons. Many astrocytes stretch between individual nerve cell bodies and capillaries. They have a characteristic perivascular end foot that is found in apposition to the capillary. The body of the same astrocyte embraces the body of the neuron.

Astrocytes respond to nerve cell activity. They may play a role in directing growing axon terminals during development, and it has been suggested that the presence of astrocytes may inhibit axon regrowth following injury in the mature brain. Astrocytes maintain a balanced extracellular ion environment for the neurons.

Microglia

Microglial cells are normally found along capillaries. If CNS tissue is damaged, microglial cells enlarge, migrate to the region of damage, and become phagocytic. When they act as phagocytes, microglial cells are called *glitter cells.*

SELECT BIBLIOGRAPHY

W. Birkmayer, and P. Riederer, *Understanding the Neurotransmitters: Key to the Workings of the Brain.* (New York: Springer-Verlag, 1989).

J. R. Cooper, F. E. Bloom, and R. H. Roth, *The Biochemical Basis of Neuropharmacology*, 6th edn. (New York: Oxford University Press, 1991).

R. Kavoussi, P. Armstead, and E. Coccaro. The neurobiology of impulsive aggression. *Anger, Aggression, and Violence. The Psychiatric Clinics of North America,* **20** (1997), 395–403.

R. A. Rhoades, and G. A. Tanner, *Medical Physiology.* (New York: Little, Brown, 1995).

A. F. Schatzberg, and C. B. Nemeroff, *Textbook of Psychopharmacology.* (Washington, D.C.: American Psychiatric Press, 1995).

T. W. Stone, ed. *CNS Neurotransmitters and Neuromodulators: Dopamine.* (Boca Raton, Fla: CRC Press, 1996).

REFERENCES

Baumgarten, H. G., and Grozdanovic, A. 1998. Role of serotonin in obsessive-compulsive disorder. *Br. J. Psychiatry* **173** (Suppl. 35):13–20.

Bjorntorp, P. 1995. Neuroendocrine abnormalities in human obesity. *Metabolism* **44** (Suppl. 2):38–41.

Blum, K., Cull, J. G., Braverman, E. R., and Comings, D. E. 1996. Reward deficiency syndrome. *Am. Sci.* **84**:132–145.

Bremner, J. D., Vythilingam, M., Ng, C. K., Vermetten, E., Nazeer, A., Oren, D. A., Berman, R. M., and Charney, D. S. 2003. Regional brain metabolic correlates of alpha-methylparatyrosine-induced depressive symptoms; implications for the neural circuitry of depression. *J. Am. Med. Assoc.* **289**(23):3125–3134.

Brewerton, T. D. 1995. Toward a unified theory of serotonin disturbances in eating and related disorders. *Psychoneuroimmunology* **20**:561–590.

Brozoski, T. J., Brown, R. M., Rosvold, H. E., and Goldman, P. S. 1979. Cognitive defect caused by regional depletion of dopamine in prefrontal cortex of rhesus monkey. *Science* **205**:929–932.

Carlsson, A., Hansson, L. O., Waters, N., and Carlsson, M. L. 1999. A glutamatergic deficiency model of schizophrenia. *Br. J. Psychiatry* **174** (Suppl. 37):2–6.

Carlsson, M., and Carlsson, A. 1990. Interactions between glutaminergic and monoaminergic systems within the basal ganglia – implications for schizophrenia and Parkinson's disease. *Trends Neurosci.* **13**:272–276.

Cloninger, R. C. 1987. A systematic method for clinical description and classification of personality variants. *Arch. Gen. Psychiatry* **44**:573–588.

Cooper, J. R., Bloom, F. E., and Roth, R. H. 1991. *The Biochemical Basis of Neuropharmacology*, 6th edn. New York: Oxford University Press.

Coyle, J. T., and Puttfarcken, P. 1993. Oxidative stress, glutamate, and neurodegenerative disorders. *Science* **262**:689–695.

Daniel, D. G., Weinberger, D. R., Jones, D. W., Zigun, J. R., Coppola, R., Handle, S., Bigelow, L. R., Goldberg, T. E., Berman, K. F., and Kelinman, J. E. 1991. The effect of amphetamine on regional blood flow during cognitive activation in schizophrenia. *J. Neurosci.* **11**:1907–1919.

Davidson, R. J., Putnam, K. M., and Larson, C. L. 2000. Dysfunction in the neural circuitry of emotion regulation – a possible prelude to violence. *Science* **289**:591–594.

Delgado, P. L., and Moreno, F. A. 1998. Different roles for serotonin in anti-obsessional drug action and the pathophysiology of obsessive-compulsive disorder. *Br. J. Psychiatry* **173** (Suppl. 35):21–25.

Depue, R. A. 1996. A neurobiological framework for the structure of personality and emotion: implications for personality disorders. In: J. F. Clarkin and M. F. Lenzenweger (eds.) *Major Theories of Personality Disorder*. New York: Guilford Press.

Desai, P., Roy, M., Roy, A., Brown, S., and Smelson, D. 1997. Impaired color vision in cocaine-withdrawn patients. *Arch. Gen. Psychiatry* **54**:696–699.

Ericsson, M., Poston, W. S. C. II, and Foreyt, J. P. 1997. Common biological pathways in eating disorders and obesity. *Addict. Behav.* **21**:733–743.

Goff, D. C. 2000. Glutamate receptors in schizophrenia and antipsychotic drugs. In: M. S. Lidow (ed.) *Neurotransmitter Receptors in Actions of Antipsychotic Medications*. Boca Raton, Fla.: CRC Press, pp. 121–136.

Goldman-Rakic, P. S., and Selemon, L. D. 1997. Functional and anatomical aspects of prefrontal pathology in schizophrenia. *Schizophr. Bull.* **23**:437–458.

Goldman-Rakic, P. S., Lidow, M. S., and Gallager, D. W. 1990. Overlap of dopaminergic, adrenergic, and serotonergic receptors and complementarity of their subtypes in primate prefrontal cortex. *J. Neurosci.* **10**:2125–2138.

Gorman, J. M., Liebowitz, M. R., Fyer, A. J., and Stein, J. 1989. A neuroanatomical hypothesis for panic disorder. *Am. J. Psychiatry* **146**:148–161.

Gurevich, E. V., and Joyce, J. N. 1997. Alterations in the cortical serotonergic system in schizophrenia: a postmortem study. *Biol. Psychiatry* **42**:529–545.

Hariri, A. R., Mattay, V. S., Tessitore, A., Kolachana, B., Fera, F., Goldman, D., Egan, M. F., and Weinberger, D. R. 2002. Serotonin transporter genetic variation and the response of the human amygdala. *Science* **297**:400–402.

Heinz, A., Higley, J. D., Gorey, J. G., Saunders, R. C., Jones, D. W., Hommer, D., Zajicek, K., Suomi, S. J., Lesch, K. P., Weinberger, D. R., and Linnoila, M. 1998. In vivo association between alcohol intoxication, aggression, and serotonin transporter availability in nonhuman primates. *Am. J. Psychiatry* **155**:1023–1028.

Holden, C. 2003. Future brightening for depression treatments. *Science* **302**:810–813.

Hubner, H. F. 1993. *Endorphins, Eating Disorders, and Other Addictive Behaviors.* New York: W. W. Norton.

Hull, E. M., Lorrain, D. S., Du, J., Matuszewich, L., Bitran, D., Nishita, J. K., and Scaletta, L. L. 1998. Organizational and activational effects of dopamine on male sexual behavior. In: L. Ellis and L. Ebertz (eds.) *Males, Females, and Behavior.* Westport, Conn.: Praeger, pp. 79–96.

Jarry, J. L., and Vaccarino, F. J. 1996. Eating disorder and obsessive-compulsive disorder: neurochemical and phenomenological commonalities. *J. Psychiatry Neurosci.* **21**:36–48.

Kalivas, P. W., Pierce, R. C., Cornish, J., and Sorg., B. A. 1998. A role for sensitization in craving and relapse in cocaine addiction. *J. Psychopharmacol.* **12**:49–53.

Knott, V. J., Bakishk, D., and Barkley, J. 1994. Brainstem evoked potentials in panic disorder. *J. Psychiatry Neurosci.* **19**:301–306.

Landwehrmeyer, B., Mengod, G., and Palacios, J. M. 1993. Dopamine D_3 receptor mRNA and binding sites in human brain. *Brain Res. Mol. Brain Res.* **18**:187–192.

Lange, K. W., Robbins, T. W., Marsden, C. D., James, M., Owen, A. M., and Paul, G. M. 1992. L-DOPA withdrawal in Parkinson's disease selectively impairs cognitive performance in tests sensitive to frontal lobe dysfunction. *Psychopharmacology* **107**:395–404.

Levant, B. 1996. Distribution of dopamine receptor subtypes in the CNS. In: T. W. Stone (ed.) *CNS Neurotransmitters and Neuromodulators: Dopamine.* Boca Raton, Fla: CRC Press, pp. 77–87.

Levitt, P., Harvey, J. A., Friedman, E., Simansky, K., and Murphy, E. H. 1997. New evidence for neurotransmitter influences on brain development. *Trends Neurosci.* **20**:269–274.

Majewska, M. D. 1996. Cocaine addiction as a neurological disorder: implications for treatment. In: M. D. Majewska (ed.) *Neurotoxicity and Neuropathology Associated with Cocaine Abuse. NIDA Research Monograph 163.* Rockville, Md.: National Institute on Drug Abuse.

Manschreck, T. C., Laughery, J. A., Weisstein, C. C., Allen, D., Humblestone, B., Neville, M., Podlewski, H., and Mitra, N. 1988. Characteristics of freebase cocaine psychosis. *Yale J. Biol. Med.* **61**:115–122.

Martial, J., Paris, J., Leyton, M., Zweig-Frank, H., Schwartz, G., Teboul, E., Thavundayil, J., Larue, S., Ng Ying King, N. M. K., and Vasavan Nair, N. P. 1997. Neuroendocrine study of serotonin function in female borderline personality disorder patients: a pilot study. *Biol. Psychiatry* **42**:737–739.

McGaugh, J. L., Cahill, L., and Roozendaal, B. 1996. Involvement of the amygdala in memory storage: interaction with other brain systems. *Proc. Natl. Acad. Sci. U.S.A.* **93**:13508–13514.

Meador-Woodruff, J. H., Mansour, A., Grandy, D., Damask, S. P., Civelli, O., and Watson, S. J. Jr. 1992. Distribution of D_5 dopamine receptor mRNA in rat brain. *Neurosci. Lett.* **145**:209–212.

Meltzer, C. C., Smith, G., DeKosky, S. T., Pollock, B. G., Mathis, C. A., Moore, R. Y., Kupfer, D. J., and Reynolds, C. F. 3rd. 1998. Serotonin in aging, late-life depression, and Alzheimer's disease: the emerging role of functional imaging. *Neuropsychopharmacology* **18**:407–430.

Menza, M. A., Golve, L. I., Cody, R. A., and Forman, N. E. 1993. Dopamine-related personality traits in Parkinson's disease. *Neurology* **43**:505–508.

Nestler, E. J. 1997. An emerging pathophysiology. *Nature* **385**:578–589.

Okubo, Y., Suhara, T., Suzuki, K., Kobayashi, K., Inoue, O., Terasaki, O., Someya, Y., Sassa, T., Sudo, Y., Matsushima, E., Iyo, M., Tateno, Y., and Toru, M. 1997. Decreased prefrontal dopamine D_1 receptors in schizophrenia revealed by PET. *Nature* **385**:634–636.

Olney, J. W., and Farber, N. B. 1995. Glutamate receptor dysfunction and schizophrenia. *Arch. Gen. Psychiatry* **52**:998–1007.

Partonen, T. 1996. Dopamine and circadian rhythms in seasonal affective disorder. *Med. Hypotheses* **47**:191–192.

Pliszka, S. R., McCracken, J. T., and Maas, J. W. 1996. Catecholamines in attention-deficit hyperactivity disorder: current perspectives. *J. Am. Acad. Child Adolesc. Psychiatry* **35**:264–272.

Posner, M., and Petersen, S. E. 1990. The attention system of the brain. *Annu. Rev. Neurosci.* **13**:25–42.

Pouwels, P. J., Brockmann, K., Kruse, B., Wilken, B., Wick, M., Hanefeld, F., and Frahm, J. 1999. Regional age dependence of human brain metabolites from infancy to adulthood as detected by quantitative localized proton MRS. *Pediatr. Res.* **46**:474–485.

Sawa, A., and Snyder, S. H. 2002. Schizophrenia: diverse approaches to a complex disease. *Science* **296**:692–695.

Schildkraut, J. J. 1965. The catecholamine hypothesis of affective disorders: a review of supporting evidence. *Am. J. Psychiatry* **122**:509–522.

Schubert, F., Gallinat, J., Seifert, F., and Rinneberg, H. 2004. Glutamate concentrations in human brain using single voxel proton magnetic resonance spectroscopy at 3 Tesla. *Neuroimage* **21**:1762–1771.

Seeman, P. H. 1992. Dopamine receptor sequences: therapeutic levels of neuroleptics occupy D_2 receptors, clozapine occupies D_4. *Neuropsychopharmacology* **7**:261–284.

Segal, M., and Bloom, F. E. 1976. The action of norepinephrine in the rat hippocampus. IV. The effects of locus coeruleus stimulation on evoked hippocampal unit activity. *Brain Res.* **107**:513–525.

Snyder, S. H., Bannerjee, S., Yamamura, H., and Greenberg, D. 1974. Drugs, neurotransmitters and schizophrenia: phenothiazines, amphetamine and enzymes synthesizing psychotomimetic drugs and schizophrenia research. *Science* **243**:398–400.

Struble, R. G., Lehmann, J., Mitchell, S. J., McKinney, M., Price, D. L., Coyle, J. T., and DeLong, M. R. 1986. Basal forebrain neurons provide major cholinergic innervation of primate neocortex. *Neurosci. Lett.* **66**:215–220.

Tamminga, C. A. 1998. Schizophrenia and glutamatergic transmission. *Crit. Rev. Neurobiol.* **12**:21–36.

— 1999. Glutamatergic aspects of schizophrenia. *Br. J. Psychiatry* **174** (Suppl. 37):12–15.

Tandon, R. 1999. Cholinergic aspects of schizophrenia. *Br. J. Psychiatry* **174** (Suppl. 37):7–11.

Thierry, A. M., Mantz, J., and Glowinski, J. 1992. Influence of dopaminergic and noradrenergic afferents on their target cells in the rat medial prefrontal cortex. *Adv. Neurol.* **57**:545–554.

Trestman, R. L., deVegvar, M., and Siever, L. J. 1995. Treatment of personality disorders. In: A. F. Schatzberg and C. B. Nemeroff (eds.) *The American Psychiatric Press Textbook of Psychopharmacology*. Washington, D.C.: American Psychiatric Press.

Tsai, G., Passani, L. A., Slusher, B. S., Carter, R., Baer, L., Kleinman, J. E., and Coyle, J. T. 1995. Abnormal excitatory neurotransmitter metabolism in schizophrenic brains. *Arch. Gen. Psychiatry* **52**:829–836.

Tucker, D. M., and Williamson, P. A. 1989. Asymmetric neural control systems in human self regulation. *Psychol. Rev.* **91**:185–215.

Unis, A. S., Cook, E. H., Vincent, J. G., Gjerde, D. K., Perry, B. D., Mason, C., and Mitchell, J. 1997. Platelet serotonin measures in adolescents with conduct disorder. *Biol. Psychiatry* **42**:553–559.

White, B. D., Dean, R. G., Edwards, G. L., and Martin, R. J. 1994. Type II corticosteroid receptor stimulation increases NPY gene expression in basomedial hypothalamus of rats. *Am. J. Physiol.* **266**:R1523–R1529.

Wolf, M. E. 1998. The role of excitatory amino acids in behavioral sensitization to psychomotor stimulants. *Prog. Neurobiol.* **54**(6):679–720.

4 Occipital and parietal lobes

Occipital lobe

Anatomy and behavioral considerations

The occipital lobe is clearly demarcated from the parietal lobe on the medial surface by the parieto–occipital sulcus and by the anterior limb of the calcarine fissure (Figure 4.1). The short section of parieto–occipital sulcus on the dorsolateral surface is used as an anchor for an imaginary line that extends ventrally to the preoccipital notch (see Figure 5.1). This imaginary line is the border between the occipital and parietal as well as the temporal lobe on the lateral cortical surface. The border between the occipital and temporal lobes on the ventral surface is less distinct (see Figure 5.2). Some authors include all of the inferior temporal and fusiform gyri (medial occipitotemporal gyrus) with the temporal lobe; others assign the caudal portions of these gyri to the occipital lobe.

The cortex of the occipital lobe consists of Brodmann's areas (BA) 17, 18, and 19 (Figures 2.2, 2.3, 4.1, 4.2). Brodmann's area 17 is the primary visual cortex (striate cortex) and occupies a large portion of the medial aspect of the occipital lobe. Much of the primary visual cortex lies within the calcarine fissure which extends approximately 2.5 cm deep into the occipital lobe. A portion of BA 17 curves around the posterior surface of the brain onto the lateral surface of the occipital lobe. Brodmann's areas 18 and 19 are recognized as secondary and tertiary visual areas, respectively. Together, BA 18 and 19 represent the visual association area.

Many direct and indirect connections exist between the occipital lobe and the frontal lobe. The superior fronto–occipital fasciculus links the occipital and temporal cortices with insular and frontal regions. The inferior fronto–occipital fasciculus interconnects lateral and ventrolateral parts of the frontal lobes with the occipital cortex. The inferior longitudinal fasciculus and the lateral occipital fasciculus also connect areas of temporal and occipital lobes. The cingulum connects limbic regions to adjacent areas of the frontal, parietal, and occipital lobes (see Figure 12.3).

Primary visual cortex (BA 17)

Fibers that originate from nerve cell bodies located in the lateral geniculate body (thalamus) project to the primary visual cortex, where they produce a retinal map. Macular areas of the retina are located close to the occipital pole and are represented over a relatively large area of visual cortex. Peripheral vision is represented more rostrally.

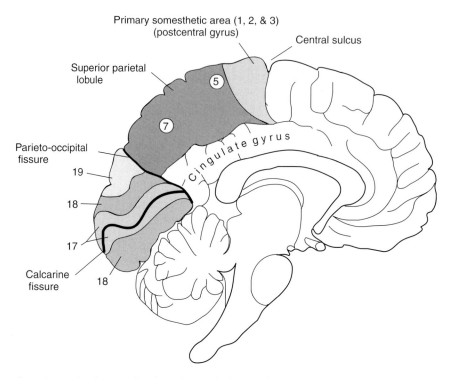

Figure 4.1.   The primary visual cortex [Brodmann's area(BA) 17] is largely buried within the calcarine fissure. A greater portion of the superior parietal lobule (BA 5 and 7) lies along the midline (compare with Figure 4.2).

Small spots of light are very effective in exciting the cells of the retina and the lateral geniculate body. In contrast, cells of the primary visual cortex respond only to visual images that have linear properties (lines and edges). The neurons of the primary visual cortex interpret contours and boundaries of a visual target in terms of line segments. Activity in the primary visual cortex was enhanced when viewing fearful faces suggesting the ability to enhance attention to fear stimuli (Pourtois *et al.*, 2004).

Three parallel pathways process visual images simultaneously. The large cell (magnocellular) system arises from large retinal ganglion cells concentrated near the periphery of the retina. The magnocellular system is responsible for defining spatial relationships and for detecting movement (the dorsal "where" pathway; see Figures 4.6 and 6.7). The small cell (parvocellular) system arises from small retinal ganglion cells that mainly serve cones located near the macula of the retina. The parvocellular system contains two parallel subsystems. The first of these is responsible for the detection of form (the ventral "what" pathway; see Figures 4.6 and 6.7). The second of these two pathways processes color.

Stimulation of the primary visual cortex produces elementary hallucinations in the contralateral visual field. These hallucinations include sparks and flashes of color or bright light. Hallucinations of object fragments (e.g., lines, corners, patterns) have been reported following a stroke in the occipital cortex (Anderson and Rizzo, 1994).

A lesion of BA 17 will produce an area of blindness (scotoma) in the contralateral visual field. Loss of an area as large as an entire quadrant of vision may go unnoticed by the patient. A lesion of the entire primary visual cortex on both sides results in cortical blindness. The patient is unable to see, but may retain "blind sight"; that is, he or she may retain a sense of the presence of a nearby object

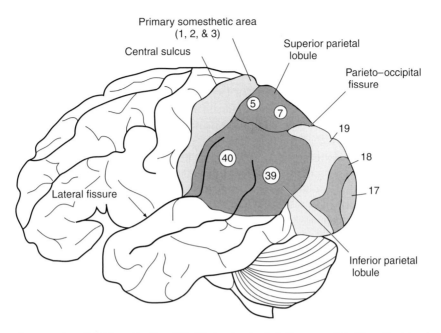

Figure 4.2.   The secondary (BA 18) and tertiary (BA 19) visual cortex is better appreciated from the lateral view. The primary somesthetic cortex coincides with BA 1, 2, and 3. The superior parietal lobule coincides with BA 5 and 7 and the inferior parietal lobule coincides with BA 39 (angular gyrus) and 40 (supramarginal gyrus).

but cannot see it. Some patients can accurately "guess" the location or identity of objects presented in their blind hemifield (Weiskrantz, 2004). It is proposed that blind sight represents the action of an accessory visual pathway involving the superior colliculus and pulvinar that projects to extrastriate dorsal ("where") visual areas (Gross *et al.*, 2004). Some patients can discriminate facial expressions. It is proposed that this is accomplished by way of extension of this system to the right amygdala (Morris *et al.*, 2001).

Clinical vignette

An 84-year-old woman had a history of craniotomy 17 years previously for the removal of a right occipital meningioma (Nagaratnam *et al.*, 1996). She presented at this time with a 3-year history of formed hallucinations, the ringing of bells, and the monotonous repetition of the same Christmas carol. The hallucinations had increased in frequency and intensity in the past few months. She reported people standing to her left, and, to her annoyance, some of them stroked her face. She had been observed brushing away imaginary objects. A computed tomographic scan revealed a 5-cm diameter mass superior to the tentorium in the right occipital region. She was treated with steroids because of an unrelated cardiac condition. The musical hallucinations continued unabated until her death a month later of left ventricular failure.

An increase was reported in the cerebral blood flow to the occipital cortex in patients who experienced procaine-induced visual hallucinations. Blood flow also was increased in limbic structures and in the lateral frontal lobe (Parekh *et al.*, 1995).

Brodmann's area 17, along with BA 9 in the frontal lobe, was found to be decreased in thickness in the brains of patients with schizophrenia. The decrease in BA 17 was not statistically significant but was consistent and was accompanied by a 10% increase in neuronal density. Although visual dysfunction is not a prominent feature of schizophrenia, it has been speculated that the decrease in neuronal density in the visual cortex may be related to poor eye tracking (Selemon *et al.*, 1995).

Secondary and tertiary visual cortex (BA 18 and 19)

Brodmann's area 18 receives binocular input and allows for the appreciation of three dimensions (stereopsis). Target distance is coded by some neurons. Some neurons of BA 19 integrate visual with auditory signals and visual with tactile signals.

The parallel visual pathways project forward into the temporal and parietal lobes from the visual cortex. Visual objects compete for attention and it is believed that emotional aspects can operate in a top-down fashion to attend to a specific target (Kastner and Ungerleider, 2001; Pessoa *et al.*, 2002). The occipitotemporal pathway (ventral pathway) is imporant in the identification of objects. Occipital neurons respond to basic cues such as edges. By the time the signals are processed in the temporal lobe more global features are recognized including shape, color, and texture. Face recognition occurs here as well (Grill-Spector *et al.*, 1998).

Electrical stimulation of BA 18 and 19 can produce complex visual hallucinations. Objects may become disproportionately large (macropsia) or distorted in shape. Images of people, animals, and various geometric shapes have been reported. Many complex hallucinations appear real to the patient (Hecaen and Albert, 1978). Complex hallucinations occur more frequently after right-sided lesions. A complete bilateral lesion of all visual cortices, which can result from occlusion of both posterior cerebral arteries, may produce denial of blindness (Anton's syndrome; Redlich and Dorsey, 1945).

Infarction of the left posterior cerebral artery involving the medial occipital lobe (see Figure 2.6) is sufficient to produce a confusional state, including disorientation, distractibility, irritability, and paranoia. Confusion and agitation may alternate with mutism. The acute confusional state presented by the patient may be misdiagnosed as a psychiatric illness (Devinsky *et al.*, 1988).

Visual agnosia sometimes occurs after lesions in the ventromedial occipital lobe. The objects are seen but cannot be named, and the patient does not know what the object can be used for (Critchley, 1964). Loss of the ability to recognize the faces of known people (prosopagnosia) may follow bilateral lesions of the ventromedial occipital lobe that extend into the ventral temporal lobe. Color naming may also be impaired with right-sided lesions (DeRenzi and Spinnler, 1967). It is hypothesized that visual agnosia results from disconnection of the visual cortex from the temporal lobe rather than from destruction of occipital lobe tissue (Joseph, 1996). Lesions restricted to BA 19 may result in loss of only color vision (achromatopsia), leaving shape detection relatively intact.

Clinical vignette

A 47-year-old right-handed woman (DF) had a severe form of agnosia resulting from carbon monoxide poisoning and was incapable of discriminating even the simplest geometric forms. She was unable to recognize objects but was able to use information about location, size, shape, and orientation to reach out and grasp the object. She was unable to copy objects but was able to draw them from memory. She was better able to recognize objects based on surface information than on outline. She could correctly identify objects with colored or gray-scale surfaces but performed poorly with line drawings. Her primary visual cortex appeared to be largely intact. The ventral stream pathway ("what") seemed to be defective (Figure 4.3). The dorsal stream pathway ("where") proved to be intact.

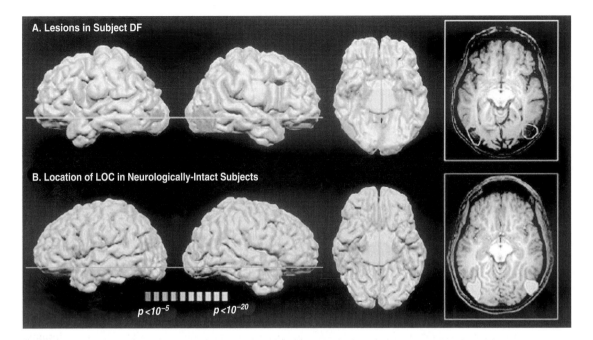

Figure 4.3.   A, B. The ventral visual stream lesions in a patient with visual agnosia (subject DF) are compared to the expected region (lateral occipital complex) for object recognition. A. Lesions in subject DF. Her lesions were traced on slices that indicated tissue damage and rendered on the pial surface in pale blue. Lateral views of the left and right hemispheres are shown, as is a ventral view of the underside of the brain. B. The expected location of the lateral occipital complex based on functional magnetic resonance imaging data from seven neurologically intact participants. The activation of the slice is shown in orange in A for comparison with the lesions in patient DF's brain. (Reproduced with permission from Oxford University Press from James *et al.*, 2003.) See also color plate.

Increased blood flow has been reported in the occipital region in patients with generalized anxiety disorder (Buchsbaum *et al.*, 1987) and with obsessive-compulsive disorder (Zohar *et al.*, 1989). Blood flow to the secondary visual cortex (BA 18 and 19) in subjects with snake phobia was increased over blood flow when they viewed a neutral image (Wik *et al.*, 1992). A more recent study indicates that the relative blood flow increase seen during visually induced anxiety is limited to BA 18 and 19 of the occipital lobe (Fredrikson *et al.*, 1997). The increase seen in the visual association area is coupled with a decrease in blood flow to the prefrontal areas (Figure 4.4). The authors propose that the increased activity reflects an externally directed vigilance function and that the secondary visual area may take control of limbic areas during visually elicited defense reactions (Fredrikson *et al.*, 1997).

The Charles Bonnet syndrome (CBS) is characterized by visual hallucinations following loss of vision often due to cataracts, glaucoma or age-related macular degeneration. The hallucinations may be simple or complex and are experienced as amusing or sometimes disturbing but are not emotionally laden events (Wilkinson, 2004). Hallucinations involving color activated the posterior fusiform area; faces, the left middle fusiform area; objects, the right middle fusiform area; and textures, the cortex bordering the collateral sulcus (ffytche *et al.*, 1998).

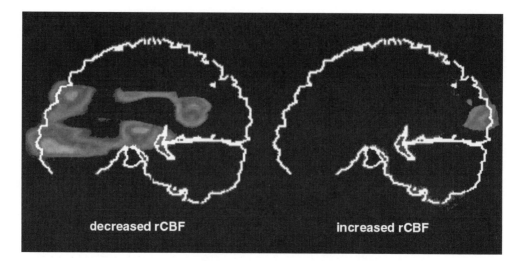

Figure 4.4.   Subjects (n =14) with phobias (snakes and spiders) were examined during exposure to videotapes of spiders and during exposure to videotapes of a neutral park scene. The positron emission tomographic image data were subtracted. Blood flow is increased to the visual association area *(right)* and decreased to the orbital prefrontal cortex *(left)* during exposure to phobia-provocative visual stimuli. rCBF, relative cerebral blood flow. (Reproduced by permission from Fredrickson, M., Fischer, H., and Wik, G. 1997. Cerebral blood flow during anxiety provocation. *J. Clin. Psychiatry* 48 (Suppl.16):16–21.)

Visual auras may occur up to an hour prior to the onset of a migraine headache. The majority are elementary hallucinations and usually consist of lights and simple geometric patterns that usually spread in a stereotyped manner across the visual field. Changes in the BOLD signal spread across the cortex beginning in foveal areas first (the most posterior region) and moving forward over areas representing the peripheral retina (Hadjikhani *et al.*, 2001). It is believed that a form of spreading depression is responsible for the spread of the hallucination across the visual field (Wilkinson, 2004).

Visual auras in epilepsy usually last only a few seconds, followed by other, more severe manifestations of the aura. The hallucinations are often seen as dots, spots or disks that may flicker, pulsate or move. More complex hallucinations, including faces, may be seen (Panayiotopoulos, 1999). Little information is available as to the neural basis largely due to the brief duration of the aura. However, Babb *et al.* (1981), used electrodes to simultaneously monitor the hippocampus and occipital lobe and found the activation occurred first in the medial occipital lobe.

Parietal lobe

Since the masterful volume by Critchley was published in 1953, the parietal lobe has come to be recognized as being heavily involved in the higher cognitive functions of the brain. The parietal lobe is integral to the perception of external space and body image. The complex and fascinating cognitive disturbances that can occur with parietal lobe lesions may at first be mistaken for hysteria. Information perceived and elaborated by the parietal lobe is submitted to the frontal association areas. It is not hard to speculate that if the information received by the frontal lobes is inaccurate, delusional perception or ideas could develop.

Anatomy and behavioral considerations

The parietal lobe underlies the parietal bone of the skull. Its anterior border is the central sulcus, and the lobe extends medially to the cingulate gyrus. Its posterior border is the parieto-occipital fissure (see Figures 2.2, 4.1, 4.2, 5.1). The parietal lobe consists of the primary somatosensory (somesthetic) cortex (BA areas 1, 2, and 3), the superior parietal lobule (BA 5 and 7), and the inferior parietal lobule (BA 39 and 40).

The anterior portion of the parietal lobe is concerned with somesthetic sensations: touch, pain, temperature, and limb position (proprioception). The posterior portion of the parietal lobe integrates somesthetic signals with signals from the visual and auditory systems.

Decreased blood flow in the parietal lobe was observed in a patient with schizoaffective disorder with catatonia and depression (Galynker *et al.*, 1997). Decreased glucose utilization in the parietal lobe was reported in a group of patients with unipolar depression (Biver *et al.*, 1994). Distortion of body image may be associated with parietal dysfunction (Sandyk, 1998). A decrease in glucose utilization was seen in both the parietal and frontal cortices of drug-free schizophrenic patients who had predominantly negative symptoms. Positive symptoms correlated with decreased glucose utilization in the anterior cingulate cortex and hippocampus (Tamminga *et al.*, 1992).

Clinical vignette

A 58-year-old right-handed woman had a 3- to 4-year history of progressive difficulty "seeing" objects. Her visual acuity and visual fields were intact, but she could not draw simple geometric figures such as a triangle or a square. Even more distressing to her was the presence of visual agnosia, or the inability to recognize objects by sight despite intact basic vision. She could not visually recognize common objects such as a cork, a thimble, or a pipe, especially if they appeared in unusual views, angles, or lighting. When she touched the objects, however, she was immediately able to identify and name them. Her performance on photographs and drawings of objects was similarly impaired.

This patient had a progressive visual agnosia from disease affecting her ventromedial occipital cortex (see Figure 4.5). Her slowly progressive history and positron emission tomography scan were consistent with the syndrome of posterior cortical atrophy. At autopsy, this syndrome has usually been a variant of Alzheimer's disease with a shift of the characteristic pathology into visual areas of the brain.

Primary somesthetic cortex

The primary somesthetic cortex occupies the postcentral gyrus (BA 1, 2, and 3). Projections to the postcentral gyrus include thalamocortical fibers from the ventral posteromedial (VPM) and ventral posterolateral (VPL) nuclei of the thalamus (see Table 9.1). These nuclei relay somesthetic signals from both sides of the face and from the contralateral body. Touch and proprioceptive signals project predominantly to BA 1. Pain signals project to BA 3. A somatotopic map of the contralateral body exists along the postcentral gyrus. The leg and genitalia are represented on the medial aspect of the cortex, with the head and remainder of the body on the lateral aspect. Corticothalamic projections from the primary somesthetic cortex terminate in the VPM and VPL thalamic nuclei.

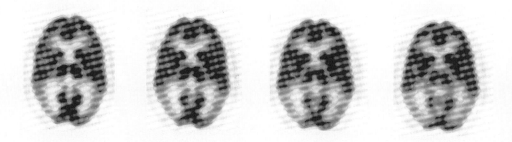

Figure 4.5.   The patient's 18-fluorodeoxyglucose positron emission tomography image revealed bilateral hypometabolism in secondary and tertiary visual cortex (posterior, lateral light areas), while sparing the primary visual cortex (posterior, mesial dark areas). (Reprinted with permission from Mendez, 2001.)

A lesion of the primary somesthetic cortex produces a temporary loss of sensation over the contralateral body. Recovery may be almost complete with time. Some loss in muscle control may remain. The parietal lobe supplies fibers of the corticospinal tract that project to the ventral region of the dorsal horn of the spinal cord. Here they are believed to regulate incoming sensory signals.

Association fibers pass through the white matter of the parietal lobe and connect the postcentral gyrus with the somesthetic association areas behind it. These higher-order association areas integrate touch and conscious proprioception with other modalities. One of these association areas is the superior parietal lobule.

Cerebral blood flow increases in the somesthetic cortex, as well as in the frontal, cingulate, insular, and temporal cortex, in subjects with simple phobia when they are provoked (snake, rodent, spider, bees). Subjects reported that tactile imagery was the most prominent sensory aspect of the phobic experience (Rauch *et al.*, 1995).

Superior parietal lobule

The superior parietal lobule coincides with BA 5 and 7 and is found on both the lateral and medial aspect of the cortex (see Figures 4.1 and 4.2). The precuneus includes BA 7 and 31 on the medial aspect. It receives heavy input from the primary somesthetic cortex. Reciprocal fibers connect the superior parietal lobule with the pulvinar and the lateral thalamic nuclei (see Chapter 9). Pyramidal cells found in the superior parietal lobule contribute heavily to fibers that project to the brainstem and to the spinal cord. Efferent fibers from the superior parietal lobule also project to motor control centers such as the red nucleus, basal ganglia, superior colliculus, and pontine tegmentum. Cortical association fibers connect the superior parietal lobule with adjacent cortex, including the temporal

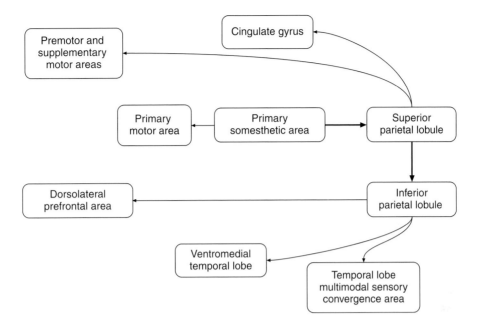

Figure 4.6.   A schematic outline of the projections of the parietal lobe. The superior parietal lobule projects to the premotor and supplementary motor areas of the frontal lobe. The inferior lobule projects to the multimodal region of the temporal lobe as well as to the ventromedial temporal lobe. Inferior lobule projections include those to the dorsolateral prefrontal area.

lobe, occipital lobe, and cingulate gyrus. Long association bundles connect the superior parietal lobule with more distant occipital and temporal regions as well as with the frontal lobe (Figure 4.6). Commissural connections through the corpus callosum interconnect the left and right superior parietal lobules.

The superior parietal lobule contains a representation of the body and limbs as well as a map of the space immediately surrounding the body (Table 4.1). This is an egocentric map as opposed to the allocentric (world-centered) map found in the hippocampus. The parietal map is created from signals from the somesthetic cortex, the visual cortex, the auditory cortex, and the middle temporal and medial superior temporal cortex (Sakata *et al.*, 1997; Colby and Goldberg, 1999). It has been suggested that the right superior temporal area also plays a role in spatial awareness (Karnath *et al.*, 2001).

The right superior parietal lobule is part of the posterior attention system. It is critical in selecting one stimulus location among many. It also disengages and shifts attention to a new target when appropriate (Posner and Dehaene, 1994; see Chapter 12). The right side attends to stimuli in both visual fields and accounts for the fact that neglect is more severe following right parietal damage (Posner and Petersen, 1990). Norepinephrine input to the right parietal region is greater than to the left, and norepinephrine primes the cortical neurons during times of heightened arousal to react to novel stimuli (Tucker and Williamson, 1984).

The superior parietal lobule integrates the sensations of touch and proprioception with vision and integrates information representing these senses with the movement of objects in the visual environment. The parietal lobe is concerned with selecting and attending to a specific target located on the skin or in the nearby extrapersonal space. Anterior superior parietal association

Table 4.1. *Simplified summary of some functions of the parietal lobe and lesions seen after the occurrence of lesions to either the dominant or nondominant side.*

	Side of lesion	
Dominant		Nondominant
Superior parietal lobule		
Function		
Spatial-motor		Spatial orientation
Lesion		
Aphasia		Spatial agnosia
Agnosia		Sensory neglect
Astereoagnosia		Astereoagnosia
Agraphesthesia		Agraphesthesia
		Dressing apraxia
Inferior parietal lobule		
Ideomotor/ideational apraxia		Aprosodia
Gerstmann's syndrome		
Bilateral		
Balint's syndrome		
Movement agnosia		

areas provide the ability to appreciate the weight and texture of an object held in the hand. The superior parietal lobe is concerned with "where" a target is located (see Figure 6.7). It provides information about the location of the target and the direction and velocity of movement of that target. It can program a plan designed to reach that target. Long association fiber bundles to the frontal cortex from the superior parietal lobule allow for the accurate execution of the developed plan.

The lateral interparietal area in the region of the intraparietal sulcus and nearby BA 7 are important in determining the relative behavioral importance of available visual objects and directing attention to a particularly salient object (Yantis *et al.*, 2002). Neurons representing various objects compete for representation and it appears that a top-down mechanism exists to bias the final selection (Bisley and Goldberg, 2003).

Lesions in the dominant superior parietal lobule can produce dysphasia and agnosia. The dysphasic patient speaks slowly, makes many errors in grammar, and may be mistakenly labeled uncooperative or confused. A lesion bordering the postcentral gyrus can produce tactile agnosia, in which the patient cannot recall the name of an object by touch alone. A patient with astereo-agnosia is unable to name (with eyes closed) a familiar object held in his/her hand based on the weight and three-dimensional characteristics of the object. A number or letter written on the patient's skin will not be recognized by touch following a lesion in the superior parietal lobule (agraphesthesia).

Lesions in the nondominant parietal lobe can result in a lack of appreciation of spatial aspects of the opposite side of the body (sensory neglect syndrome). The patient does not recognize the opposite side of his/her body and will not dress it (dressing apraxia). The patient is often unaware of the deficit (anosognosia). Astereoagnosia may also be seen after the occurrence of a lesion of the nondominant side. Inability to copy a simple drawn symmetrical figure (constructional apraxia) is common. It is theorized that since the brain cannot locate objects on the opposite side following a nondominant parietal lobe lesion, the objects cannot be attended to and therefore are ignored. Interestingly, vestibular stimulation can temporarily improve a number of elements of sensory neglect (Vallar et al., 1997) including anosognosia for left hemiplegia (Rode et al., 1998). It is proposed that anosognosia of hemiplegia is due to a loss of motor planning ability (Vallar et al., 2003).

A lesion in the nondominant posterior parietal area may produce a confusion involving location in space. The patient may be confused about his/her current location and, at the same time, be unconcerned. The patient may lose the concept of the spatial relationship of objects with the exception of objects located in his/her immediate extrapersonal space.

Bilateral involvement of the superior parietal lobule can result in the inability to see moving objects (movement agnosia). However, vision for stationary objects remains normal. A lesion bordering the superior and inferior parietal lobules, often involving the supramarginal gyrus, may eliminate the emotional content of pain.

Inferior parietal lobule

The inferior parietal lobule corresponds with the supramarginal gyrus (BA 40) and the angular gyrus (BA 39; see Figure 4.2). Like the superior parietal lobule, it has reciprocal connections with the pulvinar and the lateral thalamic nuclei. Short association fibers connect it with nearby occipital and temporal lobes, and long association fibers link it with the frontal cortex, including the frontal eye fields. The intraparietal area is the cortex associated with the intraparietal sulcus that separates the superior from the inferior parietal lobule.

Clinical vignette

A 65-year-old right-handed man had progressive difficulty locating items in space or orienting himself in familiar surroundings. The patient behaved as if blind, unable to either look at or reach for objects in his environment, such as the buttons on his clothes or utensils on eating. When presented with complex scenes, he could not recognize more than one item at a time (simultanagnosia). He could not identify two adjacent but unlinked drawings, large letters made up of smaller ones, or fragmented pictures. When commanded to move his eyes to specific visual objects in his peripheral fields, he could not do so (oculomotor apraxia). When attempting to reach out and touch objects in his peripheral fields with either arm, he would entirely miss them (optic ataxia).

In addition to the visuospatial deficits of Balint's syndrome, the patient had other impairments. Despite the absence of motor weakness, he was unable to brush his teeth or wave good-bye with his left upper extremity on verbal command (ideomotor apraxia). His attempts at performing these praxis tasks resulted in grotesque motor movements of his left upper extremity. He also had a slow, rigid gait (parkinsonism), abnormal posturing of his right hand and neck (dystonia), and spontaneous jerking of his extremities (myoclonus). Single photon emission tomography imaging showed decreased perfusion in both parietal

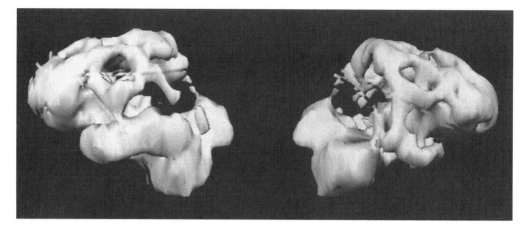

Figure 4.7.   This scan is a three-dimensional computerized reconstruction of the patient's single photon emission tomography images. The left hemisphere is on the left side. There are prominent bilateral areas of decreased perfusion in both parietal lobes consistent with his Balint's syndrome and ideomotor apraxia. (Reprinted with permission from Mendez, 2000.)

regions (Figure 4.7). This patient's illness was consistent with corticobasal degeneration, a disorder that includes cortical deficits such as Balint's syndrome and ideomotor apraxia, and basal ganglia deficits, such as parkinsonism and dystonia.

The intraparietal area is important in visual and somatosensory integration. Neurons in the ventral intraparietal area are responsive to visual targets representing spatial reference frames (maps). There appear to be multiple reference frames and some neurons react to stimuli within reaching distance (Colby and Duhamel, 1991) whereas others are closely linked to a relatively small body region (Duhamel *et al.*, 1997). The medial intraparietal area may be a source of spatial information used by the premotor cortex for visually guided movements (Caminiti *et al.*, 1996).

The inferior parietal lobule integrates the sensations of touch and proprioception with vision and integrates information representing these senses in order to determine the identity of a target (Aguirre and D'Esposito, 1997). The inferior parietal lobe is concerned with "what" a target is (see Figure 6.7). The strategic location of the angular gyrus between the occipital lobe and Wernicke's speech area results in it being "the region which turns written language into spoken language and vice versa . . ." (Geschwind, 1965).

Remembering (retrieval of specific content) and knowing (perception that processed information is from the past) activates a region of the left intraparietal area including BA 39 and 40. Remembering also activates the bilateral anterior fusiform gyrus that processes visual information related to objects (Wheeler and Buckner, 2004). The left inferior parietal lobule, premotor cortex and supplementary motor area become activated when the viewer sees body movements that are within the range of motor capability of the viewer (i.e., capable of imitation) (Blakemore and Decety, 2001). The right inferior lobule plays an important role when the self takes the perspective of others (Ruby and Decety, 2001) and may be part of a "concern mechanism" (Decety and Chaminade, 2003). The inferior parietal lobule functions to encode and retrieve a motor sequence (Rothi *et al.*, 1985). It is proposed that different areas within the inferior parietal lobule encode different types of sequences. The angular gyrus is particularly involved in transforming visual messages to the selection of a motor sequence (Ruby *et al.*, 2002).

The temporo-parietal junction includes portions of the inferior parietal lobule and superior temporal gyrus. This area is activated during egocentric perspective changes (Vallar *et al.*, 1999) as well as during caloric vestibular stimulation (Fasold *et al.*, 2002).

Lesions in the dominant inferior parietal lobule (BA 40) can produce sensory apraxia in which the patient may be able to perform one act of a series of related acts, such as lighting a match, but is unable to complete the series in order to locate and light a cigarette (ideational apraxia). The patient may be able to perform some acts spontaneously (cross arms or scratch nose) but is unable to accomplish these same acts when requested by the examiner (ideomotor apraxia; Heilman *et al.*, 1982). In contrast to deficits in short-term actions, patients with inferior parietal lobule lesions are able to engage in long-term planning (De Renzi *et al.*, 1982; Sirigu *et al.*, 1995).

Pantomime recognition (recognition of common gestures) may be lost following damage to the dominant inferior parietal lobule. A lesion involving the angular gyrus (BA 39) may produce part or all of Gerstmann's syndrome:

- Left–right confusion (left–right confusion among neurologically intact adults is seen in 9% of men and 18% of women).
- Finger agnosia – difficulty in naming fingers.
- Dysgraphia – difficulty with writing.
- Dyscalculia – difficulty with numbers.

A lesion involving the nondominant inferior parietal lobule may produce a deficit in processing the nonsyntactic component of language (aprosodia). In this situation, patients fail to appreciate aspects of a verbal message that are conveyed by the tone, loudness, and timing of the words (i.e., emotional tone).

Bilateral damage to the posterior inferior parietal lobule, often including the adjacent occipital cortex, may produce Balint's syndrome:

- Optic apraxia: eyes tend to remain fixed (stuck) on a visual target, although spontaneous eye movements are unaffected.
- Optic ataxia: a deficit in using visual guidance to grasp an object.
- Simultanagnosia: seeing only the components of a visual object; unable to see the object as a whole.

Vestibular sensations are often reported during out-of-body experiences (OBS). Lesions related to OBS include the angular gyrus. It is proposed that OBS is due to a dysfunction involving the temporo-parietal junction (Blanke *et al.*, 2004).

Volume reductions were reported for the inferior parietal lobule in patients with schizophrenia (Schlaepfer *et al.*, 1994; Goldstein *et al.*, 1999). Male but not female patients with schizophrenia showed a reversal of the normal left greater than right angular gyrus (Frederikse *et al.*, 2000; Niznikiewicz *et al.*, 2000). These regions support language and may help explain the language and thought disorders found in schizophrenia (Shenton *et al.*, 2001). Subjects at high risk for schizophrenia showed, during a verbal task, increased activation in the left inferior parietal lobule compared with controls. It was suggested that the over-activation of the inferior parietal lobule is a compensatory action related to attention to task and preparation of a suitable response.

Subjects at risk for schizophrenia who showed isolated symptoms report difficulties in focusing attention and exhibited a state-related over-activation of the intraparietal sulcus (Whalley *et al.*, 2004). The posterior parietal lobe has been implicated in distinguishing between self and others (Meltzoff and Decety, 2003).

Other symptoms

Parietal lobe seizures can produce bizarre and transient symptoms that can be confusing to both patients and clinicians. Feelings of paresthesia, numbness, heat, or cold have been described. These feelings can begin locally and spread to other contiguous body parts. Seizures beginning more posteriorly can cause pronounced distortion of body image. Limbs may feel heavier or feel as if they disappear. Even more bizarre, patients have reported feeling that someone is standing close by or the appearance of a phantom third limb. Patients with newly diagnosed schizophrenia are reported to show greater sulcal enlargement in the parietal lobe (Rubin *et al.*, 1993).

The similarities between hysteria and parietal lobe disease should again be stressed. Patients with parietal lobe lesions may show marked inconsistency in task performances such that he/she may succeed in a task that moments before appeared to be impossible.

SELECT BIBLIOGRAPHY

M. Critchley, *The Parietal Lobes.* (London: Edward Arnold, 1953).

H. Hecanen, and M. L. Albert, *Human Neuropsychology.* (New York: Wiley, 1978).

J. Hyvarinen, *The Parietal Cortex of Monkey and Man.* (New York: Springer-Verlag, 1982).

W. A. Lishman, *Organic Psychiatry*, 2nd edn. (Boston, Mass.: Blackwell Scientific, 1987).

F. Tilney, and H. A. Riley, *The Form and Functions of the Central Nervous System: An Introduction to the Study of Nervous Diseases*, 3rd edn. (New York: Hoeber, 1938).

REFERENCES

Aguirre, G. K., and D'Esposito, M. 1997. Environmental knowledge is subserved by separable dorsal/ventral neural areas. *J. Neurosci.* **17**:2512–2518.

Anderson, S. W., and Rizzo, M. 1994. Hallucinations following occipital lobe damage: the pathological activation of visual representations. *J. Clin. Exp. Neuropsychol.* **16**:651–653.

Babb, T. H., Halgren, E., Wilson, C., Engel, J., and Crandall, P. 1981. Neuronal firing patterns during the spread of an occipital lobe seizure to the temporal lobes in man. *Electroencephalogr. Clin. Neurophysiol.* **51**:104–107.

Bisley, J. W., and Goldberg, M. E. 2003. Neuronal activity in the lateral intraparietal area and spatial attention. *Science* **299**(5603):81–86.

Biver, F., Goldman, S., Delvenne, V., Luxen, A., DeMaestelaer, V., Hubain, P., Mendlewicz, J., and Lotstra, F. 1994. Frontal and parietal metabolic disturbances in unipolar depression. *Biol. Psychiatry* **36**:381–388.

Blakemore, S-J., and Decetyl, J. 2001. From the perception of action to the understanding of intention. *Nat. Rev. Neurosci.* **2**:561–567.

Blanke, O., Landis, T., Spinelli, L., and Seeck, M. 2004. Out-of-body experience and autoscopy of neurological origin. *Brain* **127**:243–258.

Buchsbaum, M. S., Wu, J., Haier, R., Hazlett, E., Ball, R., Katz, M., Sokolski, K., Lagunas-Solar, M., and Langer, D. 1987. Positron emission tomography assessment of effects of benzodiazepines on regional glucose metabolic rate in patients with anxiety disorder. *Life Sci.* **40**:2393–2400.

Caminiti, R., Ferranina, S., and Johnson, P. B. 1996. The sources of visual information to the primate frontal lobe: a novel role for the superior parietal lobule. *Cereb. Cortex* **6**:319–328.

Colby, C. L., and Duhamel, J.-R. 1991. Heterogeneity of extrastriate visual areas and multiple parietal areas in the macaque monkey. *Neuropsychologia* **29**:517–537.

Colby, C. L., and Goldberg, M.E. 1999. Space and attention in parietal cortex. *Annu. Rev. Neurosci.* **22**:319–349.

Critchley, M. 1953. *The Parietal Lobes.* London: Edward Arnold.
   1964. The problem of visual agnosia. *J. Neurol. Sci.* **1**:274–290.

Decety, J., and Chaminade, T. 2003. Neural correlates of feeling sympathy. *Neuropsychologia* **41**:127–138.

DeRenzi, E., and Spinnler, H. 1967. Impaired performance on color tasks in patients with hemispheric damage. *Cortex* **3**:194–216.

DeRenzi, E., Faglioni, P., and Sorgato, P. 1982. Modality-specific and supramodal mechanisms of apraxia. *Brain* **105**:301–312.

Devinsky, O., Bear, D., and Volpe, B. T. 1988. Confusional states following posterior cerebral artery infarction. *Arch. Neurol.* **45**:160–163.

Duhamel, J.-R., Bremmer, F., BenHamed, S., and Graf, W. 1997. Spatial invariance of visual receptive fields in parietal cortex neurons. *Nature* **389**:845–848.

Fasold, O., von Brevern, M., Kuhberg, M., Ploner, C. J., Villringer, A., Lempert, T., and Wenzel, R. 2002. Human vestibular cortex as identified with caloric stimulation in functional magnetic resonance imaging. *Neuroimage* **17**(3):1384–1393.

ffytche, D. H., Howard, R. J., Brammer, M. J., David, A., Woodruff, P., and Williams, S. 1998. The anatomy of conscious vision: an fMRI study of visual hallucinations. *Nat. Neurosci.* **1**:1247–1260.

Frederikse, M., Lu, A., Aylward, E., Barta, P., Sharma, T., and Pearlson, G. 2000. Sex differences in inferior parietal lobule volume in schizophrenia. *Am. J. Psychiatry* **157**:422–427.

Fredrikson, M., Fischer, H., and Wik, G. 1997. Cerebral blood flow during anxiety provocation. *J. Clin. Psychiatry* **58**(Suppl. 16):16–21.

Galynker, I. I., Weiss, J., Ongseng, F., and Finestone, H. 1997. ECT treatment and cerebral perfusion in catatonia. *J. Nucl. Med.* **38**:251–254.

Geschwind, N. 1965. Disconnection syndromes in animals and man. Part I and II. *Brain* **88**:237–294, 585–644.

Goldstein, J. M., Goodman, J. M., Seidman, L. J., Kennedy, D. N., Makris, N., Lee, H., Tourville, J., Caviness, V. S. Jr., Faraone, S. V., and Tsuang, M. T.1999. Cortical abnormalities in schizophrenia identified by structural magnetic resonance imaging. *Arch. Gen. Psychiatry* **56**:537–547.

Grill-Spector, K., Kushnir, T., Hendler, T., Edelman, S., Itzchat, Y., and Malach, R., 1998. A sequence of object-processing stages revealed by fMRI in the human occipital lobe. *Hum. Brain Mapp.* **6**:316–328.

Gross, C. G., Moore, T., and Rodman, H. R. 2004. Visually guided behavior after V1 lesions in young and adult monkeys and its relation to blindsight in humans. *Prog. Brain Res.* **144**:279–294.

Hadjikhani, N., Sanchez del Rio, M., Wu, O., Schwartz, E., Bakker, D., Fischl, B., Kwong, K. K., Cutrer, F. M., Rosen, B. R., Tootel, R. H., Sorensen, A. G., and Moskowitz, M. A. 2001. Mechanisms of migraine aura revealed by functional MRI in human visual cortex. *Proc. Natl. Acad. Sci. U.S.A.* **98**:4687–4692.

Hecaen, H., and Albert, M.L. 1978. *Human Neuropsychology.* New York: Wiley.

Heilman, K.M., Rothi, L.J., and Valenstein, E. 1982. Two forms of ideomotor apraxia. *Neurology* **32**:342–346.

James, T. W., Culham, J., Humphrey, G. K., Milner, A. D., and Goodale, M. A. 2003. Ventral occipital lesions impair object recognition but not object-directed grasping: an fMRI study. *Brain* **126**:2463–2475.

Joseph, R. 1996. *Neuropsychology, Neuropsychiatry, and Behavioral Neurology.* Baltimore, Md.: Williams and Wilkins.

Karnath, H. -O., Ferber, S., and Himmelbach, M. 2001. Spatial awareness is a function of the temporal not the posterior parietal lobe. *Nature* **411**:950–953.

Kastner, A., and Ungerleider, L. G. 2001. The neural basis of biased competition in human visual cortex. *Neuropsychologia* **39**(12):1263–1276.

Mendez, M. F. 2000. Corticobasal ganglionic degeneration with Balint's syndrome. *J. Neuropsychiatry Clin. Neurosci.* **12**:273–275.

     2001. Visuospatial deficits and preserved reading ability in a patient with posterior cortical atrophy. *Cortex* **37**(4):535–543.

Meltzoff, A. N., and Decety, J. 2003. What imitation tells us about social cognition: a rapprochement between developmental psychology and cognitive neuroscience. *Philos. Trans. R. Soc. Lond. B Biol. Sci.* **358**:491–500.

Morris, J. S., DeGelder, B., Weiskrantz, L., and Dolan, R. J. 2001. Differential extrageniculostriate and amygdala responses to presentation of emotional faces in a cortically blind field. *Brain* **124**:1241–1252.

Nagaratnam, N., Virk, S., and Brdarevic, O. 1996. Musical hallucinations associated with recurrence of a right occipital meningioma. *Br. J. Clin. Pract.* **50**:56–57.

Niznikiewicz, M., Donnino, R., McCarley, R. W., Nestor, P. G., Iosifescu, D. V., O'Donnell, B., Levitt, J., and Shenton, M. E. 2000. Abnormal angular gyrus asymmetry in schizophrenia. *Am. J. Psychiatry* **157**:428–437.

Panayiotopoulos, C.P. 1999. Visual phenomena and headache in occipital epilepsy: a review, a systematic study and differentiation from migraine. *Epileptic Disord.* **1**:205–216.

Parekh, P. I., Spencer, J. W., George, M. S., Gill, D. S., Ketter, T. A., Andreason, P., Herscovitch, P., and Post, R. M. 1995. Procaine-induced increases in limbic rCBF correlate positively with increases in occipital and temporal EEG fast activity. *Brain Topogr.* **7**:209–216.

Pessoa, L., Kastner, S., and Ungerleider, L. 2002. Attentional control of the processing of neural and emotional stimuli. *Brain Res.* **15**(1):31–45.

Pourtois, G., Grandjean, D., Sander, D., and Vuilleumier, P. 2004. Electrophysiological correlates of rapid spatial orienting towards fearful faces. *Cereb. Cortex* **14**(6):619–633.

Posner, M. I., and Dehaene, S. 1994. Attentional networks. *Trends Neurosci.* **17**:75–79.

Posner, M., and Petersen, S. E. 1990. The attention system of the brain. *Annu. Rev. Neurosci.* **13**:25–42.

Rauch, S. L., Savage, C. R., Alpert, N. M., Miguel, E. C., Baer, L., Breiter, H. C., Fischman, A. J., Manzo, P. A., Moretti, C., and Jenike, M. A. 1995. A positron emission tomographic study of simple phobic symptom provocation. *Arch. Gen. Psychiatry* **52**:20–28.

Redlich,F. C., and Dorsey, J. E. 1945. Denial of blindness by patients with cerebral disease. *Arch. Neurol. Psychiatry* **53**:407–417.

Rode, G., Perenin, M. T., Honoré, J., and Boisson, D. 1998. Improvement of the motor deficit of neglect patients through vestibular stimulation: evidence for a motor neglect component. *Cortex* **34**:253–261.

Rothi, L. J., Heilman, K. M., and Watson, R. T. 1985. Pantomime comprehension and ideomotor apraxia. *J. Neurol. Neurosurg. Psychiatry* **48**:207–210.

Rubin, P., Karle, A., Moller-Madsen, S., Hertel, C., Povlsen, U. J., Noring, U., and Hemmingsen, R. 1993. Computerised tomography in newly diagnosed schizophrenia and schizophreniform disorder. A controlled blind study. *Br. J. Psychiatry* **163**:604–612.

Ruby, P., and Decety, J. 2001. Effect of subjective perspective taking during simulation of action: a PET investigation of agency. *Nature Neurosci.* **4**:546–550.

Ruby, P., Sirigu, A., and Decety, J. 2002. Distinct areas in parietal cortex involved in long-term and short-term action planning: a PET investigation. *Cortex* **38**:321–339.

Sakata, H., Taira, M., Kuisunoki, M., Murata, A., and Tanaka, Y. 1997. The parietal association cortex in depth perception and visual control of hand action. *Trends Neurosci.* **20**:350–357.

Sandyk, R. 1998. Reversal of a body image disorder (macrosomatognosia) in Parkinson's disease by treatment with AC pulsed electromagnetic fields. *Int. J. Neurosci.* **93**:43–54.

Schlaepfer, T. E., Harris, G. J., Tien, A. Y., Peng, L. W., Lee, S., Federman, E. B., Chase, G. A., Barta, P. E., and Pearlson, G. D. 1994. Decreased regional cortical gray matter volume in schizophrenia. *Am. J. Psychiatry* **151**:842–848.

Selemon, L. D., Rajkowska, G., and Goldman-Rakic, P. S. 1995. Abnormally high neuronal density in two widespread areas of the schizophrenic cortex. A morphometric analysis of prefrontal area 9 and occipital area 17. *Arch. Gen. Psychiatry* **52**:808–818.

Shenton, M. E., Dickey, C. C., Frumin, M., and McCarley, R. W. 2001. A review of MRI findings in schizophrenia. *Schizophr. Res.* **49**:1–52.

Sirigu, A., Zalla, T., Pillon, B., Grafman, J., Dubois, B., and Agid, Y. 1995. Planning and script analysis following prefrontal lobe lesions. *Ann. N. Y. Acad. Sci.* **769**:277–288.

Tamminga, C. A., Thaker, G. K., Buchanan, R., Kirkpatrick, B., Alphs, L. D., Chase, T. N., and Carpenter, W. T. 1992. Limbic system abnormalities identified in schizophrenia using positron emission tomography with fluorodeoxyglucose and neocortical alterations with deficit syndrome. *Arch. Gen. Psychiatry* **49**:522–530.

Tucker, D. M., and Williamson, P. A. 1984. Asymmetric neural control systems in human self regulation. *Psychol. Rev.* **91**:185–215.

Vallar, G., Guariglia, C., and Rusconi, M. L. 1997. Modulation of the neglect syndrome by sensory stimulation. In: P. Thier and H. -O. Karnath (eds.) *Parietal Lobe Contributions to Orientation in 3D Space.* Heidelberg: Spinger-Verlag, pp. 555–578.

Vallar, G., Lobel, E., Galati, G., Berthoz, A., Pizzamiglio, L., and Le Bihan, D. 1999. A fronto-parietal system for computing the egocentric spatial frame of reference in humans. *Exp. Brain Res.* **124**:281–286.

Vallar, G., Bottini, G., and Sterzi, R. 2003. Anosognosia for left-sided motor and sensory deficits, motor neglect, and sensory hemi-inattention: is there a relationship? *Prog. Brain Res.* **142**:289–301.

Weiskrantz, L. 2004. Roots of blindsight. *Prog. Brain Res.* **144**:229–241.

Whalley, H. C., Simonotto, E., Flett, S., Marshall, L., Ebmeier, K. P., Owens, D. G. C., Goddard, N. H., Johnstone, E. C., and Lawrie, S. M. 2004. fMRI correlates of state and trait effects in subjects at genetically enhanced risk of schizophrenia. *Brain* **127**:478–490.

Wheeler, M. E., and Buckner, R. L. 2004. Functional-anatomic correlates of remembering and knowing. *Neuroimage* **21**:1337–1349.

Wilkinson, F. 2004. Auras and other hallucinations: windows on the visual brain. *Prog. Brain Res.* **144**:305–320.

Wik, G., Fredrikson, M., Ericson, K., Eriksson, L., Stone-Elander, S., and Grieitz, T. 1992. A functional cerebral response to frightening visual stimulation. *Psychiatry Res. Neuroimag.* **50**:15–24.

Yantis, S., Schwarzbach, J., Serences, J. T., Carlson, R. L., Steinmetz, M. A., Pekar, J. J., and Courtney, S. M. 2002. Transient neural activity in human parietal cortex during spatial attention shifts. *Nat. Neurosci.* **5**(10):995–1002.

Zohar, J., Insel, T. R., Berman, K. F., Foa, E. B., Hill, J. L., and Weinberger, D. R. 1989. Anxiety and cerebral blood flow during behavioral challenge: dissociation of central from peripheral and subjective measures. *Arch. Gen. Psychiatry* **46**:505–510.

Temporal lobe – neocortical structures

Emil Kraepelin (1919) suggested that abnormalities in the frontal lobe were responsible for problems in reasoning and that damage to the temporal lobe resulted in delusions and hallucinations in patients with dementia praecox (schizophrenia). The classical findings of Kluver and Bucy in the 1930s clearly and strongly linked the temporal lobes to behavior. Their work provided the basis from which the concept of the limbic system has developed.

The temporal lobe can be divided into two regions: lateral and ventromedial. The lateral region supports cognitive functions associated with several sensory systems. It is recognized as neocortex and is the focus of this chapter. The ventromedial region of the temporal lobe contains major portions of the limbic system and thus contributes significantly to emotional tone. The ventromedial, limbic temporal lobe is discussed in Chapter 11.

It is now accepted that dysfunction of the dorsolateral region of the temporal lobe may be associated with several psychopathological states. Temporal lobe lesions due to a variety of neurological insults can lead a patient to present with signs and symptoms that are more consistent with a psychiatric diagnosis than with a traditional neurological one.

Anatomy and behavioral considerations

The temporal lobe lies ventral to the lateral fissure (of Sylvius) and the parietal lobe. It is rostral to the occipital lobe (Figure 5.1). The superior temporal sulcus and the lateral fissure lie above the superior temporal gyrus and are particularly deep.

The transverse gyri (of Heschl; BA 41 and 42) are located on the superior surface of the superior temporal gyrus (see Figure 2.3). The superior, middle, and inferior temporal gyri roughly correspond with BA 22, 21, and 20, respectively. The cortex of the temporal pole is BA 38. The caudal portion of the middle and inferior temporal gyri, which lie inferior to the parietal lobe, constitutes BA 37. If the lips of the lateral fissure are pulled apart, the insular cortex is seen to lie deep within the lateral fissure.

Gyri and sulci are more variable on the inferior surface of the temporal lobe (Figure 5.2). Three parallel gyri can be recognized; the most lateral consists of the inferior temporal gyrus rostrally and the lateral occipitotemporal gyrus caudally. The medial

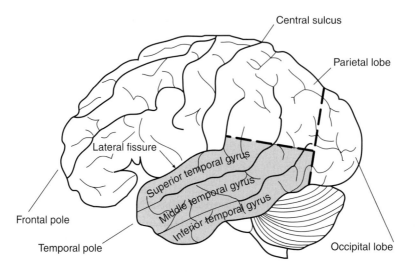

Figure 5.1.   The dashed lines indicate the imaginary boundaries between the parietal, occipital, and temporal lobes. The temporal lobe lies below the lateral fissure, below the parietal lobe, and to the front of the occipital lobe. The dashed line that demarcates the occipital from the parietal and temporal lobes is an imaginary line that runs from the parieto–occipital sulcus above to the preoccipital notch below.

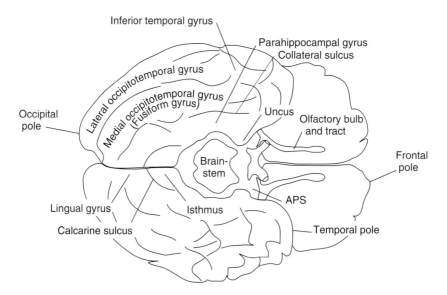

Figure 5.2.   The boundary between the temporal lobes and the occipital lobe is indistinct on the ventral surface of the brain. The isthmus of the cingulate gyrus is continuous with the parahippocampal gyrus. APS, anterior perforated substance.

occipitotemporal gyrus (fusiform gyrus) is separated from the lateral occipitotemporal gyrus by the inferior temporal sulcus. The collateral sulcus and its rostral extension, the rhinal fissure, mark the lateral extent of the parahippocampal (hippocampal) gyrus. The caudal continuation of the parahippocampal gyrus into the occipital lobe is the lingual gyrus. The parahippocampal gyrus expands at its rostral pole to form the uncus (see Chapter 11).

Clinical vignette

A 68-year-old left-handed man had difficulty understanding speech after a stroke sustained during coronary artery bypass surgery. When he awoke from anesthesia, he could not understand what people were saying, as if they were "speaking too fast or in Chinese." His own speech was not affected, and he could read and write perfectly. In addition, environmental sounds became indistinct and difficult to understand. On examination, he was very talkative, but, when spoken to, he appeared confused and perplexed. His audiometry testing was adequate, and he could discriminate pure tones based on frequency, intensity, or duration. In contrast, he had difficulty understanding spoken commands, and he could not understand simple sounds, such as a birdcall or a train whistle.

This patient had auditory agnosia for spoken words (word deafness) and environmental sounds. These problems were consequent to a stroke involving the right temporal auditory cortex (Figure 5.3). Whereas right temporal lesions can produce auditory agnosia for environmental sounds, the presence of the additional word deafness was probably due to a greater right hemisphere role in auditory-language pathways in this left-handed person.

Clinical vignette

A 71-year-old language teacher complained of a progressive loss of the ability to use and understand Spanish and German. The patient had difficulty understanding even common nouns in Spanish, and he was no longer able to understand any German words. His English was impaired as well. The patient had lost the meaning of many words such as cuff, lapel, and eyelashes and, on an aphasia battery, his word comprehension was moderately impaired. Moreover, the patient was losing the ability to identify many of the objects that he could not name.

This patient's presentation was compatible with the syndrome of semantic dementia characterized by early loss of word comprehension followed by more pervasive inability in the identification of objects. His magnetic resonance imaging (MRI) studies showed anterior inferior temporal atrophy in the left hemisphere (Figure 5.4).

Superior and middle temporal gyrus

Auditory cortex

Brodmann's area 41 of the transverse gyri corresponds with the primary auditory cortex. It receives projections from the medial geniculate body of the thalamus. Brodmann's area 42 constitutes the secondary auditory cortex (see Figure 2.3). The auditory association area extends rostrally from BA 41 and 42 along the superior temporal gyrus, caudally to the parietal/temporal junction, and medially to include the temporal cortex located on the upper surface of the lateral fissure. In right-handed persons, the planum temporale, part of

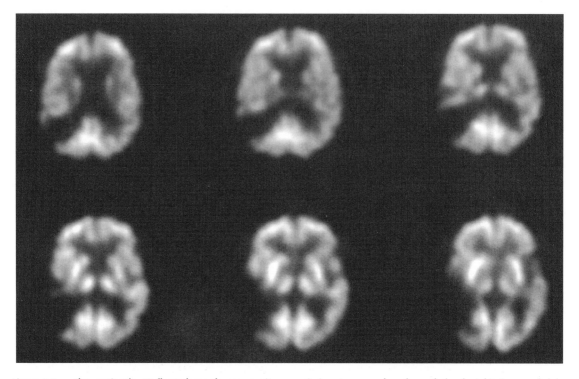

Figure 5.3.   The patient's 18-fluorodeoxyglucose positron emission tomography showed focal right temporal lobe hypometabolism affecting his auditory cortex. (Reprinted with permission from Mendez, 2001.)

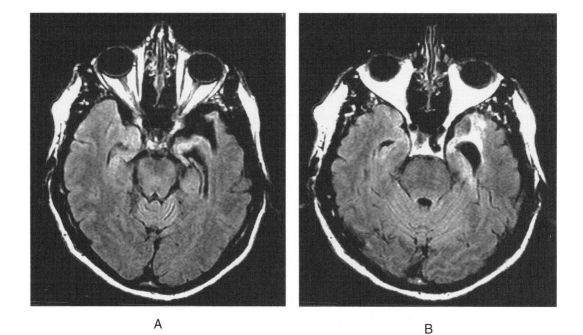

A   B

Figure 5.4.   A, B. T2-weighted magnetic resonance images showed bilateral anterior inferior temporal atrophy disproportionately affecting the left temporal lobe. (Reprinted with permission from Mendez and Cummings, 2003.)

the auditory association area, is larger on the left side of the brain. The lateral fissure on the left is also longer. The planum temporale is larger at birth in girls than in boys and remains larger in females throughout life although the degree of left–right asymmetry is not as great in females (Kulynych *et al.*, 1994).

The primary auditory area contains a tonotopic map that reflects the distribution of frequency-dependent cells along the organ of Corti. The auditory cortex consists of cell columns in an arrangement similar to that of other sensory cortical areas. Biaural input to these columns may be related to sound localization. Speech sounds are analyzed by the left temporal lobe. Tonal differences (e.g., musical scale) are analyzed by the right temporal lobe. There is evidence from animal experimentation that some auditory area neurons respond only to species-specific sounds (Wolberg and Newman, 1972). *It can be speculated that neurons sensitive to specific sounds such as crying or angry voices may also exist.*

Language is related to the posterior superior temporal gyrus and is lateralized to the left (dominant) side. Information processed in the anterosuperior temporal gyrus is projected to the orbital prefrontal cortex. Pauses during speech, used in speech planning and word retrieval, were associated with activation of the left superior temporal sulcus (BA 22 and 39) (Kircher *et al.*, 2004).

Electrical stimulation of the primary auditory region produces elementary hallucinations, including ringing, buzzing, or whispering. On the rare occasion when tumors involve this area, there is often a repetitive quality that makes the experience more disagreeable. Word deafness may result if the pathway from the primary auditory cortex to the auditory association cortex is interrupted. Occasionally, in patients with complex partial seizures, more meaningful sounds such as footsteps or music can be experienced.

The left lateral fissure is larger in schizophrenics than in normal individuals (Rubin *et al.*, 1993), and the planum temporale is reduced in volume in this population (Kwon *et al.*, 1999). Schizophrenia is associated with a decrease in the normal left–right asymmetry in the planum temporale (McCarley *et al.*, 1993a) and with a reversal of normal left–right asymmetry (Petty *et al.*, 1995; Kwon *et al.*, 1999). Schizophrenia may involve an anomaly in language processing related to the failure of the proper development of the normal left–right asymmetry (Crow, 1997). Schizophrenic patients compared with controls using fMRI showed reduced coupling between the left dorsolateral prefrontal cortex and the left superior temporal gyrus (frontotemporal connectivity). The coupling was reduced further in patients experiencing auditory hallucinations. It was hypothesized that reduced frontotemporal connectivity is responsible for the failure of normal constraint of inner speech (Lawrie *et al.*, 2002).

Temporal association areas

Posterior temporal cortex adjacent to the occipital cortex is a visual association area. Temporal cortex adjacent to the primary and secondary auditory cortex is an auditory association area. The cortex deep within the superior temporal sulcus is a multimodal sensory convergence area and receives input from auditory, visual, and somatosensory association cortices, as well as from limbic cortex (Figure 5.5).

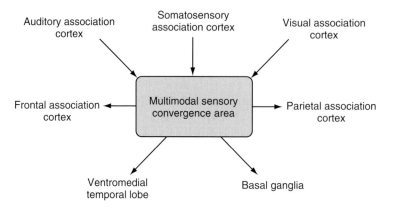

Figure 5.5.   The multimodal sensory convergence area receives input from all sensory association areas and projects to the frontal and parietal association areas as well as to the basal ganglia and to the ventromedial temporal cortex.

The temporal multimodal sensory convergence area gives rise to efferent projections to parietal and frontal association areas as well as to the limbic system (see Figure 11.3) and the basal ganglia (Figure 5.5). The corpus callosum and the anterior commissure interconnect the left and right temporal lobes (see Chapter 14). Both of these fiber bundles serve the neocortical regions. A large number of commissure fibers interconnect the parahippocampal gyrus, the rostral parts of the middle and inferior temporal gyri, and the amygdala.

Projections from the temporal multimodal sensory convergence area include fibers that terminate in the pulvinar and the mediodorsal nucleus of the thalamus (Pandya *et al.*, 1994). The mediodorsal nucleus projects to the prefrontal lobe. The pulvinar projects to the posterior cingulate gyrus. The posterior cingulate gyrus is known to be important in the memory and recall of the location of significant targets located in the extrapersonal space (see Chapter 12).

The multimodal sensory convergence area integrates information that arrives from sensory association regions. It distributes the integrated information to other vital brain regions for emotional (ventromedial temporal lobe), cognitive (frontal association area), or motor (basal ganglia) processing for elaboration or response preparation. Fibers that project from the multimodal sensory convergence area to the prefrontal lobe parallel those from the amygdala. The similarity in connectivity undoubtedly accounts for the fact that damage to either the amygdala or the multimodal sensory convergence area in monkeys produces many of the behavioral changes seen in Kluver–Bucy syndrome (see Chapter 13; Gloor, 1997).

Posterior portions of the middle and inferior temporal gyri adjacent to the occipital lobe are heavily involved with visual processing. Visual signals that enter the posterior temporal lobe are matched with embedded constructs for object recognition (e.g., box, sphere, face; Figure 5.6). Lesions in this area in rhesus monkeys render them unable to distinguish one complex visual

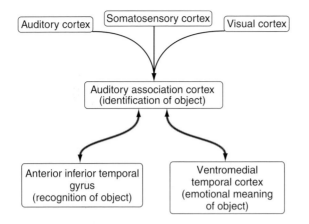

Figure 5.6.   The predominant flow of information is from the auditory association cortex to the anteroinferior temporal gyrus (recognition of object) and to the ventromedial temporal cortex (emotional meaning of object).

image from another (as a human would distinguish one face from another) and unable to continue to attend to a specific visual image (Ungerleider and Mishkin, 1982). Reciprocal connections with the anterior inferior temporal gyrus and temporal pole provide recognition of the object (e.g., edible, predator). These same posterior gyri also have extensive reciprocal connections with the ventromedial temporal cortex. It is through these connections that emotional values are assigned to visual objects. The inferior temporal area is bilaterally activated during sexual arousal and is hypothesized to relate to the perception of the visual stimuli as sexual in nature (Stoléru *et al.*, 1999).

The left posterior inferior temporal area (BA 37) functions to process letters and words and is an association area that integrates input from several areas. This area is activated in blind as well as in sighted subjects processing a variety of word forms (Büchel *et al.*, 1998). There is reduced activation of the same area in subjects with dyslexia (Brunswick *et al.*, 1999).

Cortex surrounding the superior temporal sulcus is important in social perception using visual cues such as movements of the hands, mouth and eyes. For example, animated visual images clearly identified with head, hand and leg movements (biological motion) activate cortex of the posterior portion of the superior temporal sulcus, with the right more prominently activated (Blakemore and Decety, 2001).

The fusiform gyrus is part of the ventral "what" pathway and is strongly activated when subjects view images of human faces (Figure 5.7). This area has been called the fusiform face area (FFA). This area responds to objects other than faces and appears to be sensitive to complex attributes common to both faces and objects (Haxby *et al.*, 2001; Hasson *et al.*, 2004). It is hypothesized to detect motion related to facial expression (Cipolotti *et al.*, 1999; Blair *et al.*, 2002).

The observation that patients in complex partial seizure status (continuous complex partial seizures) can be awake and even responsive can be explained (at least partially) by the existence of anatomical connections between the two temporal lobes that do not involve most of the other brain regions (noncallosal connections). If a seizure is generalized through the corpus callosum, it is very likely that consciousness will be totally lost (e.g., generalized seizures). One patient, while undergoing electrical stimulation of the left superior temporal gyrus as she counted out

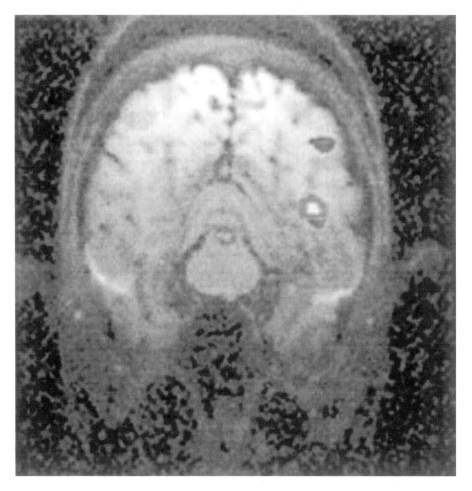

Figure 5.7.   This functional magnetic resonance image shows activation of the "fusiform face area" responsive to human faces. The right hemisphere appears on the left. The brain images at the left show in color the voxels that produced a significantly higher magnetic resonance signal intensity during the epochs containing faces than during those containing objects. These significance images are overlaid on a T1-weighted anatomical image of the same slice. In each image, the region of interest is shown outlined in green. (Reproduced with permission Kanwisher *et al.*, 1997.) See also color plate.

loud, reported that she heard her speech as an "echo" and at the same time felt "frightened" (Fried, 1997).

A reduction in volume of the superior temporal gyrus in schizophrenia has been suspected for some time (Southard, 1910) and has been confirmed more recently (Barta *et al.*, 1990). The effect appears to be lateralized to the dominant cortex, especially in males (Reite *et al.*, 1997). There is a strong correlation between the increase of thought disorder and volume reduction in the left posterosuperior temporal gyrus (McCarley *et al.*, 1993a). By comparison, there is a close association between auditory hallucinations and volume reduction in more anterior regions of the superior temporal gyrus (Barta *et al.*, 1990). These findings are consistent with the finding that there is greater impairment in auditory processing than in visual processing in schizophrenia.

Clinical vignette

A 27-year-old man with a 10-year history of partial complex seizures developed progressive interpersonal difficulties and became socially withdrawn. After suffering a complex partial seizure with secondary generalization, he behaved in a suspicious manner towards his wife, stating that he knew that she was not who she claimed to be but rather was an impostor who had abducted and replaced his wife. He had many similar subsequent episodes. Electroencephalography showed intermittent, irregular right anterior temporal theta slowing and right anterior and anteromedial temporal spikes and sharp waves. A computed tomographic scan revealed a mild enlargement of the right lateral fissure, suggesting right temporal atrophy. The syndrome responded well to carbamazepine therapy (Drake, 1987).

Abnormalities in P300 latency suggest dysfunction in the left superior temporal gyrus (O'Donnell *et al.*, 1995). Listening tests that show a left hemisphere advantage in normal individuals reveal a significantly reduced left hemisphere advantage in schizophrenic patients. These findings support the contention that left temporal lobe dysfunction is present in schizophrenia (Bruder *et al.*, 1995). It has been speculated that the loss of superior temporal gyrus may result in the loss of a proper gradient of associational linkages (Shenton *et al.*, 1992). Relative metabolism in the posterosuperior temporal region is decreased in schizophrenic patients as they hallucinate (Cleghorn *et al.*, 1992). Blood flow to the left superior temporal cortex increases in schizophrenic patients as they experience auditory hallucinations and then decreases as the hallucinations resolve (Suzuki *et al.*, 1993).

Bands of dopamine (D_2) receptors form a distinct modular and laminar pattern in portions of the temporal lobe. The D_2 bands are found in greatest frequency in the auditory association cortex (BA 22, 39, and 42) and in the next highest frequency in the auditory-visual areas (BA 20 and 37). Postmortem analysis of tissue from schizophrenic patients demonstrated a disruption in the pattern of D_2 receptor bands in the superior and inferior temporal gyri, with the greatest difference from controls seen in the superior temporal gyrus (Goldsmith *et al.*, 1997). Disturbances in D_2 receptor distribution correlate with auditory hallucinations, reduced tissue volume and altered auditory-evoked potentials reported by other authors (Shenton *et al.*, 1992; McCarley *et al.*, 1993b).

Intravenous procaine administration produces emotional responses as well as auditory and visual hallucinations. Regional blood flow studies localize the auditory hallucinations to superior temporal activation. It is hypothesized that hallucinations are secondary to activation of the amygdala (Ketter *et al.*, 1996).

Clinical vignette

A 58-year-old man suffered a right hemisphere stroke that produced a left-sided weakness. The weakness improved progressively over a few days, and the patient was discharged. Over a number of weeks, his wife noticed that he was different but could not tell how. She complained that he was no longer paying attention to her. They started having repeated fights. The marital discord brought them to a family counselor who referred them to a neuropsychiatry clinic. On examination it was found that the man suffered from receptive aprosodia with a complete inability to perceive any emotions displayed either by voice or by facial expression.

Lesions of the posterior parts of the left temporal lobe with extension into the ventral parietal lobe can cause a receptive aphasia (Wernicke's aphasia) in which a severe comprehension deficit to spoken language develops. Extension of the lesion up into the parietal lobe can produce a similar deficit in the appreciation of written language. Expressive speech may become hyperfluent, with the patient using nonsense words. Such patients can be mistaken for being acutely psychotic, particularly if they have a past psychiatric history. The arcuate fasciculus connects Wernicke's area with Broca's area in the frontal lobe. Lesions limited to the arcuate fasciculus cause a form of aphasia characterized by difficulty with repetition (conduction aphasia).

Patients with lesions involving the right (nondominant) temporal/parietal region may lose their capacity to discern the emotional content of speech (receptive aprosodia). These patients misperceive paralinguistic social-emotional messages, and after the onset of the lesion they may notice that the voices of friends and relatives are different. Patients then may become progressively paranoid and delusional.

Temporal lobe seizures involving the posterolateral cortex are characterized by aphasia if the seizure is localized to the dominant lobe, and there are also auditory, visual, and vestibular disturbances. In contrast, mesial temporal seizures are characterized by the presence of an aura, followed by staring and behavioral arrest. Oroalimentary automatism is common (Fried, 1997).

Inferior temporal and fusiform gyrus

The inferior temporal gyrus, and particularly BA 20, is the last processing step for the ventral visual system devoted to object feature analysis. It is concerned with images projected onto the fovea of the retina. The anteroinferior temporal gyrus projects to the orbital prefrontal cortex (Mega et al., 1997). The relationship between the inferior temporal gyrus and orbital prefrontal cortex provides continuity between the lateral temporal lobe and the limbic system (Carmichael and Price, 1995).

The posterior lateral fusiform gyrus, described as the fusiform face area (FFA), is an extrastriate visual area that becomes activated when viewing faces (Narumoto et al., 2001), even in 2-month-old infants (Tzourio-Mazoyer et al., 2002). The FFA is activated whether the face is clearly defined or is implied by surrounding, contextual cues (Cox et al., 2004). The right side is more sensitive to emotional than to neutral expressions (Vuilleumier et al., 2001) and activation of the amygdala can potentiate responses of the fusiform gyrus (Tabert et al., 2001). The FFA is sensitive to faces but also distinguishes between consciously remembered and forgotten faces(Lehmann et al., 2004).

One patient, while being stimulated in the left inferotemporal cortex, reported familiar music and vivid visual images of personal importance but was aware that they were unreal (Fried, 1997).

Clinical vignette

A 28-year-old right-handed stockbroker with no prior psychiatric history suffered traumatic brain injury to the right temporoparietal and, to a lesser extent, right frontal lobe. On recovery, he had the delusion that he was dead. None of his surroundings looked familiar. This delusion of death is called a Cotard delusion (Young et al., 1992).

Epileptic discharges in the middle and inferior temporal gyri can result in complex hallucinations or confusional episodes or may cause an abnormal attribution of emotional significance to otherwise neutral thoughts and external stimuli. Hallucinations become increasingly complex as the disturbance expands from primary to more complex association areas. A variety of emotional reactions can occur during the course of a temporal lobe seizure. Fear is the most frequently reported emotion during a seizure. Other reported emotions include anxiety, pleasure, displeasure, depersonalization, depression, familiarity, and unfamiliarity.

A lower glucose metabolic rate in the ventral stream, including the right inferotemporal area and fusiform gyrus, was reported in schizophrenic subjects with predominantly negative symptoms (Potkin *et al.*, 2002). This is consistent with difficulties seen in this group in correctly identifying and expressing the emotional content of both faces and scenes (Borod *et al.*, 1993; Bryson *et al.*, 1998).

Further behavioral considerations

Lesions of the left temporo–occipital and right frontoparietal areas as well as the pontine tegmentum have been reported to produce musical sounds. Deafness greatly facilitates the emergence of this type of hallucination. Electrical stimulation applied during surgery to the lateral or superior surfaces of the superior temporal gyrus produces musical hallucinations (Keshavan *et al.*, 1992). Electroencephalographic studies showed abnormal patterns in frontal and temporal cortical regions in hyperactive children (Mann *et al.*, 1992).

The proximity of the anterior temporal regions (temporal pole) to bony protrusions and cavities increases its vulnerability to injury, particularly when rotational acceleration is imparted to the freely moving head (Levin and Kraus, 1994). Such injury can result in white matter damage that may be diffuse and may not be detectable by structural imaging.

Blood flow studies revealed that the visual processing of images of faces is performed in different regions depending on the category of face (old versus young; male versus female) or whether the face has just recently been viewed or is a familiar face that is from several weeks' experience. Categorization of a face is dependent on the left occipital cortex, inferior temporal cortex, and frontal cortex. The ability to recognize a familiar face also involves the inferior temporal cortex. Damage to the inferior occipitotemporal gyrus and lingual gyrus produces prosopagnosia (Andreasen *et al.*, 1996).

Reduplicative paramnesia is a delusional belief that a place has been duplicated. It is postulated that a combined right posterior parietal lesion and frontal pathology leads to the development of this syndrome. The posterior right hemisphere lesion causes visuoperceptual dysfunction involving identification of person or place, and the frontal pathology makes it impossible to resolve the conflicting information, resulting in delusional ideas. The following related syndromes may involve the temporal lobe more directly.

As many as 40% of schizophrenic patients exhibit symptoms of a delusional misidentification syndrome (Cutting, 1994). These syndromes include Capgras' delusion. A patient suffering from Capgras' syndrome believes that well-known persons, including family members, are impostors or may be identical doubles, or both. Two lesions may be needed to produce this syndrome. Right temporal lobe lesions may cause distortion in the sense of familiarity of a person. Frontal damage (usually bilateral) results in the inability to resolve the conflict and hence the feeling of unfamiliarity that results in the belief that the loved one is an impostor (Malloy *et al.*, 1992). The Cotard delusion is an extreme example of depersonalization in a misidentification syndrome (Sno, 1994); see previous Clinical vignette.

The insula

The insular cortex lies deep within the lateral fissure (see Figure 9.1). It consists of several long gyri located more caudally, paralleling the lateral fissure, and five short gyri located more rostrally. It is made up of an anterior and a posterior region divided by the middle cerebral artery that passes across the surface of the insular cortex. It has connections with many limbic-related structures, including the entorhinal area, hippocampus, amygdala, and prefrontal cortex, as well as with the motor cortex and basal ganglia. The insular cortex also has interconnections with the sensory association areas and is considered the cortical viscerosensory area. It has been suggested to be a gateway between the somatosensory areas and the limbic system and has been included as a component of the limbic integration cortex (Augustine, 1996). The temporal pole, the orbital prefrontal cortex, and the insula are recognized as components of the paralimbic cortex (Moran *et al.*, 1987).

The anterior insula along with adjacent frontal opercular cortex, especially on the dominant side, represents a primary gustatory area. This area corresponds closely with BA 43 (Ogawa, 1994). The anterior insula is activated during sexual arousal in men (Stoléru *et al.*, 1999). The anterior insula on the right supports conscious awareness of visceral activity (heart beat) and provides a basis for subjective feelings of visceral awareness (Critchley *et al.*, 2004), including taste (Kringelbach *et al.*, 2004). The left anterior insula was activated in response to all odors whereas the right insula was activated specifically by disgusting odors (Heining *et al.*, 2003). The posterior insula has been identified as the cardiac control cortex (Oppenheimer, 1993). It plays a role in the appreciation of emotional aspects of pain (Geschwind, 1965). The insula is also a component of the articulatory loop, which is important in processing verbal material (Paulesu *et al.*, 1993) and is activated during inner-speech generation (Shergill *et al.*, 2000).

Insular tumors have been reported to elicit partial seizures that begin with sensations of butterflies in the throat or tingling in the arm followed by a warm flush (Roper *et al.*, 1993). Patients who develop panic symptoms with lactate infusion exhibit a blood flow increase bilaterally in the temporal lobes, insular cortex, brainstem superior colliculus, and putamen (Reiman *et al.*, 1989). Blood flow has been reported to increase during anticipatory anxiety in the anterior insular area, which is postulated to serve as an internal alarm center (Reiman, 1997). Recalled sadness in normal subjects produces activation of the anterior insula (Lane *et al.*, 1997). Results suggest that the anterior insular cortex participates in the emotional response to particularly distressing cognitive or interoceptive sensory stimuli (Reiman *et al.*, 1997). Activation of the insular cortex may reflect its role in cardiac control (Oppenheimer, 1993). The insula also responds to gustatory stimuli (Small *et al.*, 1999).

SELECT BIBLIOGRAPHY

H. D. Ellis, J.-P. Luaute, and N. Retterstol, Delusional misidentification syndromes. *Psychopathology* **27** (1994), 117–120, (1 of 25 articles on this topic in this issue of *Psychopathology*.)

W. A. Lishman, *Organic Psychiatry*. (Oxford: Blackwell Scientific, 1987.)

J. Rhawn, *Neuropsychology, Neuropsychiatry, and Behavioral Neurology*. (New York: Plenum Press, 1989.)

W. Willis, Jr., and R. Grossman, *Medical Neurobiology*. (St. Louis, Mo.: Mosby, 1977.)

REFERENCES

Andreasen, N. C., O'Leary, D. S., Arndt, S., Cizadlo, T., Hurtig, R., Rezai, K., Watkins, G. L., Ponto, L. B., and Hichwa, R. D. 1996. Neural substrates of facial recognition. *J. Neuropsychiatry Clin. Neurosci.* **8**:139–146.

Augustine, J. R. 1996. Circuitry and functional aspects of the insular lobe in primates including humans: a full-length review. *Brain Res. Brain Res. Rev.* **22**:229–244.

Barta, P. E., Pearlson, G. D., Powers, R. E., Richards, S. S., and Tune, L. E. 1990. Auditory hallucinations and smaller superior temporal gyral volume in schizophrenia. *Am. J. Psychiatry* **147**:1457–1462.

Blair, R. J., Frith, U., Smith, N., Abell, F., and Cipolotti, L. 2002. Fractionation of visual memory: agency detection and its impairment in autism. *Neuropsychologia* **40**:108–118.

Blakemore, S.-J., and Decety, J. 2001. From the perception of action to the understanding of intention. *Nature Rev. Neurosci.* **2**:561–567.

Borod, J. C., Martin, C. C., Alpert, M., Brozgold, A., and Welkowitz, J. 1993. Perception of facial emotion in schizophrenic and right brain-damaged patients. *J. Nerv. Ment. Dis.* **181**:494–502.

Bruder, G., Rabinowicz, E., Towey, J., Brown, A., Kaufmann, C. A., Amador, X., Malaspina, D., and Gorman, J. M. 1995. Smaller right ear (left hemisphere) advantage for dichotic fused words in patients with schizophrenia. *Am. J. Psychiatry* **152**:932–935.

Brunswick, N., McCrory, E., Price, C., Frith, C. D., and Frith, U. 1999. Explicit and implicit processing of words and pseudowords by adult developmental dyslexics: a search for Wernicke's Wortschatz? *Brain* **122**:1901–1917.

Bryson, G., Bell, M., Kaplan, E., Greig, T., and Lysaker, P. 1998. Affect recognition in deficit syndrome schizophrenia. *Psychiatry Res.* **77**:113–120.

Büchel, C., Price, C. J., and Friston, K. J. 1998. A multimodal language area in the ventral visual pathway. *Nature* **394**:274–277.

Carmichael, S. T., and Price, J. L. 1995. Limbic connections of the orbital and medial prefrontal cortex in macaque monkeys. *J. Comp. Neurol.* **363**:615–641.

Cipolotti, L., Robinson, G., Blair, J., and Frith, U. 1999. Fractionation of visual memory: evidence from a case with multiple neurodevelopmental impairments. *Neuropsychologia* **37**:329–332.

Cleghorn, J. M., Franco, S., Szechtman, B., Kaplan, R. D., Szechtman, H., Brown, G. M., Nhmias, C., and Garnett, E. S. 1992. Toward a brain map of auditory hallucinations. *Am. J. Psychiatry* **149**:1062–1069.

Cox, D., Meyers, E., and Sinha, P. 2004. Contextually evoked object-specific responses in human visual cortex. *Science* **304**:115–117.

Critchley, H. D., Wiens, S., Rothshtein, P., Ohman, A., and Dolan, R. J. 2004. Neural systems supporting interoceptive awareness. *Nature Neurosci.* **7**(2): 189–195.

Crow, T. J. 1997. Schizophrenia as failure of hemispheric dominance for language. *Trends Neurosci.* **20**:339–343.

Cutting, J. 1994. Evidence for right hemisphere dysfunction in schizophrenia. In: A. S. David and J. C. Cutting (eds.) *The Neuropsychology of Schizophrenia.* Hove, England: Erlbaum, pp. 321–242.

Drake, M. E. 1987. Postictal Capgras syndrome. *Clin. Neurol. Neurosurg.* **89**:4

Fried, I. 1997. Auras and experiential responses arising in the temporal lobe. *J. Neuropsychiatry. Clin. Neurosci.* **9**:420–428.

Geschwind, N. 1965. Disconnexion syndromes in animals and man. *Brain* **88**:269–272.

Gloor, P. 1997. *The Temporal Lobe and Limbic System.* New York: Oxford University Press.

Goldsmith, S. K., Shapiro, R. M., and Joyce, J. N. 1997. Disrupted pattern of D_2 dopamine receptors in the temporal lobe in schizophrenia. *Arch. Gen. Psychiatry* **54**:649–658.

Hasson, U., Nir, Y., Levy, I., Fuhrmann, G., and Rafael, M. 2004. Intersubject synchronization of cortical activity during natural vision. *Science* **303**(5664):1634–1640.

Haxby, J. V., Gobbini, M. I., Furey, M. L., Ishai, A., Schouten, J. L., and Pietrini, P. 2001. Distributed and overlapping representations of faces and objects in ventral temporal cortex. *Science* **293**(5539):2425–2430.

Heining, M., Young, A. W., Ioannou, G., Andrew, C. M., Brammer, M. J., Gray, J. A., and Phillips, M. L. 2003. Disgusting smells activate human anterior insula and ventral striatum. *Ann. N. Y. Acad. Sci.* **1000**:380–384.

Kanwisher, N., McDermott, J., and Chun, M. M. 1997. The fusiform face area: a module in human extrastriate cortex specialized for face perception. *J. Neurosci.* **17**(11):4302–4311.

Keshavan, M. S., David, A. S., Steingard, S., and Lishman, W. A. 1992. Musical hallucinations: a review and synthesis. *Neuropsychiatry Neuropsychol. Behav. Neurol.* **5**:211–223.

Ketter, T. A., Andreason,P. J., George, M. S., Lee, C., Gill, D. S., Parekh, P. I., Willis, M. W., Herscovitch, P., and Post, R. M. 1996. Anterior paralimbic mediation of procaine-induced emotional and psychosensory experiences. *Arch. Gen. Psychiatry* **53**:59–69.

Kircher, T. T. J., Brammer, M. J., Levelt, W., Bartels, M., and McGuire, P. K. 2004. Pausing for thought: engagement of the left temporal cortex during pauses in speech. *Neuroimage* **21**:84–90.

Kraepelin, E. 1919/1971. *Dementia Praecox.* Barclay, E., and Barclay, S. (trans.). New York: Churchill Livingstone.

Kringelbach, M. L., de Araujo, I. E. T., and Rolls, E. T. 2004. Taste-related activity in the human dorsolateral prefrontal cortex. *Neuroimage* **21**:781–788.

Kulynych, J. J., Vladar, K., Jones, D. W., and Weinberger, D. R. 1994. Gender differences in the normal lateralization of the supratemporal cortex: MRI surface-rendering morphometry of Heschl's gyrus and the planum temporale. *Cereb. Cortex* **4**:107–118.

Kwon, J. S., McCarley, R. W., Hirayasu, Y., Anderson, J. E., Fischer, I. A., Kikinis, R., Jolesz, F. A., and Shenton, M. E. 1999. Left planum temporale volume reduction in schizophrenia. *Arch. Gen. Psychiatry* **56**:142–148.

Lane, R., Reiman, E. M., Ahern, G. L., Schwartz, G. E., and Davidson, R. J. 1997. Neuroanatomical correlates of happiness, sadness, and disgust. *Am. J. Psychiatry* **154**:926–933.

Lawrie, S. M., Buechel, C., Whalley, H. C., Frith, C. D., Friston, K. J., and Johnstone, E. C. 2002. Reduced frontotemporal functional connectivity in schizophrenia associated with auditory hallucinations. *Biol. Psychiatry* **51**:1008–1011.

Lehmann, C., Mueller, T., Federspiel, A., Hubl, D., Schroth, G., Huber, O., Strik, W., and Dierks, T. 2004. Dissociation between overt and unconscious face processing in fusiform face area. *Neuroimage* **21**:75–83.

Levin, H., and Kraus, M. F. 1994. The frontal lobes and traumatic brain injury. *J. Neuropsychiatry Clin. Neurosci.* **6**:443–454.

Malloy, P., Cimino, C., and Westlake, R. 1992. Differential diagnosis of primary and secondary Capgras delusions. *Neuropsychiatry Neuropsychol. Behav. Neurol.* **5**:83–96.

Mann, C. A., Lubar, J. R., Zimmerman, A. W., Miller, C. A., and Muenchen, R. A. 1992. Quantitative analysis of EEG in boys with attention deficit hyperactivity disorder: controlled study with clinical implications. *Pediatr. Neurol.* **8**:20–36.

McCarley, R. W., Shenton, M. E., O'Donnell, B. F., and Nestor, P. G. 1993a. Uniting Kraepelin and Bleuler: the psychology of schizophrenia and the biology of temporal lobe abnormalities. *Harv. Rev. Psychiatry* **1**:36–56.

McCarley, R. W., Shenton, M. E., O'Donnell, B. F., Gaux, S. F., Kikinis, R., Nestor, G., and Jolesz, F. A. 1993b. Auditory 300 abnormalities and left superior temporal gyrus volume reduction in schizophrenia. *Arch. Gen. Psychiatry* **50**:190–197.

Mega, M. S., Cummings, J. L., Salloway, S., and Malloy, P. 1997. The limbic system: an anatomic, phylogenetic, and clinical perspective. *J. Neuropsychiatry Clin. Neurosci.* **9**:315–330.

Mendez, M. F. 2001. Generalized auditory agnosia with spared music recognition in a left-hander. Analysis of a case with a right temporal stroke. *Cortex* **37**:139–150.

Mendez, M. F., and Cummings, J. L. 2003. *Dementia: A Clinical Approach*, 3rd edn. New York: Butterworth-Heineman, p. 206.

Moran, M. Z., Mufson, E. J., and Mesulam, M. M. 1987. Neural inputs into the temporopolar cortex of the rhesus monkey. *J. Comp. Neurol.* **256**:88–103.

Narumoto, J., Ikada, T., Sadato, N., Fukui, K., and Yonekura, Y. 2001. Attention to modulate fMRI activity in human right superior temporal sulcus. *Brain Res. Cogn. Brain Res.* **12**:225–231.

O'Donnell, B. F., Faux, S. F., McCarley, R. W., Kimble, M. O., Salisbury, D. F., Nestor, P. G., Kikinis, R., Jolesz, F. A., and Shenton, M. E. 1995. Increased rate of P300 latency prolongation with age in schizophrenia. *Arch. Gen. Psychiatry* **52**:544–549.

Ogawa, H. 1994. Gustatory cortex of primates: anatomy and physiology. *Neurosci. Res.* **20**:1–13.

Oppenheimer, S. 1993. The anatomy and physiology of cortical mechanisms of cardiac control. *Stroke* **24**(Suppl. 12):I3–I5.

Pandya, D. N., Rosene, D. L., and Doolittle, A. M. 1994. Corticothalamic connections of auditory-related areas of the temporal lobe in the rhesus monkey. *J. Comp. Neurol.* **345**(3):447–471.

Paulesu, E., Frith, C. D., and Frackowiak, R. S. J. 1993. The neural correlates of the verbal component of working memory. *Nature* **362**:342–344.

Petty, R. G., Barta, P. E., Pearlson, G. D., McGilchrist, I. K., Lewis, R. W., Tien, A. Y., Pulver, A., Vaughn, D. D., Casanova, M. F., and Powers, R. E. 1995. Reversal of asymmetry of the planum temporale in schizophrenia. *Am. J. Psychiatry* **152**(5):715–721.

Potkin, S. G., Alva, G., Fleming, K., Anand, R., Keator, D., Carreon, D., Doo, M., Jin, Y., Wu, J. C., and Fallon, J. H. 2002. A PET study of the pathophysiology of negative symptoms in schizophrenia. Positron emission tomography. *Am. J. Psychiatry* **159**(2):227–237.

Reiman, E. M. 1997. The application of positron emission tomography to the study of normal and pathologic emotions. *J. Clin. Psychiatry* **58**(Suppl. 16):4–12.

Reiman, E. M., Raichle, M. E., Robins, E., Mintun, M. A., Fusselman, M. J., Fox, P. T., Price, J. L., and Hackman, K. A. 1989. Neuroanatomical correlates of a lactate-induced anxiety attack. *Arch. Gen. Psychiatry* **46**:493–500.

Reiman, E. M., Lane, R. D., Ahern, G. L., Schwartz, G. E., Davidson, R. J., Friston, K. J., Yun, L.-S., and Chen, K. 1997. Neuroanatomical correlates of externally and internally generated human emotion. *Am. J. Psychiatry* **154**(7):918–925.

Reite, M., Sheeder, J., Teale, P., Adams, M., Richardson, D., Simon, J., Jones, R. H., and Rojas, D. C. 1997. Magnetic source imaging evidence of sex differences in cerebral lateralization in schizophrenia. *Arch. Gen. Psychiatry* **54**:433–440.

Roper, S. N., Levesque, M. F., Sutherling, W. W., and Engel, J. Jr. 1993. Surgical treatment of partial epilepsy arising from the insular cortex. *J. Neurosurg.* **79**:266–269.

Rubin, P., Karle, A., Moller-Madsen, S., Hertel, C., Povlsen, U. J., Noring, U., and Hemmingsen, R. 1993. Computerised tomography in newly diagnosed schizophrenia and schizophreniform disorder. A controlled blind study. *Br. J. Psychiatry* **163**:604–612.

Shenton, M. E., Kikinis, R., Jolesz, F. A., Pollack, S. D., LeMay, M., Wible, C. G., Hokama, H., Martin, J., Metcalf, D., Coleman, M., and McCarley, R. W. 1992. Abnormalities of the left temporal lobe and thought disorder in schizophrenia: a quantitative magnetic resonance imaging study. *N. Engl. J. Med.* **327**:604–612.

Shergill, S. S., Bullmore, E., Simmons, A., Murray, R., and McGuire, P. 2000. Functional anatomy of auditory verbal imagery in schizophrenic patients with auditory hallucinations. *Am. J. Psychiatry* **157**:1691–1693.

Small, D. M., Zald, D. H., Jones-Gotman, M., Zatorre, R. J., Pardo, J. V., Frey, S., and Petrides, M. 1999. Human cortical gustatory areas: a review of functional neuroimaging data. *Neuroreport* **10**:7–14.

Sno, H. N. 1994. A continuum of misidentification symptoms. *Psychopathology* **27**:144–147.

Southard, E. E. 1910. A study of the dementia praecox group in the light of certain cases showing anomalies or scleroses in particular brain regions. *Am. J. Insanity* **67**:119–176.

Stoléru, S., Grégoire, M.-C., Gérard, D., Decety, J., Lafarge, E., Cinotti, L., Lavenne, F., LeBars, D., Vernet-Maury, E., Rada, H., Collet, C., Mazoyer, B., Forest, M. G., Magnin, F., Spira, A., and Comar, D. 1999. Neuroanatomical correlates of visually evoked sexual arousal in human males. *Arch. Sex. Behav.* **28**(1):1–21.

Suzuki, M., Yuasa, S., Minabe, Y., Murata, M., and Kurachi, M. 1993. Left superior temporal blood flow increases in schizophrenia and schizophreniform patients with auditory hallucination: a longitudinal case study using ^{123}I-IMP SPECT. *Eur. Arch. Psychiatry Clin. Neurosci.* **242**:257–261.

Tabert, M. H., Borod, J. C., Tang, C. Y., Lange, G., Wei, T. C., Johnson, R., Nusbaum, A. O., and Buchsbaum, M. S. 2001. Differential amygdala activation during emotional decision and recognition memory tasks using unpleasant words: an fMRI study. *Neuropsychologia* **39**:556–573.

Tzourio-Mazoyer, N., Schonen, S. D., Crivello, F., Reutter, B., Aujard, Y., and Mazoyer, B. 2002. Neural correlates of woman face processing by 2-month-old infants. *Neuroimage* **15**:454–461.

Ungerleider, L. G., and Mishkin, M. 1982. Two cortical visual systems. In: D. J. Ingle, M. H. Goodale, and R. J. W. Mansfield (eds.) *The Analysis of Visual Behavior*. Cambridge, Mass: M.I.T. Press.

Vuilleumier, P., Armong, J. L., Driver, J., and Dolan, R. J. 2001. Effects of attention and emotion of face processing in the human brain: an event-related fMRI study. *Neuron* **30**(3):829–841.

Wolberg, Z., and Newman, J. D. 1972. Auditory cortex of squirrel monkey: response patterns of single cells to species-specific vocalizations. *Science* **175**:212–214.

Young, M. W., Robinson, I. H., Hellavell, D. J., dePauw, K. E., and Pentland, B. 1992. Cotard delusion after brain injury (case study). *Psychol. Med.* **21**:799–804.

6 Frontal lobe

The elusive functions of the frontal lobe continue to fascinate the neuroscientist and the neuropsychologist. The frontal lobe is impressively developed in humans and makes up more than one-third of the entire cortical area (Damasio and Anderson, 1993). It controls actions of our body through its motor areas. It also appears to be responsible for shaping our attitudes and organizing our repertoire of behaviors through the actions of the prefrontal areas. Functions that are hallmarks of human behavior, such as intentionality, self-regulation, and self-awareness, are thought to be under the executive control of the frontal lobe.

An ongoing controversy among the prefrontal cortex researchers is whether this region contains regions with discrete functions subservient to an overall executive module that provides an integrated output of the system, or whether the entire prefrontal region is involved in this integrative function. The latter hypothesis requires the neural modules of the prefrontal regions to be highly dynamic. Evidence for both theories exists and the truth is likely to have elements of both schemas where both specialization and versatility contribute to the proper functioning of this most fascinating of brain regions. Different competing, and not necessarily mutually exclusive, theories will be introduced in this chapter.

Anatomical subdivisions

The frontal lobe lies rostral (anterior) to the central sulcus and is made up of three anatomically distinct regions: the dorsolateral aspect, the medial aspect, and the orbital (inferior) aspect. The motor cortex (BA 4, 6, 8, 44, and 45) makes up the posterior portion of both the dorsolateral and medial aspects. The frontal lobe rostral to the motor area, including the orbital cortex, is the prefrontal cortex (Figures 6.1–6.3).

The motor cortex is responsible for the origin of the majority of the axons that make up the corticobulbar and corticospinal (pyramidal) tracts. The corticobulbar tract projects to the brainstem (the bulb is the lower brainstem). The corticospinal tract projects to the spinal cord. The motor cortex consists of the:

- Primary motor cortex
- Premotor cortex
- Supplementary motor cortex
- Frontal eye fields
- Broca's speech area.

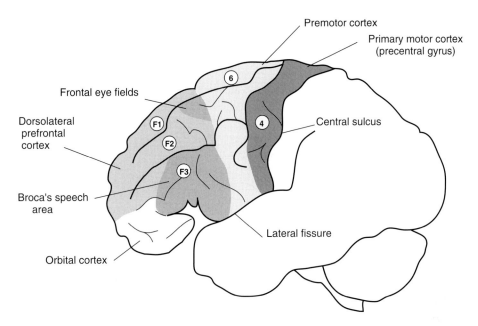

Figure 6.1.   Lateral view of the frontal cortex indicating gyri, sulci, and functional areas. The prefrontal cortex is represented in this view by the dorsolateral prefrontal cortex and the orbital cortex. The remainder of frontal cortex seen here is motor cortex. F1, superior frontal gyrus; F2, middle frontal gyrus; F3, inferior frontal gyrus.

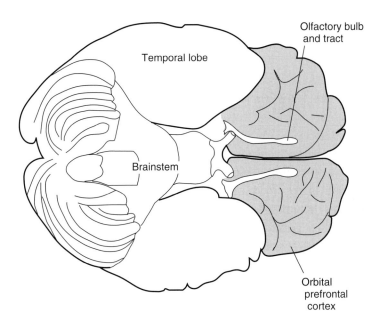

Figure 6.2.   Inferior aspect of the frontal cortex.

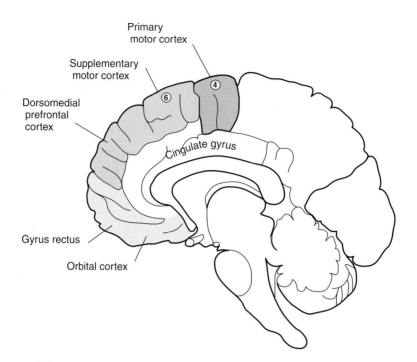

Figure 6.3.   Medial view of the frontal cortex. The prefrontal cortex is represented in this view by the dorsomedial prefrontal cortex and the orbital prefrontal cortex, including the gyrus rectus. The premotor cortex and supplementary motor cortex represent the motor cortex on the medial surface.

The prefrontal cortex is served by axons that arise from the mediodorsal (MD) thalamic nucleus and consists of the:

- Dorsolateral prefrontal cortex
- Medial prefrontal cortex
- Orbital prefrontal cortex.

The anterior cingulate gyrus is also served by the MD thalamic nucleus and is often included as part of the prefrontal cortex (see Figures 6.3 and 12.1). Distinct clinical syndromes can be identified with lesions of each of the three prefrontal areas, but in practice there is often overlap in resulting symptomatology. The medial prefrontal cortex and anterior supplementary motor cortex may overlap in function.

The gray and white matter of the prefrontal cortex develop at different rates. The gray matter increases in volume until somewhere between 4 and 12 years of age after which it decreases gradually (Giedd *et al.*, 1999). Synaptic density decreases as gray matter increases (Huttenlocher, 1979) and white matter volume continues to increase beyond adolescence into early adulthood (Sowell *et al.*, 2001). It is believed that primary motor and sensory areas myelinate before association areas (Fuster, 2002).

Motor cortex

Primary motor cortex

The primary motor cortex (BA 4) corresponds with the precentral gyrus on the lateral surface of the cortex and extends medially into the longitudinal cerebral fissure that separates the left from the right cerebral hemisphere (see Figures 6.1 and 6.3). About a third of the fibers that make up the corticospinal (pyramidal) tract arise from nerve cell bodies found in BA 4. The remainder of the pyramidal tract originates from cell bodies located in other areas of the cortex, including the premotor, supplementary motor, and somesthetic (parietal) cortex. Axons from BA 4 also terminate in the cranial nerve motor nuclei of the brainstem, the basal ganglia, the reticular formation and the red nucleus. Projections from the red nucleus (rubrospinal tract) along with the corticospinal tract make up the major lateral descending motor system.

A pattern of the body is represented by neurons distributed across the primary motor cortex, producing a "homunculus." The extent of each body part over the cortex corresponds with the degree of motor control over each of the represented parts. The fingers, lips, and tongue are represented by large regions of cortex, whereas toes are represented by a relatively small region. The primary motor cortex located along the midline controls the body below the waist. The primary motor cortex located on the lateral surface of the brain controls the muscles of the body found above the waist. Control exerted by the primary motor cortex by way of the pyramidal tract is greatest over the musculature of the hand. Note that in contrast to the legs, which function in locomotion, the face, head, and hands are more commonly used to transmit signals that express emotion.

A lesion of the primary motor cortex will result in paralysis of contralateral musculature. The affected muscles are flaccid at first; then, over the course of several days, the reflexes become brisk and the muscles exhibit spasticity. Gross movement control reappears after several weeks or months, but fine movements are usually lost permanently (Brodal, 1981).

Premotor cortex

The premotor cortex (BA 6 on the lateral surface; see Figure 6.1) receives the majority of its input from the superior parietal cortex (Wise *et al.*, 1997). Most axons that leave the premotor cortex terminate in the primary motor cortex. A smaller contingent of axons descends from the premotor cortex through the internal capsule to the reticular formation, which gives rise to the reticulospinal tracts. The reticulospinal tracts are part of the major medial descending motor system, which functions in support of body posture and locomotion through control of axial and proximal limb musculature.

Premotor areas are activated when new motor programs are initiated or when learned motor programs are modified. Premotor neurons increase their activity in anticipation of limb movement. Premotor areas appear to be involved in the generation of a motor sequence from memory that requires precise timing (Halsband *et al.*, 1993). In addition, the premotor area appears to be particularly involved with visuomotor activity, since lesions of the premotor area produce deficits in visually guided movements.

Passive viewing of faces led to activation of the right ventral premotor area, whereas imitative viewing produced bilateral activation. This suggests that the right hemisphere may play a key role in the production of empathetic facial movements (Dimberg and Petterson, 2000; Leslie *et al.*, 2004). Individuals who score high on empathy tests also demonstrate the chameleon effect (Sonnby-Borgström, 2002). That is they unconsciously tend to mimic the facial expressions of the individual with whom they are speaking and even experience the mood of their interactive partner (Levenson *et al.*, 1990).

Clinical vignette

Mr. C. C., a 65-year-old man, suffered a right hemisphere stroke that resulted in left arm paralysis. After discharge from the hospital he noted that his wife as well as other people around him were not as responsive to him as they were before the stroke. He found that just being angry or trying to look or sound angry had no effect on people. He had to explode in a rage in order to get his point across. His wife demanded that he see a psychiatrist. On examination Mr. C. C. was found to have severe expressive aprosodia. He was totally unable to express anger, happiness, sadness, surprise, or even inquisitiveness.

Clinical studies suggest that the descending influence of the premotor cortex is over axial and proximal limb musculature. Unilateral lesions of the premotor cortex result in moderate weakness of contralateral shoulder and pelvic muscles. Forearm strength remains unaffected, but grasping movements are impaired when they are dependent on the supporting action of the shoulder. Movements are slow, and there is a disturbance of their kinetic structure. Windmilling movements of the arms below shoulder level are normal in the forward direction but abnormal when attempted in the backward direction. Bicycling movements of the legs are unaffected (Freund and Hummelsheim, 1984).

Supplementary motor area

The supplementary motor area (SMA) is found on the medial side of the frontal lobe along the longitudinal cerebral fissure (see Figure 6.3). It corresponds approximately with BA 6 on the medial surface, although the exact boundaries are debated (Wise *et al.*, 1996). fMRI studies recognize two distinct regions: anterior SMA (pre-SMA) and the posterior SMA (SMA proper, or SMA) (Picard and Strick, 1996). The SMA receives afferents from the primary somesthetic area of the parietal lobe (see Chapter 4) as well as from the superior parietal lobule, the prefrontal cortex, and the cingulate gyrus. Afferent fibers from the thalamus arise from both the ventral anterior and ventral lateral nuclei (VA and VL), making the SMA a recipient of feedback from both the basal ganglia and the cerebellum. Efferent fibers from the SMA include transcortical fibers to the premotor and primary motor areas as well as to the basal ganglia, red nucleus, and directly to the spinal cord. The SMA can be subdivided into two components. The more caudal of the two is related to movement execution. The more rostral component appears to function as a clearing house for cognitive and motivational information that arrives from the prefrontal and cingulate areas before distribution to more caudal SMA and then on to premotor areas (Rizzolatti *et al.*, 1996).

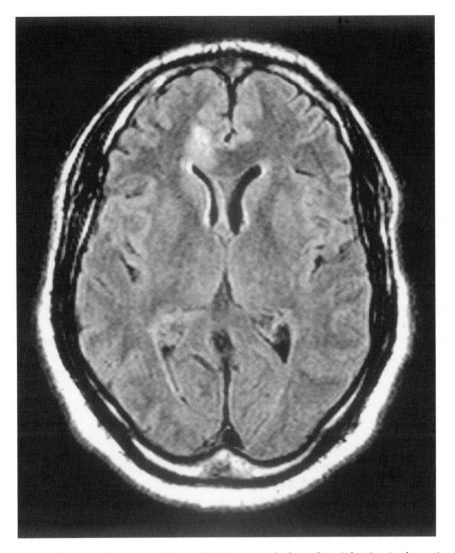

Figure 6.4.   Horizontal magnetic resonance image (FLAIR sequence) showed an infarction in the region of the right supplementary motor area. Reprinted with permission from Mendez and Clark (2004).

Clinical vignette

A 55-year-old right-handed man had an acute onset of hesitant, effortful speech. Examination showed predominant difficulty with articulatory fluency. His forward flow of speech was disrupted by speech sound repetitions and by lengthy pauses while preparing for the next utterance. He also had frequent vowel distortions and substitutions, fluctuating resonance, and a halting and harsh vocal quality. In contrast, his language abilities were preserved, including reading and writing.

This patient had difficulty due to a right supplementary area lesion. Neuroimaging revealed a right hemisphere stroke of probable embolic origin involving the pericallosal branch of the right anterior cerebral artery (Figure 6.4). His deficit illustrated the disruption of complex motor routines for speech from a supplementary area lesion.

Clinical vignette

The relationship between actual frontal lobe ictal activity and the exhibited psychopathology is complex, as exemplified by the following case reported by Boone and associates in 1988. A 13-year-old girl was admitted to a psychiatric hospital for deteriorating behavior. Before hospitalization she was becoming increasingly inattentive and was sexually active with a number of partners. She was becoming progressively more volatile and unpredictable with verbal and physical aggressiveness. She also exhibited pressured speech with periodic incoherent and bizarre output. She had one episode in which she cut the superficial skin over her wrists with a razor. Concurrent with the deteriorating behavior, spells developed during which she turned briefly to the right, stared and picked at her clothes. The episode was usually followed by urinary incontinence. Computed tomography and magnetic resonance imaging were normal. Electroencephalography demonstrated ictal activity of 2.5 Hz spike and slow wave complexes that originated primarily in the left frontal lobe but also occasionally in the right frontal regions.

Functional neuroimaging studies show that the SMA activates before the primary motor area (i.e., when the patient imagines performing an activity or intends to perform an activity) and is activated during complex motor subroutines. It is suggested that the SMA assembles a sequence of motor actions into a motor plan and that it is involved in the intentional preparation of movement (Grafton *et al.*, 1992a). The SMA and anterior cingulate cortex become active in preparation for cued movements indicating involvement with motor planning (Sahyoun *et al.*, 2003). Activity in the pre-SMA is enhanced when subjects attended to the task to be performed ("attention to intention") (Lau *et al.*, 2004). Activation of the pre-SMA was more extensive for self-initiated movements as opposed to visually triggered movements. Activation of the SMA proper was more extensive when sequential rather than fixed movements were elicited (Deiber *et al.*, 1999).

The SMA may be involved in procedural memory, which is the process responsible for the acquisition and recall of motor programs (e.g., how a novice learns to grip and swing a golf club). Blood flow studies have led to the suggestion that the SMA may act as an executor in the acquisition and articulation of new motor skills (Grafton *et al.*, 1992b).

Clinical deficits due to surgery or to anterior cerebral artery infarction produce a lesion of the SMA as well as surrounding structures that may include the dorsomedial prefrontal area, the anterior corpus callosum, and the cingulate gyrus (see Chapter 12). Such a lesion of the SMA, right or left, produces mutism or a severe reduction in speech (speech arrest), usually in association with profound contralateral motor deficit (akinetic syndrome). Comprehension remains normal and speech returns; however, spontaneous and propositional speech are reduced. Initial effects are profound, but rapid recovery ensues over several months, with speech defects recovering more slowly. Recovery may appear complete in several years. Even after this time, however, mistakes may be observed in repeated complex movements of the hand (alternating supination and pronation), with the hand hesitating to reverse movement (Bleasel *et al.*, 1996). The alien hand sign has been reported in some cases (see Chapter 14; Feinberg *et al.*, 1992).

Frontal eye fields

The frontal eye fields are found on the dorsolateral frontal cortex and correspond with Brodmann's area 8 (see Figures 2.3 and 6.1). The eye fields contribute to voluntary eye movements but are not necessary for initiation of all types of eye movements. The frontal eye field projects to the superior colliculus, to the caudate nucleus, and to the paramedian pontine reticular formation (PPRF), which is the pontine center for lateral gaze.

Saccadic eye movements are the only voluntary conjugate eye movements and direct the eyes toward an attractive object in the visual environment (Buttner-Ennever, 1988). The posterior parietal cortex plots the position and movement ("where") of all visual targets simultaneously and provides this information to the brainstem (superior colliculus). The parietal and temporal cortex also provide the frontal eye field with information about the identity ("what") of each of the targets.

The frontal eye field acts as the executive and selects one target out of all the available visual targets and commands the brainstem to move the eyes on to the selected target.

Eye tracking dysfunction (ETD) appears to be a genetically determined trait marker of schizophrenia. One hypothesis suggests that ETD reflects frontal lobe dysfunction (Gooding et al., 1994).

Broca's speech area

Broca's speech area occupies BA 44 and 45 on the inferior frontal gyrus (see Figures 2.3 and Figure 6.1). It is considered to be part of the prefrontal cortex and consists of both heteromodal prefrontal cortex and premotor cortex. This region is specialized on the dominant side of the cortex for the production of speech. The major input to this region is from Wernicke's area by way of the arcuate fasciculus. Wernicke's area corresponds with the posterior region of the superior temporal gyrus (BA 22). Fibers that originate from cells in Broca's area project to the facial region of the primary motor cortex, which directly controls the muscles of speech. The area comparable to Broca's on the nondominant cortex is responsible for the emotional/melodic component of speech (Joseph, 1988).

Broca's speech area is activated during the production of both overt and covert speech as well as when an individual imitates another person's speech (Figure 6.5; Smith et al., 1992; Sukhwinder et al., 2000). Evidence indicates that this region is active during inner speech in normal subjects and may be critical in verbal hallucinations experienced by schizophrenics (McGuire et al., 1993, 1996). Impairment in verbal fluency ("say as many words beginning with 's'" – in the next 30 seconds) is seen in patients with lesions in Broca's area as well as in other regions of the dorsolateral prefrontal cortex. Broca's area is involved in word retrieval as well as in verbal fluency (Caplan et al., 2000). Word fluency activates both left BA 44 and 45 whereas semantic processing preferentially activates BA 45 (Amuts et al., 2004).

A lesion of Broca's area on the dominant side results in an inability to produce speech (motor or expressive aphasia). The patient retains the ability to understand the written and spoken word. With recovery, the patient learns to speak with difficulty, producing only key nouns and verbs and leaving out modifying adjectives and adverbs. The same cortex on the nondominant side is believed to be responsible for the musical intonation of speech (prosody). A lesion on the nondominant side results in expressive aprosodia in which the patient is unable to effectively modulate speech (i.e., speech becomes monotonic without facial expressions).

Depression is often observed during Broca's and other nonfluent aphasia. Some of the depression is a result of left hemisphere damage, not just a reaction to the psychosocial loss (Benson and Ardila,

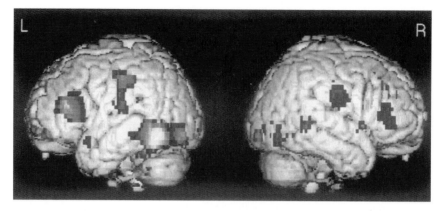

Figure 6.5. Functional magnetic resonance images demonstrating greater activation to words than to consonant letter strings during a nonlinguistic visual feature detection task. The images illustrate a left hemisphere language network for reading probably including temporal–occipital visual word form and lexical regions, an inferior parietal phonological encoding region, and Broca's area in the inferior frontal lobe. The right hemisphere also participates but to a much smaller degree than the left hemisphere. (Reproduced with permission from Price *et al.*, 1996.) See also color plate.

1993). Severe depression correlates with deep left frontal lesions, especially if the lesion includes the anterior limb of the internal capsule (Starkstein *et al.*, 1987). Blood flow to Broca's area is decreased in patients with posttraumatic stress disorder when provoked (see Figure 11.7; Rauch *et al.*, 1996). A significant volume reduction was reported in only BA 44 and 45 on both the left and right side in patients with schizophrenia when the entire prefrontal cortex was compared (Buchanan *et al.*, 1998).

Prefrontal cortex

The prefrontal cortex is divided into the dorsolateral region (see Figure 6.1), the medial region (see Figure 6.3), and the orbital (inferior) region (see Figure 6.2). All three regions receive fibers from the mediodorsal thalamic nucleus, which relays information from the temporal cortex, the pyriform cortex, and the amygdaloid nucleus. The orbital and dorso-medial subdivisions of the prefrontal cortex are included as part of the limbic association cortex. The prefrontal cortex also receives projections from the substantia nigra, indicating a role for the prefrontal region in motor behavior. Direct prefrontal input (which bypasses the thalamus) from the pons, hypothalamus, and amygdala also exists. Connections with the amygdala are reciprocal. The functional difference between the indirect input through the thalamus and the direct input is unknown.

The prefrontal cortex is extensively connected bidirectionally to the nonlimbic cortical sensory association areas. It receives highly processed sensory information (visual, auditory, and somato-sensory) that constantly updates it on the state of the environment. It monitors not only the external environment (nonlimbic cortical input) but also the internal environment (limbic input). It is specialized to organize and direct behavior by the internalized representation of the facts and events. In this way the prefrontal lobes are necessary for intrinsically generated behavior. One scheme

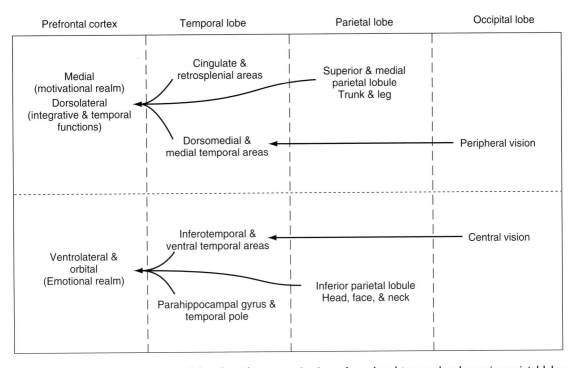

Figure 6.6.   The dorsolateral and medial prefrontal areas receive input from dorsal temporal and superior parietal lobes and portions of the occipital lobe that mediate peripheral vision. This dorsal system appears to function in the motivational and planning realm, closely associated with the trunk and lower limb, and with the location of an object in space ("where"). The ventrolateral and orbital prefrontal areas receive input from inferior temporal and inferior parietal lobes and portions of the occipital cortex that mediate central vision. This ventral system appears to function in the emotional realm, closely associated with the head, face, and neck, and with the identification of an object ("what"). (After Pandya, D.N., and Yeterian, E.H. 1990. Prefrontal cortex in relation to other cortical areas in rhesus monkey: architecture and connections. In: H.B.M. Uylings, C.G. Van Eden, J.P.C. DeBruin, M.A. Corner, and M.G.P. Feenstra (eds.) *The prefrontal cortex: its structure, function and pathology*. Amsterdam: Elsevier, pp.63–94.)

separates input to the prefrontal area into a dorsal stream and a ventral stream based on architectonics, connections, and function (Figure 6.6). The dorsal stream includes information from the peripheral retina and somatosensory input from the trunk and leg region. This information feeds forward from the striate and extrastriate cortex through the inferior parietal lobule and intraparietal sulcus area. The dorsal stream provides spatial information for working memory active in the superior dorsolateral prefrontal cortex and superior frontal sulcus area. The dorsal system allows for integration and temporal sequencing of behavior. Its links with the trunk and lower limb underscore its importance in regulating behavior in three-dimensional space. In contrast, ventrally processed information includes signals from the central retina and inferotemporal region that imply object identification. Input from the parahippocampal gyrus adds emotional tone that is projected to the orbital and ventrolateral prefrontal areas. Convergence of internal and external environmental information enables the prefrontal cortex to create plans to deal with any changes that necessitate action (Courtney *et al.*, 1998).

   Prefrontal neurons respond in situations that reflect learned associative relationships between goal-relevant tasks. They appear to form ensembles that represent commonalities across past experiences that have proven to be effective in achieving a particular goal (Miller, 2000). Prefrontal areas are involved in the storage and retrieval related to sequential and temporal aspects of planning (Goel *et al.*, 1997). This planning and the ability of the prefrontal cortex to rearrange the sequence and complexity of planning has earned the prefrontal cortex the title "organ of creativity" (Fuster, 2002).

Clinical observations parallel the anatomical division of the prefrontal lobes into dorsal and ventral trends. Damage to the ventral prefrontal areas typically results in perseveration, emotional lability, and personality changes. In contrast, damage to the dorsomedial regions results in deficits in the ability to initiate behavior as well as deficits in motivation, attention to task, and communication.

Prefrontal output to the basal ganglia and to the frontal motor regions (BA 6 and 4) further indicates a significant role of the prefrontal cortex in motor behavior. Output from the prefrontal cortex to the limbic system takes both direct and indirect routes. The indirect route exits via the cingulate gyrus, and these prefrontal fibers distribute to many cortical regions throughout their long course around the corpus callosum.

An increase in blood flow in the frontal lobes has been associated with introversion. Extraverts show lower blood flow in the frontal lobes and hippocampus. These results suggest that introverts are engaged in frontally based cognition, including remembering events from their past, making plans for the future, or solving problems (Johnson *et al.*, 1999).

Patients with lesions in the left frontal cortex demonstrate a higher frequency of depression than patients with more posterior lesions or patients with either anterior or posterior right hemisphere lesions (Morris *et al.*, 1992; Starkstein and Robinson, 1993). Glucose metabolism studies in both teenagers and adults with a history of attention-deficit hyperactivity disorder show decreased metabolism in the left anterior frontal areas (Zametkin *et al.*, 1990; Ernst *et al.*, 1994).

The inhibition of glutamatergic transmission in the prefrontal lobes correlates with cognitive dysfunction seen in patients with schizophrenia. It is hypothesized that this inhibition is responsible for dysregulation of dopamine in the corpus striatum (Breier, 1999).

Generalized, bilateral damage to the prefrontal lobes can produce severe behavioral changes. Characteristically these patients become apathetic and exhibit disinhibition of impulsive behavior. They appear unconcerned (abulia) and exhibit slowness and lack of spontaneity in speech and slowness in thought and in emotional expression. The movements of frontal lobe patients are slow (bradykinesia), and they exhibit a slow, uncertain "magnetic" gait (frontal ataxia or gait apraxia). In contrast, their behavior may change, and they may become irritable and euphoric.

An intriguing prefrontal syndrome is the environmental dependency syndrome, or EDS (Lhermitte, 1986). Two patients with focal unilateral frontal lobe lesions were observed in a doctor's office, in a lecture room, in a car, in a garden, and while visiting an apartment. In each situation the patients assumed behavior appropriate to the environment, including treating the physician as a patient. The patient's behavior was striking, as though implicit in the environment was an order to respond to the situation in which they found themselves. EDS implies a disorder in personal autonomy.

Frontal lobe seizures are particularly difficult to diagnose. Frontal lobe seizures are common and are usually secondary to head trauma. They can be brief, odd, or misleading. They can be misinterpreted as pseudoseizures. Extensive connections of the orbital prefrontal cortex to limbic structures (mainly amygdala and hippocampus) via the uncinate fasciculus help in understanding the difficulty in differentiating between ictal events that occur in those areas. Laughter, crying, moaning, and verbal automatisms have been described with lesions of the superior frontal gyrus and cingulate gyrus. In addition, complex gestures such as body rubbing, rearrangement of clothes, sexual auto-matism, mood changes, wandering, and agitation have all been reported with frontal lobe lesions. Finally, nonconvulsive frontal seizure states can produce prolonged behavioral disturbances (Riggio and Harner, 1992).

Orbital prefrontal cortex

The orbital cortex is intimately related through the uncinate fasciculus to the anterior insula, temporal pole, inferior parietal lobe, and amygdala. These connections place it in a position to evaluate and regulate information from the limbic system that can be used by the motor cortex to effect a response. The orbital cortex plays a dominant role in mediating arousal (Joseph, 1996). It is also postulated to regulate the experience of anxiety (Gray, 1987). Inhibitory control arises from the orbital and medial prefrontal cortex. Inhibition can help prevent distraction and support the focusing component of selective sensory attention (Fuster, 2002).

The orbital region provides a critical facility to the feeling of familiarity based on processing both interoceptive and exteroceptive inputs and the ability to inhibit drive. A primary role of the orbital cortex is the acquisition of appropriate behaviors and the inhibition of inappropriate ones based on reward contingencies (Elliot *et al.*, 2000). The medial orbital cortex is related to cognitive and emotional processes and the sense of reward when making the correct choice. It plays a key role in the circuitry of positive emotion. Lateral orbital regions are more involved with inhibiting the more familiar response when the novel, less familiar response produces a reward (Zald and Kim, 1996). Activity increased bilaterally when mothers viewed pictures of their own 3- to 5-month infants over activity when viewing pictures of other 3- to 5-month infants (Nitschke *et al.*, 2004). A particular feature of the orbital and medial regions is suppression of distracting internal and external signals during the performance of current behavior (Fuster, 1996).

Olfactory signals converge with taste signals in the orbital prefrontal cortex to create the represen-tations of flavor. Other sensory signals converge with flavor in the orbital prefrontal cortex and visual-to-taste associations occur here as well (Rolls, 1997a). The orbital cortex is activated by pleasant and painful touch, rewarding and aversive taste and by odor (Rolls, 2000).

The orbitofrontal cortex also receives inputs from the visual system, taste, olfaction, and somatosensory regions. Included in this region are BA 11, 12, 13, and 14. This region is poorly developed in rodents but is well developed in primates (including humans). The secondary taste cortex was localized to the lateral part of the orbitofrontal cortex (Rolls, 1990). Medial to the taste region a smell (olfactory) region was also described (Rolls and Baylis, 1994). Visual input seems to reach this region via temporal lobe structures. Somatosensory and auditory input also arrive from the primary sensory regions. The insula is similarly connected to the orbitofrontal cortex. The more posterior (caudal) regions receive strong input from the amygdala (Price *et al.*, 1991).

The orbitofrontal cortex projects back to the cingulate cortex and temporal lobe regions including the entorhinal cortex (gateway to hippocampus) (Insausti *et al.*, 1987). Importantly also, the orbitofrontal region projects to the preoptic and lateral hypothalamic regions, and the ventral tegmental area.

Examination of the functions of the orbitofrontal region in humans is very difficult. A significant portion of our knowledge of this area comes from primate studies. Data from Macaque monkeys with orbitofrontal cortical lesions suggest that this region is important for learning about which stimuli are rewarding and which are not. Even more importantly, this region seems to be important for mediating behavioral change when reinforcement contingencies change (Jones and Mishkin, 1972). Physiological studies showed that activity of the orbitofrontal taste neurons are modulated by hunger (they stop responding to the taste of food after satiety) while taste neurons of the primary taste region do not stop responding to the taste stimulus. The convergence of sensory modalities on this region (auditory, somatosensory, visual, taste, and smell) strongly suggest this area plays the major role in mediating stimulus-reinforcement association learning.

The orbitofrontal cortex also receives information about faces. Face-responsive neurons in this region seem to behave differently than, for example, face-responsive neurons of the temporal lobe. Face-responsive neurons of the orbitofrontal region may convey information about which face is being seen (Rolls and Baylis, 1994). Attractive faces produced activation of the medial orbitofrontal cortex which was enhanced by a smiling expression (O'Doherty *et al.*, 2003). Some of the orbitofrontal face-responsive neurons seem to be responsive to facial gestures and movements. These findings would strongly relate to the function of social reinforcement as facial expressions are crucial for conveying approval or disapproval. It is likely that most of the associations developed in this region occur in a subconscious or unconscious (automatic) fashion.

The different reinforcements developed would naturally have different strength (based on neural or synaptic connections developed in response to the particular association) (Rolls 1997b). In a complex societal situation the strongest association will be the one capable of effecting a response among a number of competing possible responses. A different mechanism for response selection is labeled "somatic marker theory" discussed below. Acts of imagined social embarrassment produced significant activation of the left orbitofrontal cortex (BA 10 and 47) (Berthoz *et al.*, 2002). The same region was activated by viewing angry faces (Blair *et al.*, 1999; Kesler-West *et al.*, 2001).

Clinical vignette

A 67-year-old right-handed man with frontotemporal dementia (FTD) was hospitalized with a gradual personality change. He sold his successful business, stopped paying the bills, and ran up large debts on merchandise from a television home shopping network. He became impulsive and disinhibited, fondled his wife in public, sexually propositioned his daughters, and uttered uncharacteristic racial slurs at social gatherings. At the same time, he became distractable and hyperactive, with compulsive behaviors such as repeatedly pulling the hair of his arms (trichotillomania) and exhibited hyperoral behavior such as overeating.

The patient met criteria for FTD, probably of a familial nature. His family history was positive for a similar dementing illness in his father and in a paternal grandparent. Single photon emission tomography scans showed extensive hypoperfusion in both frontal lobes, more extensive in the right hemisphere (Figure 6.7). His initial personality changes, including poor judgment, disinhibition, and inappropriate behaviors, were consistent with involvement of the orbital prefrontal cortex.

Clinical vignette

Ms. A.C., a 17-year-old female student, was involved in competitive piano and ballet. Her grades were consistently outstanding. She had no personal or family history of psychiatric problems. She was out with friends on a Saturday night when she was involved in an accident. She fell off the back of a pickup truck and

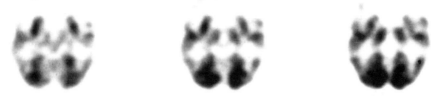

Figure 6.7.   The patient's 18-fluoro deoxyglucose positron emission tomography scan showed prominent hypometabolism of the frontal lobes. Note the near absence of activity in the anterior part of the brain. (Reprinted with permission from Mendez *et al.*, 1997.)

landed on her head. At the accident scene she was alert and oriented but felt dazed. In the emergency room, CT and neurological examinations were normal. She was observed for 2 h and released. The patient's mother was told that her daughter was fine and that she should return to school and full activity on Monday. For the following few weeks, Ms. A.C. was unable to perform either piano or ballet at school, although she had no problem practicing at home. Her grades deteriorated. She became depressed and attempted suicide. Neuropsychological testing showed that the patient had a problem performing in the presence of interference (i.e., difficulty in maintaining a mental set). This is evidence of damage in the prefrontal region. The patient responded well to antidepressant therapy. Her frontal lobe deficit resolved spontaneously over time with continued nonpressured practice.

Lesions in the orbital region result in a syndrome that is characterized by disinhibition, which varies from lack of social tact to the commission of antisocial acts. The nature of this behavior indicates that these patients no longer recognize the inappropriateness of their actions. They are emotionally labile, irritable, and impulsive. The patient with an orbital prefrontal lesion may be hyperactive, even hypomanic, especially if the lesion involves the posterior orbital cortex. Although overt sexual aggression is rare, sexual preoccupation and improper sexual comments are frequent. Patients are easily distracted, and often they are unable to complete tasks because they are distracted by ordinarily insignificant stimuli. Patients with orbital cortex lesions have been compared with drug users. They choose instant reward over waiting. Lesions early in life had greater effects. This area plays a role in re-experiencing emotions. Most patients with lesions found it difficult to re-experience emotions with the exception of fear and had difficulty in attaching emotional tone to images (Bechara *et al.*, 2000).

The pathology in Frontotemporal dementia (FTD) is more localized to the frontal and anterior temporal regions as compared to Alzheimer's disease (AD). Consequently, more behavioral disturbances (e.g., disinhibition, hypersexuality, irritability, depression, apathy) are seen in association with FTD as compared to AD.

The ventromedial prefrontal cortex (VMPC)

The VMPC is contiguous with the orbitofrontal cortical region discussed above and credited with stimulus-reinforcement association learning. This cortical region (based on nonhuman primate neuroanatomy) receives input from all sensory modalities (Pandya and Yeterian, 1996). On the other hand, evidence suggests that this is the only frontal cortical region with projections to central autonomic control structures (Nauta, 1971) with demonstrated influence on visceral sensations (Hall *et al.*, 1977). Moreover, the VMPC region has bi-directional connections with hippocampus and amygdala (Goldman-Rakic *et al.*, 1984).

Based on the nature of the connections of the VMPC region with sensory input and output to autonomic-visceral control and to other limbic as well as other frontal cortical regions a hypothesis known as the "somatic marker hypothesis" was advanced by Antonio Damasio (1994) to shed light on the process of decision-making by humans. The somatic marker hypothesis suggests that structures in the VMPC region hold representations of the associations between certain complex situations and the visceral sensations or emotions previously linked to that situation. The actual memories are not held here thus damage to this region will not affect the memories themselves but the link between them. When a similar (or related) situation arises the ventromedial region is activated and the visceral/emotional experience is recalled. The recalling could be an actual visceral re-experiencing of emotions and feelings or just a cognitive representation of such. This evocation process functions as a constraint over the process of reasoning over multiple options and response choices. Certain choices can be rapidly eliminated or endorsed, thus decreasing the number of choices available. In the absence of this hypothesized process, options and outcomes become more equalized and the process of choosing will depend entirely on logical processes. This strategy would be slower and may fail to take into account previous experiences.

Patients with damage to the VMPC present with severe impairment of social and personal decision-making (Damasio, 1994). These patients have largely preserved intellectual abilities. Patients may have difficulty planning their workday as well as difficulty choosing suitable friends, partners or activities. Their choices are not personally advantageous, inadequate, and usually lead to financial losses, losses in social standing, and losses to family and friends.

Metabolism is increased throughout the brain during non rapid eye movement (REM) sleep in major depression (+30%), which supports the hyperarousal theory of depression. Regional increases are seen in the occipital, temporal, parietal, and frontal lobes. In contrast, depressed patients exhibit hypofrontality, with the effect more marked in the medial orbital region than in the dorsolateral region (Ho *et al.*, 1997). Decreased blood flow to the medial frontal pole appears to be the critical abnormality in depression-related cognitive impairment (depressive pseudodementia; Figure 6.8) and may be associated with emotional states such as withdrawal and apathy (Dolan *et al.*, 1992; Ho *et al.*, 1997). Decreased metabolic activity is seen in the orbital prefrontal cortex and particularly in the left hemisphere during protracted cocaine abstinence (Volkow *et al.*, 1992). A decrease in cerebral blood flow in both the orbital prefrontal and the dorsolateral prefrontal cortex is reported in patients with depression. Decreased blood flow is seen in the orbital prefrontal cortex in phobic patients when they are presented with visual phobogenic stimuli (see Figure 4.4). In contrast, an increase in blood flow is seen during transient sadness in healthy subjects (Mayberg, 1997) and in patients with simple phobia during provocation (Rauch *et al.*, 1995). A dramatic decrease in perfusion was reported in the inferior frontal lobe of a woman who developed catatonia during a depressive episode (Galynker *et al.*, 1997).

Clinical vignette

A 52-year-old woman presented with personality change over 2–3 weeks characterized by disinterest, disengagement, and decreased ability to solve problems. She was a school teacher and could no longer plan her lessons, process feedback from her students, or follow-through on her assignments. Her general and

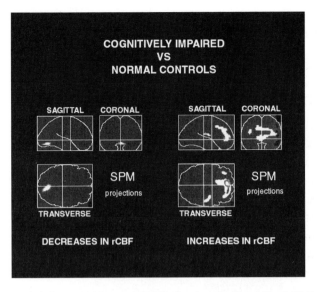

Figure 6.8.   Statistical parametric maps (SPM) showing significant ($p<0.05$ Bonferroni corrected) decreases (left) and increases (right) in relative cerebral blood flow. The light areas represent mathematical differences between patients with depression-related cognitive impairment and control subjects. The pixels at which there is a significant change have been projected onto sagittal, coronal, and transverse renderings of the standard brain volume of Talairach and Tournoux. (Reproduced by permission from Dolan, R. J., Bench, C. J., Brown, R. G., Scott, L. C., Friston, K. J., and Frackowiak, R. S. J. 1992. Regional cerebral blood flow abnormalities in depressed patients with cognitive impairment. *J. Neurol. Neurosurg. Psychiatry* **55**:768–773.)

neurological examinations were normal except for mental status testing which showed decreased verbal output, diminished motor initiation, lack of concern, and poor sequencing and set-shifting abilities. Magnetic resonance imaging showed an enhancing dural mass over the left cerebral convexities with effacement of the sulci in both frontal lobes (see Figure 6.9). Biopsy of the lesion revealed changes consistent with dural neurosarcoidosis.

Her personality changes resulted from pressure of the neurosarcoid mass on her dorsolateral prefrontal cortex. The patient was treated for neurosarcoidosis with corticosteroids (prednisone). One month after initiation of therapy, a second MRI scan showed decreases in the dural lesion, and repeat neuropsychological testing showed coincident improvements in all measures of frontal functions.

Metabolism is increased in the orbital prefrontal cortex along with the whole cerebral hemispheres, caudate nuclei, and cingulate gyri in patients with obsessive-compulsive disorder (see Figure 12.7; Baxter, 1992; Swedo *et al.*, 1992; Rauch *et al.*, 1994). This increase may be in response to reduced striatal inhibition and therefore reflects an attempt on the part of the patient to inhibit obsessions and compulsions (Baxter *et al.*, 1990). A significant decrease in orbital prefrontal metabolism was seen after successful drug treatment, and the decrease in the right orbital prefrontal region correlated directly with two measures of obsessive-compulsive improvement (Swedo *et al.*, 1992). Lesions in the orbital prefrontal cortex are difficult to evaluate utilizing procedures such as EEG due to their proximity to the eye. Eye movements cause major artifacts that mask EEG abnormalities.

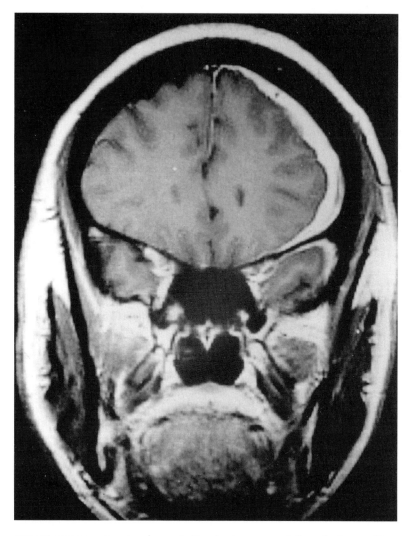

Figure 6.9.   Magnetic resonance imaging demonstrating dural mass over left cerebral convexities resulting in dorsolateral frontal personality changes (Mendez and Zander, 1992).

Patients with depression and Parkinson's disease or Huntington's disease have diminished metabolism in both the orbital prefrontal cortex and the caudate nucleus. Depression has been diagnosed in 60% of patients with anterior frontal lesions (Cummings, 1993). This is consistent with a neuropsychiatry principle that suggests a contingent but not an obligatory anatomical relationship for specified behavioral syndromes. Left anterior lesions increase the patient's vulnerability to depression, but the occurrence of depression may also require environmental or psychosocial factors. This is in contrast to most neurological syndromes, in which an obligatory relationship is typical (Cummings, 1993). Decreased left prefrontal activity on positron emission tomography (PET) scans is consistently found in actively depressed patients. The decrease is more pronounced if the patient reports being more depressed on the day of scanning (Ketter *et al.*, 1994).

The orbitofrontal region, like the anterior temporal region (Chapter 4), is in close proximity to bony protrusions. Both are vulnerable to injury, particularly when rotational acceleration is imparted to the freely moving head (Levin and Kraus, 1994). The injury may include white matter damage that may be diffuse and not detectable using structural imaging. Orbitofrontal damage alone or combined with temporal pole damage can result in complex behavioral changes. The orbital prefrontal cortex may be damaged by trauma or tumors (e.g., meningiomas). Since lesions in this area impact on complex psychological functions, neuropsychological impairment may go unnoticed for years. Subtle personality changes may be the only early clue before the eventual development of signs of increased intracranial pressure, including seizures in the case of a space-occupying lesion. Extensive orbital cortex damage blunts emotional reactions, and the patient may sit quietly and silently. If sufficiently stimulated, animals and humans respond in an irritable and aversive manner (Butter *et al.*, 1968). Social responses are lacking or inappropriate. Human mothers with orbital lesions neglect or beat their children or both without provocation (Broffman, 1950). Monkeys with orbital lesions separate themselves from their social group (Myers *et al.*, 1973).

The pseudopsychopathic subject usually has sustained an orbital prefrontal lesion. The patient's attention is easily distracted by irrelevant stimuli. There is also excessive and aimless motility, disinhibition, and hypomanic stance. Paranoid tendencies may develop.

Dorsomedial prefrontal cortex

The dorsomedial component of the prefrontal cortex (DMPFC) extends in an arc from the supplementary motor cortex downward to the orbital component of the prefrontal cortex. It lies dorsal and rostral to the cingulate gyrus, and many authors include the anterior cingulate gyrus as part of the dorsomedial prefrontal area (see Figures 6.3 and 12.1). This region is supplied mainly by the anterior cerebral artery. Aneurysms of this artery are a common cause of medial frontal lobe damage, and the involved cortex may include the supplementary motor area as well.

The DMPFC is important in motivation and the initiation of activity (see Figure 6.6). It is sensitive to gaze and was activated when subjects evaluated the emotional aspect of gaze (Wicker *et al.*, 2003). A more ventral area appeared to be involved in the emotion processing. These two areas are closely linked with the anterior cingulate gyrus. The DMPFC is often activated by "theory of mind" tasks (Happé *et al.*, 1996; Brunet *et al.*, 2000).

The patient with a dorsomedial prefrontal lesion is apathetic. He or she exhibits a lack of spontaneous movement. Immediately after the onset of the lesion, the patient often presents with akinetic mutism. Paresis of the lower limb may be seen if the lesion extends posteriorly to infringe on the primary motor cortex. The patient often fails to respond to commands. Incontinence is frequently seen, and the patient appears indifferent to the problem.

When control subjects viewed images of people, the DMPFC was activated bilaterally, whereas when schizophrenic patients viewed the same images there was no activation of the DMPFC from either side (Brunet *et al.*, 2003).

The pseudodepressed subject usually has sustained a lesion to the dorsomedial prefrontal region. There is a general decrease of awareness, and a state of apathy with basic lack or weakness of drive. In extreme cases, this can lead to an akinetic–abulic syndrome and mutism.

The medial prefrontal cortex (BA 9) along with the thalamus was activated when a group of 12 women were asked to recall recent emotional events. Additional brain areas were activated when they viewed an emotion-evoking filmstrip. Activation was independent of the nature of the emotion – happiness, sadness, or disgust. A similar experiment revealed activation in the medial prefrontal cortex and cingulate cortex, but only on the right side (Teasdale *et al.*, 1999). The authors suggest that the medial prefrontal cortex and thalamus are important in the appreciation of emotion in the absence of concurrent sensory input (Lane *et al.*, 1997; Reiman *et al.*, 1997).

Dorsolateral prefrontal cortex

The dorsolateral prefrontal cortex (DLPFC) extends between the longitudinal cerebral fissure above and the lateral fissure below on the lateral surface of the brain. It receives input from the motor cortex as well as from the multimodal sensory convergence areas of the parietal and temporal lobes. In contrast to the orbital cortex, the connections of the DLPFC place it in a position to evaluate and regulate information from the somatic sensory system that can be used by the motor cortex to effect a response.

The DLPFC has been described as a place "where past and future meet." It looks backward in time to create memories from sensory input. It looks forward in time to assemble a motor plan of action (Fuster, 1995).

The DLPFC is heavily involved in working memory. Working memory is the act of bringing to mind and processing limited amounts of information, for example reading and recalling a telephone number or solving a math problem "in your head" (Baddeley, 1992; Goldman-Rakic, 1997). Studies indicate that the events that take place in the DLPFC make up what is considered working memory (Goldman-Rakic, 1996a). Brodmann's areas 6, 8, and 9 become preferentially activated when a working memory task must be continuously updated and revised for temporal sequence (Wager and Smith, 2003).

Two components of working memory are recognized. The short-term component operates on the order of seconds. The second represents executive processes and operates on information retrieved from storage. Different frontal regions are associated with the storage of different kinds of information. Use of verbal material activates Broca's area and left supplementary and premotor areas. Use of spatial information activates the right premotor area. Two forms of executive processes are selective attention and task management. Both activate the anterior cingulate and dorsolateral prefrontal cortex (Smith and Jonides, 1999). Working memory and attention are closely related. For example, if we anticipate a friendly face within a crowd of strangers, we must hold the visual memory of the familiar face at the ready as we attend to the different individuals in the crowd.

The DLPFC samples and regulates the flow of information to the motor cortex by way of direct connections with the motor cortex and indirect connections with the mediodorsal and reticular nuclei of the thalamus. The reticular thalamic nucleus regulates and directs sensory information to the cortex (Yingling and Skinner, 1977). In contrast, the projections from the orbital region to the motor cortex regulate arousal and control the degree to which the limbic system influences motor behavior. The DLPFC monitors and adjusts behavior. The more superior portions of the

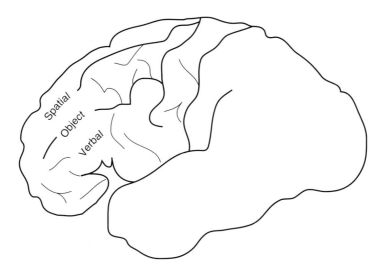

Figure 6.10. The approximate location of working memory for visuospatial processing (spatial), for features of faces or objects (object), and for semantic encoding and verbal processes (verbal), on the prefrontal cortex. Compare with Figure 6.6.

dorsolateral prefrontal cortex direct behavior in terms of sequential or temporal cues (Knight *et al.*, *1995*). More inferior portions regulate behavior in terms of spatial cues. Neurons involved with memory (~40% of total) decrease their firing rate over time after a stimulus. In contrast, neurons involved with encoding a motor response (~60% of total) increase their firing rate as the time to act approaches (Quintana and Fuster, 1992).

Symbolic representations retrieved from long-term memory as well as from current sensory cues are "sketched out" in the DLPFC in what has been described as working memory (Figure 6.10). Working memory allows the representations to be manipulated and associated with other ideas and with incoming information in order to guide behavior. There appears to be no one locus of a central executive processor. Instead, visuospatial processing takes place in the dorsolateral prefrontal cortex. The working memory for faces and objects takes place in more lateral and inferior regions of the prefrontal cortex. Semantic encoding and verbal representations are found in more inferior, insular, and anterior prefrontal regions (Goldman-Rakic and Selemon, 1997). Activity in the left inferior prefrontal cortex correlated with retrieval of words and was more active for remembered versus forgotten words. The more active the region, the better the memory performance (Reynolds *et al.*, 2004).

A second hypothesis recognizes a similar dorsoventral gradient, but distinguishes between types of processing rather than material types. In this second view the superior frontal cortex is involved in monitoring and manipulation of information whereas the more ventral dorsolateral cortex is responsible for rehearsal during short-term storage (Owen, 2000). More recent evidence supports this second hypothesis (Wager and Smith, 2003).

Goal-directed behaviors related to short-term planning (e.g., hammering) activated left middle frontal gyrus, supramarginal gyrus, inferior temporal gyrus and middle occipital gyrus. Activity in BA 46 was associated with willed actions including finger movements and freely generated words. It is hypothesized that activation of the DLPFC reflects selection of a single action out of a number of potential actions (Lau *et al.*, 2004).

Lesions of the dorsolateral area cause abnormalities in complex psychological functions which are classified as executive function deficits. The patient demonstrates difficulties in planning, feedback, learning, sequencing, establishing, maintaining, and changing a set behavior. The ability to organize events in temporal sequence is most affected. Perseveration, stimulus-bound behavior, and echopraxia may be seen (Sandson and Albert, 1987). The Wisconsin Card Sorting Test is valuable in evaluating the status of the dorsolateral area (Drewe, 1974). Performance on this test is more adversely affected with high dorsolateral or dorsomedial lesions (Milner, 1995). The patient may present with a general disinterest, apathy, shortened attention span, lack of emotional reactivity, and difficulty in attending to relevant stimuli. The patient often finds comfort in following established routines and thought processes (Fuster, 1996). A reduction in verbal fluency may be seen if involvement of the left dorsolateral area is significant. Verbal fluency is reduced in patients with Parkinson's disease (Gurd and Ward, 1989). It is believed this is a result of impaired dopaminergic projections to the DLPFC in this population (Amuts et al., 2004).

Patients with dorsolateral lesions (BA 46) are able to order words within a sentence but fail to properly sequence words when describing a plan of action. Prefrontal lesions seem to produce impairments in long-term planning whereas inferior parietal lesions produce impairments in short-term sequence execution (Sirigu et al., 1998). Semantic speech which requires searching within a category (e.g., naming fruits or cars) is affected following lesions of the left dorsolateral area (Gurd et al., 2002). In contrast, over-learned sequence speech (e.g., naming days of the week) does not activate the dorsolateral prefrontal cortex but does activate Broca's area on the left (Bookheimer et al., 2000).

Blood flow to the dorsolateral prefrontal cortex increases during the performance of the Wisconsin Card Sorting Test. This increase is not seen in schizophrenic patients (Weinberger et al., 1986). The decrease in metabolism seen in the dorsolateral prefrontal cortex of patients with borderline personality disorder is speculated to correspond with chronic feelings of depersonalization and unreality (De La Fuente et al., 1997).

Subjects successful in repressing unwanted nonemotional memories showed bilateral dorsolateral prefrontal cortical activation coupled with right hippocampal deactivation. The degree of hippocampal deactivation correlated with the magnitude of forgetfulness. These results support the concept of an active process of forgetting (Anderson et al., 2004). Successful suppression of emotional memories also showed bilateral prefrontal activation but was coupled with suppression of activity in the amygdala (Ochsner et al., 2002). Transcranial magnetic stimulation focused on the right dorsolateral prefrontal cortex had a therapeutic effect on 10 patients with posttraumatic stress disorder (Cohen et al., 2004).

Blood flow to the brain is decreased in major depression in elderly patients to about the same extent as in Alzheimer's disease (Baxter et al., 1985). Reductions are particularly evident in the parietal, superior temporal, and frontal cortex (Sackeim et al., 1990). Positron emission tomographic scanning in patients with major depression reveals decreased metabolism in the dorsolateral prefrontal cortex. Both blood flow and metabolism have been reported to be decreased in the dorsolateral prefrontal cortex in patients with primary depression (Baxter et al., 1989; Bench et al., 1992; Dolan et al., 1992). Increases in hypometabolism and hypoperfusion to normal levels have been reported following successful drug therapy but not after unsuccessful drug therapy (Mayberg, 1997). The dorsolateral prefrontal cortex is usually easy to evaluate by CT scans and is the region of the prefrontal lobe

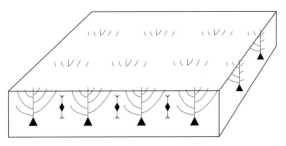

Normal prefrontal cortex

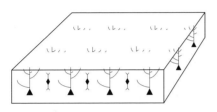

Schizophrenic prefrontal cortex

Figure 6.11.   An increase in density is seen in prefrontal neurons in postmortem tissue of schizophrenic patients. (Reproduced by permission from Selemon, L. D., Rajkowska, G., and Goldman-Rakic, P. W. 1995. Abnormally high neuronal density in the schizophrenic cortex. A morphometric analysis of prefrontal area 9 and occipital area 17. *Arch. Gen. Psychiatry* **52**:805–818.)

sampled by routine EEG. Depressed patients exhibit hypometabolism in the left anterolateral pre-frontal cortex (Baxter *et al.*, 1989).

Schizophrenics show abnormal prefrontal activation, particularly in response to tasks that require executive function such as working memory (Manoach, 2003). Alcoholics, compared with normals, showed diminished activation of BA 9, 10, and 45 in a visual spatial task requiring working memory. At the same time the alcoholics showed increased activation in BA 47 suggesting they are using the more inferior "what" stream and declarative memory as compared with the more dorsal "where" stream used by controls (Pefferbaum *et al.*, 2001). Subjects at high risk for alcoholism showed decreased bilateral activation of BA 40 and 44 and the inferior frontal gyrus when compared with low risk subjects (Rangaswamy *et al.*, 2004).

Information processing in the dorsolateral prefrontal lobes of schizophrenics is deficient. This correlates with the finding that an abnormally high density of neurons is found in the prefrontal cortex of schizophrenic brains (Figure 6.11). The increased density corresponds with a slight (non-significant) decrease in cortical thickness (Selemon *et al.*, 1995). The left dorsolateral region has been shown to have decreased cerebral blood flow corresponding with psychomotor poverty in schizophrenics (Liddle *et al.*, 1992). Negative symptoms of schizophrenia correlate with a decrease in glucose utilization in the frontal and parietal cortex (Tamminga *et al.*, 1992). Thought disorder in schizophrenia may represent the breakdown of working memory and is hypothesized to correlate with abnormalities in the dorsolateral prefrontal cortex (Goldman-Rakic, 1996a). It has been hypothesized that the increased density is due to a reduction of the neuropil, suggesting a decrease in the number of synapses (i.e., excessive synaptic pruning; Glantz and Lewis, 1993; Tamminga, 1999).

Synaptic pruning in the frontal cortex is seen normally in adolescence, preceded somewhat by cell death (Huttenlocher, 1979). More efficient word processing may be the natural result of pruning. Excessive synaptic pruning is hypothesized to result in the hallucinated speech of schizophrenia (Hoffman and McGlashan, 1997). Protection provided by estrogens may account for the later age of onset of schizophrenia in women (Seeman, 1997).

A decrease in interstitial neurons found in the white matter of the middle frontal gyrus of the dorsolateral prefrontal cortex of schizophrenics has been reported (Akbarian *et al.*, 1996). It was proposed that this decrease may reflect an abnormal migration pattern during the second trimester of pregnancy.

There is no longer any doubt that the intactness of prefrontal function is essential for our normal function in society. Through the integration of sensory input, emotional tone, and motivation of cortical, subcortical, and limbic sources, the prefrontal cortex critically intervenes in the initiation and guidance of behavior.

Neurotransmitters in the prefrontal cortex

Dopaminergic tracts to the prefrontal areas originate in the ventral tegmental area of the midbrain (see Chapter 3 and Figure 10.3). The targets of these mesencephalic tracts include the periamygdalar and entorhinal limbic regions (mesolimbic tract), as well as all areas of the frontal cortex (mesocortical tract). The prefrontal dopamine system differs from other cerebral dopamine systems in that it has a higher dopamine turnover rate, decreased responsiveness to dopamine agonists and antagonists, more irregular neuronal activity, and a lack of auto receptors. Auto receptors are sites on the presynaptic membrane sensitive to dopamine that, when stimulated, inhibit the release of more dopamine. The dopamine fibers project preferentially to the medial regions of the prefrontal cortex (Goldman-Rakic, 1995), where they terminate preferentially on the distal dendrites and spinous processes of pyramidal neurons (Goldman-Rakic, 1996b). Dopamine connections in the PFC are typically triadic as revealed by electron microscopy studies with connections to pyramidal cells, excitatory afferents, and inhibitory interneurons (Williams and Goldman-Rakic, 1993). This pattern of connection suggests that dopamine can modulate both afferent input and local inhibition. It has been hypothesized that excessive dopamine activity is detrimental to cognitive functions mediated by the prefrontal cortex (Murphy *et al.*, 1996).

Norepinephrine pathways originate from the nucleus locus ceruleus in the brainstem reticular formation (see Chapter 10). The cerulocortical fibers enter the prefrontal areas through the frontal poles, then extend caudally within the gray matter to innervate the adjacent cortical areas. Norepinephrine is more concentrated in the anterior regions. It is also highly concentrated in the postcentral parietal lobe area and in the prefrontal region. This raises the possibility that norepinephrine plays a role in the cognitive processing of somatosensory information. The reticular origin of the cerulocortical fibers to the prefrontal cortex also indicates the possibility that norepinephrine may play a role in cortical arousal.

The serotonin system originates in the raphe nuclei of the pons and mesencephalon (see Chapter 10). Serotonin is found in relatively low concentrations and seemingly plays a more minor role in the prefrontal region than does either dopamine or norepinephrine. Serotonergic axons terminate preferentially on interneurons rather than on pyramidal neurons in the prefrontal cortex (Smiley and Goldman-Rakic, 1996).

The concentration of serotonin [(5-hydroxytryptamine $(HT)_{2A,C}$)] receptors is decreased in the supplementary and dorsal premotor motor cortex of schizophrenics and correlates with negative symptoms. In contrast, the concentration of serotonin($5\text{-}HT_{1A}$) receptors is increased, especially in the prefrontal and premotor areas (Gurevich and Joyce, 1997).

A cholinergic system originates from the basal brain regions (diencephalon, ventral pallidum, nucleus basalis; see Chapters 7 and 8). Acetylcholine fibers project diffusely to the neocortex including the prefrontal regions. This tract has been shown to be affected in Alzheimer's disease.

Gamma-aminobutyric acid (GABA) is the most abundant inhibitory transmitter in the brain. Through lateral inhibition, it enhances the saliency of the excitatory patterns of prefrontal regions. The excitatory glutamic and aspartic acids have also been identified in the prefrontal regions.

It is important to note that the prefrontal neurotransmitter system develops early in life and matures progressively through infancy and adolescence.

It has been theorized that the positive symptoms of schizophrenia are caused by an overactivity of the mesolimbic system or an excessive number of D_2-like dopamine receptors. (D_2-like receptors include D_2-, D_3-, and D_4-receptor subtypes; see Chapter 3.) This is because all clinically effective antipsychotic drugs are antagonists of D_2-like dopamine receptors (Nestler, 1997). The negative symptoms may be due to a loss of function of the mesocortical system. It is hypothesized that there is: (1) an increase in activity of the mesolimbic system, which responds to antipsychotic drugs (D_2-like receptors), and (2) a decrease in activity in the prefrontal area, which does not respond to antipsychotic drugs.

There are reduced numbers of the D_1-like dopamine receptors, which include D_1- and D_5-receptor subtypes, in the prefrontal cortex of schizophrenics (Okubo *et al.*, 1997). Dopamine is believed to be important in working memory largely through action on the D_1-like receptors. The reduced number of D_1-like receptors may underlie cognitive deficiencies common to schizophrenic patients. Reduction in the density of D_1-like receptors which are found on the dendrites of pyramidal cells may be responsible for the reduction in cortical thickness (Selemon *et al.*, 1995).

SELECT BIBLIOGRAPHY

P. F. Buckley ed. Schizophrenia. *Psychiatric Clinics of North America*, **21** (1998).

E. Perecman ed. *The Frontal Lobes Revisited*. (New York: IRBN Press, 1987.)

J. M. Fuster *The Pre-Frontal Cortex: Anatomy, Physiology, and Neuropsychology of the Frontal Lobe*, 2nd edn. (New York: Raven Press, 1989.)

H. H. Jasper, S. Riggio, and P. S. Goldman-Rakic eds. Epilepsy and the Functional Anatomy of the Frontal Lobe. *Advances in Neurology*, **66** (1995).

H. O. Lunders ed. Supplementary Sensorimotor Area. *Advances in Neurology*, **70** (1996).

A. C. Roberts, T. W. Robbins, and L. Weiskrantz, *The Prefrontal Cortex. Executive and Cognitive Functions.* (New York: Oxford University Press, 2000.)

D. T. Stuss, and D. F. Benson, *The Frontal Lobes.* (New York, Raven Press, 1986.)

H. B. M. Uylings, C. G. Van Eden, J. P. C. DeBruin, M. A. Corner, and M. G. P. Feenstra eds. The Prefrontal Cortex. Its Structure, Function and Pathology. *Progress in Brain Research*, **85** (1990).

REFERENCES

Akbarian, S., Kim, J. J., Potkin, S. G., Hetrick, W. P., Bunney, W. E., and Jones, E. G. 1996. Maldistribution of interstitial neurons in prefrontal white matter of the brains of schizophrenic patients. *Arch. Gen. Psychiatry* **53**:425–436.

Amuts, K., Weiss, P. H., Mohlberg, H., Pieperhoff, P., Eickhoff, S., Gurd, J. M., Marshall, J. C., Shah, N. J., Fink, G. R., and Zilles, K. 2004. Analysis of neural mechanisms underlying verbal fluency in cytoarchitectonically defined stereotaxic space – the roles of Brodmann's areas 44 and 45. *Neuroimage* **22**:42–56.

Anderson, M. C., Ochsner, K. N., Kuhl, B., Cooper, J., Robertson, E., Gabrieli, S. W., Glover, G. H., and Gabrieli, J. D. E. 2004. Neural systems underlying the suppression of unwanted memories. *Science* **303**(5655):232–235.

Baddeley, A. 1992. Working memory. *Science* **255**:556–559.

Baxter, L. R. Jr. 1992. Neuroimaging studies of obsessive compulsive disorder. *Psychiatr. Clin. North Am.* **15**(4):871–884.

Baxter, L. R. Jr., Phelps, M. E., Mazziotta, J. C., Schwartz, J. M., Gerner, R. H., Selin, C. E., and Sumida, R. M. 1985. Cerebral metabolic rates for glucose in mood disorders – studies with positron emission tomography and fluorodeoxyglucose F18. *Arch. Gen. Psychiatry* **42**:441–447.

Baxter, L. R. Jr., Schwartz, J. M., Phelps, M. E., Mazziotta, J. C., Guze, B. H., Selin, C. E., Gerner, R. H., and Sumida, R. M. 1989. Reduction of prefrontal cortex glucose metabolism common to three types of depression. *Arch. Gen. Psychiatry* **46**:243–250.

Baxter, L. R. Jr., Schwartz, J. M., Guze, B. H., Bergman, K., and Szuba, M. P. 1990. PET imaging in obsessive compulsive disorder with and without depression. *J. Clin. Psychiatry* **51**(Suppl.):61–69.

Bechara, A., Damasio, H., and Damasio, A. R. 2000. Emotion, decision making and the orbitofrontal cortex. *Cerebr. Cortex* **10**:295–307.

Bench, C. J., Dolan, R. J., Friston, K. J., Brown, R., and Scott, L. 1992. The anatomy of melancholia: a positron emission tomography study of primary depression. *Psychol. Med.* **3**:602–615.

Benson, D. F., and Ardila, A. 1993. Depression in aphasia. In: S. E. Starkstein and R. G. Robinson (eds.) *Depression in Neurologic Disease.* Baltimore, Md.: Johns Hopkins Press, pp. 152–164.

Berthoz, S., Armony, J. L., Blair, R. J. R., and Dolan, R. J. 2002. An fMRI study of intentional and unintentional (embarrassing) violations of social norms. *Brain* **125**:1696–1708.

Blair, R. J., Morris, J. S., Frith, C. D., Perrett, D. I., and Dolan R. J. 1999. Dissociable neural responses to facial expressions of sadness and anger. *Brain* **122**:883–893.

Bleasel, A., Comair, Y., and Luders, H. O. 1996. Surgical ablations of the mesial frontal lobe in humans. In: H. O. Lunders (ed.) *Supplementary Sensorimotor Area.* Philadelphia, Pa.: Lippincott–Raven, pp. 217–235.

Bookheimer, S. Y., Zetiro, T. A., Blaxton, T. A., Gaillard, P. W., and Theodore, W. H. 2000. Activation of language cortex with automatic speech tasks. *Neurology* **55**:1151–1157.

Boone, K. B., Miller, B. L., Rosenberg, L., Durazo, A., McIntrye, M., and Weil, M. 1988. Neuro psychological and behavioral abnormalities in an adolescent with frontal lobe seizure. *Neurology* **38**:583–586.

Breier, A. 1999. Cognitive deficit in schizophrenia and its neurochemical basis. *Br. J. Psychiatry* **174**(Suppl. 37):16–18.

Brodal, A. 1981. *Neurological Anatomy*. New York: Oxford University Press.

Broffman, M. 1950. The lobotomized patient during the first year at home. In: M. Greenblatt, R. Arnot, and H. C. Solomon (eds.) *Studies in Lobotomy*. Orlando, Fla.: Grune and Stratton.

Brunet, E., Sarfati, Y., Hardy-Bayle, M. C., and Decety, J. 2000. A PET investigation of the attribution of intentions with a nonverbal task. *Neuroimage* **11**:157–166.

— 2003. Abnormalities of brain function during a nonverbal theory of mind task in schizophrenia. *Neuropsychologia* **41**:1574–1582.

Buchanan, R. W., Vladar, K., Barta, P. E., and Pearlson, G. D. 1998. Structural evaluation of the prefrontal cortex in schizophrenia. *Am. J. Psychiatry* **155**:1049–1055.

Butter, C. M., Mishkin, M., and Mirsky, A. F. 1968. Emotional response toward humans in monkeys with selective frontal lesions. *Psychol. Behav.* **4**:163–171.

Buttner-Ennever, J. A. (ed.) 1988. Neuroanatomy of the oculomotor system. *Reviews of Oculomotor Research*, vol. **2**. New York: Elsevier.

Caplan, D., Alpert, N., Waters, G., and Olivieri, A. 2000. Activation of Broca's area by syntactic processing under conditions of concurrent articulation. *Hum. Brain Map.* **9**(2):65–71.

Cohen, H., Kaplan, Z., Kotler, M., Kouperman, I., Moisa, R., and Grisaru, N. 2004. Repetitive transcranial magnetic stimulation of the right dorsolateral prefrontal cortex in posttraumatic stress disorder: a double-blind, placebo-controlled study. *Am. J. Psychiatry* **161**:515–524.

Courtney, S. M., Petit, L., Haxby, J. V., and Ungerleider, L. G. 1998. The role of prefrontal cortex in working memory: examining the contents of consciousness. *Philos. Trans. R. Soc. Lond. B. Biol. Sci.* **353**:1819–1828.

Cummings, J. L. 1993. The neuroanatomy of depression. *J. Clin. Psychiatry* **54** (Suppl.):14–20.

Damasio, A. R. 1994. *Descartes' Error: Emotion, Reason, and the Human Brain*. New York: Grist/Putnam.

Damasio, A. R., and Anderson, S. W. 1993. The frontal lobes. In: K. M. Heilman and E. Valenstein (eds.) *Clinical Neuropsychology*, 3rd edn. New York: Oxford University Press.

De La Fuente, J. M., Goldman, S., Stanus, E., Vizuete, C., Morlan, I., Bobes, J., and Mendlewicz, J. 1997. Brain glucose metabolism in borderline personality disorder. *J. Psychiatr. Res.* **31**:531–541.

Deiber, M. -P., Honda, M., Ibañez, V., Sadato, N., and Hallett, M. 1999. Mesial motor areas in self-initiated versus externally triggered movements examined with fMRI: effect of movement type and rate. *J. Neurophysiol.* **81**:3065–3077.

Dimberg, U., and Petterson, M. 2000. Facial reactions to happy and angry facial expressions: evidence for right hemisphere dominance. *Psychophysiology* **37**(5):693–696.

Dolan, R. J., Bench, C. J., Brown, R. G., Scott, L. C., Friston, K. J., and Frackowiak, R. S. J. 1992. Regional cerebral blood flow abnormalities in depressed patients with cognitive impairment. *J. Neurol. Neurosurg. Psychiatry* **55**:768–773.

Drewe, E. A. 1974. The effect of type and area of brain lesion on Wisconsin Card Sorting Test performance. *Cortex* **10**:159–170.

Elliott, R., Dolan, R. J., and Frith, D. D. 2000. Dissociable functions in the medial and lateral orbitofrontal cortex: evidence from human neuroimaging studies. *Cerebr. Cortex* **10**(3):308–317.

Ernst, M., Liebenauer, L. L., King, C., Fitzgerald, G. A., Cohen, R. M., and Zametkin, A. J. 1994. Reduced brain metabolism in hyperactive girls. *J. Am. Acad. Child Adolesc. Psychiatry* **33**:858–868.

Feinberg, T. E., Schindler, R. J., Flanagan, N. G., and Haber, L. D. 1992. Two alien hand syndromes. *Neurology* **42**:19–24.

Freund, H.-J., and Hummelsheim, H. 1984. Premotor cortex in man: evidence for innervation of proximal limb muscles. *Exp. Brain Res.* **53**:479–482.

Fuster, J. M. 1995. Memory and planning. Two temporal perspectives of frontal lobe function. *Adv. Neurol.* **66**:9–20.

— 1996. Frontal lobe syndromes. In: B. Fogel, R. B. Schiffer, and S. M. Rao (eds.) *Neuropsychiatry.* Baltimore, Md.: Williams & Wilkins, pp. 407–413.

— 2002. Frontal lobe and cognitive development. *J. Neurocytol.* **31**:373–385.

Galynker, I. I., Weiss, J., Ongseng, F., and Finestone, H. 1997. ECT treatment and cerebral perfusion in catatonia. *J. Nucl. Med.* **38**:251–254.

Giedd, J. N., Blumenthal, J., Jeffries, N. O., Castelleanos, F. X., Liu, H., Zijdenbos, A., Paus, T., Evans, A. C., and Rapaport, J. L. 1999. Brain development during childhood and adolescence: a longitudinal MRI study. *Nature Neurosci.* **2**:861–863.

Glantz, L. A., and Lewis, D. A. 1993. Synaptophysin immunoreactivity is selectively decreased in the prefrontal cortex of schizophrenic subjects (abstract). *Soc. Neurosci. Abstr.* **19**:201.

Goel, V., Grafman, J., Tajik, J., Gana, S., and Danto, D. 1997. A study of the performance of patients with frontal lobe lesions in a financial planning task. *Brain* **120**:1805–1822.

Goldman-Rakic, P. S. 1995. Anatomical and functional circuits in prefrontal cortex of nonhuman primates: Relevance to epilepsy. *Adv. Neurol.* **66**:51–65.

— 1996a. Dissolution of cerebral cortical mechanisms in subjects with schizophrenia. In: S. J. Watson (ed.) *Biology of Schizophrenia and Affective Disease.* Washington D.C.: American Psychiatric Press.

— 1996b. Regional and cellular fractionation of working memory. *Proc. Natl. Acad. Sci. U.S.A.* **93**:13473–13480.

— 1997. Space and time in the mental universe. *Nature* **386**:559–560.

Goldman-Rakic, P. S., and Selemon, L. D. 1997. Functional and anatomical aspects of prefrontal pathology in schizophrenia. *Schizophr. Bull.* **23**(3):437–458.

Goldman-Rakic, P. S., Selemon, L. D., and Schwartz, M. L. 1984. Dual pathways connecting the dorsolateral prefrontal cortex with the hippocampal formation and parahippocampal cortex in the rhesus monkey. *Neuroscience* **12**:719–743.

Gooding, S. R., Iacono, W. G., and Grove, W. M. 1994. Frontal lobe deficits and eye tracking dysfunction. Presented at the 34th Annual Meeting of the Society for Psychophysiological Research, Atlanta, Ga., 6 October, 1994.

Grafton, S. T., Mazziotta, J. C., Woods, R. P., and Phelps, M. E. 1992a. Human functional anatomy of visually guided finger movements. *Brain* **115**:565–587.

Grafton, S. T., Mazziotta, J. C., Presty, S., Friston, K. J., Frackowiak, R. S. J., and Phelps, M. E. 1992b. Functional anatomy of human procedural learning determined with regional cerebral blood flow and PET. *J. Neurosci.* **12**:2542–2548.

Gray, J. A. 1987. *The psychology of fear and stress.* New York: Oxford University Press.

Gurd, J. M., and Ward, C. D. 1989. Retrieval from semantic and letter-initial categories in patients with Parkinson's disease. *Neuropsychologia* **27**:743–746.

Gurd, J. M., Amunts, K., Weiss, P. H., Zafiris, O., Zilles, K., Marshall, J. C., and Fink, G. R. 2002. Posterior parietal cortex is implicated in continuous switching between verbal fluency tasks: an fMRI study with clinical implications. *Brain* **125**:1024–1038.

Gurevich, E. V., and Joyce, J. N. 1997. Alterations in the cortical serotonergic system in schizophrenia: a postmortem study. *Biol. Psychiatry* **42**:529–545.

Hall, R. E., Livingston, R. B., and Bloor, C. M. 1977. Orbital cortical influences on cardiovascular dynamics and myocardial structure in conscious monkeys. *J. Neurosurg.* **46**:638–647.

Halsband, U., Ito, N., Tanji, J., and Freund, H. J. 1993. The role of premotor cortex and the supplementary motor area in the temporal control of movement in man. *Brain* **116**:243–266.

Happé, F., Ehlers, S., Fletcher, P., Frith, U., Johansson, M., and Gillberg, C. 1996. Theory in the mind of the brain. Evidence from a PET scan study of Asperger syndrome. *Neuroreport* **8**:197–201.

Ho, A. P., Gillis, J. C., Buchsbaum, M. S., Wu, J. C., Abel, L., and Bunney, W. E. 1997. Brain glucose metabolism during non-rapid eye movement sleep in major depression: a positron emission tomography study. *Arch. Gen. Psychiatry* **53**:645–652.

Hoffman, R. E., and McGlashan, T. H. 1997. Synaptic elimination, neurodevelopment, and the mechanism of hallucinated "voices" in schizophrenia. *Am. J. Psychiatry* **154**:1683–1689.

Huttenlocher, P. R. 1979. Synaptic density in the human frontal cortex – developmental changes and effects of aging. *Brain Res.* **163**:195–205.

Insausti, R., Amaral, D. G., and Cowan, W. M. 1987. The entorhinal cortex of the monkey. II Cortical afferents. *J. Comp. Neurol.* **264**:356–395.

Jones, B., and Mishkin, M. 1972. Limbic lesions and the problem of stimulus reinforcement associations. *Exp. Neurol.* **36**:362–377.

Johnson, D. L., Wiebe, J. S., Gold, S. M., Andreasen, N. C., Hichwa, R. D., Watkins, G. L., and BolesPonto, L. L. 1999. Cerebral blood flow and personality: a positron emission tomography study. *Am. J. Psychiatry* **156**:252–257.

Joseph, R. 1988. The right cerebral hemisphere: emotion, music, visual-spatial skills, body-image, dreams and awareness. *J. Clin. Psychol.* **44**:630–673.

— 1996. *Neuropsychology, Neuropsychiatry, and Behavioral Neurology*, 2nd edn. New York: Plenum Press.

Kesler-West, M. L., Andersen, A. H., Smith, C. D., Avison, M. J., Davis, C. E., Kryscio, R. J., and Blonder, L. X. 2001. Neural substrates of facial emotion processing using fMRI. *Cogn. Brain Res.* **11**:213–226.

Ketter, T., George, M., Ring, H., Pazzaglia, P., Marangel, L., Kimbrell, T., and Post, R. 1994. Primary mood disorders: structural and resting functional studies. *Psychiatr. Ann.* **24**:642–647.

Knight, R. T., Grabowecky, M. F., and Scabini, D. 1995. Role of human prefrontal cortex in attention control. *Adv. Neurol.*, **66**:21–36.

Lane, R. D., Reiman, E. M., Ahern, G. L., Schwartz, G. E., and Davidson, R. J. 1997. Neuroanatomical correlates of happiness, sadness, and disgust. *Am. J. Psychiatry* **154**:926–933.

Lau, H. C., Rogers, R. D., Haggard, P., and Passingham, R. E. 2004. Attention to intention. *Science* **303**:1208–1210.

Leslie, K. R., Johnson-Frey, S. H., and Grafton, S. T. 2004. Functional imaging of face and hand imitation; towards a motor theory of empathy. *Neuroimage* **21**:601–607.

Levenson, R. W., Ekman, P., and Friesen, W. V. 1990. Voluntary facial action generates emotion-specific autonomic nervous system activity. *Psychophysiology* **27**(4):363–384.

Levin, H., and Kraus, M. F. 1994. The frontal lobes and traumatic brain injury. *J. Neuropsychiatry Clin. Neurosci.* **6**:443–454.

Lhermitte, F. 1986. Human autonomy and the frontal lobes. *Ann. Neurol.* **19**:335–343.

Liddle, P. R., Friston, K. J., Frith, C. D., Hirsch, S. R., Jones, T., and Frackowiak, R. S. J. 1992. Patterns of cerebral blood flow in schizophrenia. *Br. J. Psychiatry* **160**:179–186.

Manoach, D. S. 2003. Prefrontal cortex dysfunction during working memory performance in schizophrenia: reconciling discrepant findings. *Schizophr. Res.* **60** (2–3): 285–298.

Mayberg, H. S. 1997. Limbic-cortical dysregulation: a proposed model of depression. *J. Neuropsychiatry Clin. Neurosci.* **9**:471–481.

McGuire, P. K., Shah, G. M. S., and Murray, R. M. 1993. Increased blood flow in Broca's area during auditory hallucinations in schizophrenia. *Lancet* **342**:703–706.

McGuire, P. K., Silberswieg, D. A., Murray, R. M., David, A. S., Frackowiak, R. S. J., and Firth, C. D. 1996. Functional anatomy of inner speech and auditory verbal imagery. *Psychol. Med.* **26**:29–38.

Mendez, M. F., and Clark, D. G. 2004. Aphemia-like syndrome from a right supplementary motor area lesion. *Clin. Neurol. Neurosurg.* **106**(4): 337–339.

Mendez, M. F., and Zander, B. A. 1992. Reversible frontal lobe dysfunction from neurosarcoidosis. *Psychosomatics* **33**:215–217.

Mendez, M. F., Bagart, B., and Edwards-Lee, T. 1997. Self-injurious behavior in frontotemporal dementia. *Neurocase* **3**:231–236.

Miller, E. K. 2000. The prefrontal cortex and cognitive control. *Nat. Rev. Neurosci.* **1**:59–65.

Milner, B. 1995. Aspects of human frontal lobe function. In: H. H. Jasper, S. Riggio, and P. W. Goldman-Rakic (eds.) *Epilepsy and the Functional Anatomy of the Frontal Lobe.* New York: Raven Press.

Morris, P. L. P., Robinson, R. G., and Raphael, B. 1992. Lesion location and depression in hospitalized stroke patients. *Neuropsychiatry Neuropsychol. Behav. Neurol.* **5**:75–82.

Murphy, B. L., Arnsten, A. F., Goldman-Rakic, P. S., and Roth, R. H. 1996. Increased dopamine turn-over in the prefrontal cortex impairs spatial working memory performance in rats and monkeys. *Proc. Natl. Acad. Sci. U.S.A.* **93**:1325–1339.

Myers, R. E., Swett, C., and Miller, M. 1973. Loss of social group affinity following prefrontal lesions in free-ranging macaques. *Brain Res.* **64**:257–269.

Nauta, W. J. H. 1971. The problem of the frontal lobe: a reinterpretation. *J. Psychiatr. Res.* **8**:167–187.

Nestler, E. J. 1997. An emerging pathophysiology. *Nature* **385**:578–579.

Nitschke, J. B., Nelson, E. E., Rusch, B. D., Fox, A. S., Oakes, T. R., and Davidson, R. J. 2004. Orbitofrontal cortex tracks positive mood in mothers viewing pictures of their newborn infants. *Neuroimage* **21**:583–592.

Ochsner, K. N., Bunge, S. A., Gross, J. J., and Gabrieli, J. D. E. 2002. Rethinking feelings: an fMRI study of the cognitive regulation of emotion. *J. Cogn. Sci.* **14**(8):1215–1229.

O'Doherty, J., Winston, J., Critchley, H., Perrett, D., Burt, D. M., and Dolan, R. J. 2003. Beauty in a smile: the role of medial orbitofrontal cortex in facial attractiveness. *Neuropsychologia* **41**(2):147–155.

Okubo, Y., Suhara, T., Suzuki, K., Kobayashi, K., Inoue, O., Terasaki, O., Someya, Y., Sassa, T., Sudo, Y., Matsushima, E., Iyo, M., Tateno, Y., and Toru, M. 1997. Decreased prefrontal dopamine D1 receptors in schizophrenia revealed by PET. *Nature* **385**:634–636.

Owen, A. M. 2000. The role of the lateral frontal cortex in mnemonic processing: the contribution of functional neuroimaging. *Exp. Brain Res.* **133**:33–43.

Pandya, D. N., and Yeterian, E. H. 1990. Prefrontal cortex in relation to other cortical areas in rhesus monkey: architecture and connections. In: H. B. M. Uylings, C. G. Van Eden, J. P. C. DeBruin, M. A. Corner, and M. G. P. Feenstra (eds.) *The Prefrontal Cortex: Its Structure, Function and Pathology.* Amsterdam: Elsevier, pp. 63–94.

—1996. Morphological correlations of human and monkey frontal lobe. In: A. R. Damasio, H. Damasio, and Y. Christen (eds.), *Neurobiology of Decision Making.* New York: Springer-Verlag, pp. 13–46.

Pfefferbaum, A., Desmond, J. E., Galloway, C., Menon, V., Glover, G. H., and Sullivan, E. V. 2001. Reorganization of frontal systems used by alcoholics for spatial working memory: an fMRI study. *Neuroimage* **14**:7–20.

Picard, N., and Strick, P. L. 1996. Motor areas of the medial wall: a review of their location and functional activation. *Cereb. Cortex* **6**:342–353.

Price, C. J., Wise, R. J. S., and Frackowiak, R. S. J. 1996. Demonstrating the implicit processing of visually presented words and pseudo words. *Cerebr. Cortex* **6**:62–70.

Price, J. L., Carmichael, S. T., Carnes, K. M. *et al.* 1991. Olfactory input to the prefrontal cortex. In: J. L. Davis and H. Eichenbaum (eds.) *Olfaction: A Model System for Computational Neuroscience.* Cambridge, Mass.: MIT Press, pp. 101–120.

Quintana, J., and Fuster, J. M. 1992. Mnemonic and predictive functions of cortical neurons in a memory task. *Neuro report* **3**:721–724.

Rangaswamy, M., Porjesz, B., Ardekani, B. A., Choi, S. J., Tanabe, J. L., Lim, K. O., and Begleiter, H. 2004. A functional MRI study of visual oddball: evidence for frontoparietal dysfunction in subjects at risk for alcoholism. *Neuroimage* **21**:329–339.

Rauch, S. L., Jenike, M. A., Alpert, N. M., Baer, L., Breiter, H. C., Savage, C. R., and Fischman, A. J. 1994. Regional cerebral blood flow measured during symptom provocation in obsessive-compulsive disorder using oxygen 15-labeled carbon dioxide and positron emission tomography. *Arch. Gen. Psychiatry* **51**:62–70.

Rauch, S. L., Savage, C. R., Alpert, N. M., Miguel, E. C., Baer, L., Breiter, H. C., Fischman, A. J., Manzo, P. A., Moretti, C., and Jenike, M. A. 1995. A positron emission tomographic study of simple phobic symptom provocation. *Arch. Gen. Psychiatry* **52**:20–28.

Rauch, S. L., van der Kolk, B. A., Fisler, R. E., Alpert, N. M., Orr, S. P., Savage, C. R., Fischman, A. J., Jenike, M. A., and Pitman, R. K. 1996. A symptom provocation study of posttraumatic stress disorder using positron emission tomography and script-driven imagery. *Arch. Gen. Psychiatry* **53**:380–387.

Reiman, E. M., Lane, R. D., Ahern, G. L., Schwartz, G. E., Davidson, R. J., Friston, K. J., Yun, L.-S., and Chen, K. 1997. Neuroanatomical correlates of externally and internally generated human emotion. *Am. J. Psychiatry* **154**:918–925.

Reynolds, J. R., Donaldson, D. I., Wagner, A. D., and Braver, T. S. 2004. Item- and task-level processes in the left inferior prefrontal cortex: positive and negative correlates of encoding. *Neuroimage* **21**:1472–1483.

Riggio, S., and Harner, R. N. 1992. Frontal lobe epilepsy. *Neuropsychiatry Neuropsychol. Behav. Neurol.* **5**:283–293.

Rizzolatti, G., Luppino, G., and Matelli, M. 1996. The classic supplementary motor area is formed by two independent areas. In: H. O. Lunders (ed.) *Supplementary Sensorimotor Area.* Philadelphia, Pa.: Lippincott–Raven, pp. 45–56.

Rolls, E. T. 1990. A theory of emotion, and its applications to understanding the neural basis of emotions. *Cognit. Emot.* **4**:161–1990.

— 1997a. Taste and olfactory processing in the brain and its relation to the control of eating. *Crit. Rev. Neurobiol.* **11**:263–287.

— 1997b. Brain mechanisms of vision, memory, and consciousness. In: M. Ito, Y. Miyashita, and E. T. Rolls (eds.) *Cognition, Computation, and Consciousness.* Oxford: Oxford University Press, pp. 81–120.

— 2000. The orbitofrontal cortex and reward. *Cerebr. Cortex* **10**:284–294.

Rolls, E. T., and Baylis, L. L. 1994. Gustatory, olfactory and visual convergence within the primate orbitofrontal cortex. *J. Neurosci.* **14**:5437–5452.

Sackeim, H. A., Prohovnik, I., Moeller, J. R., Brown, R. P., Apter, S., Prudic, J., Devanand, D. P., and Mukherjee, S. 1990. Regional cerebral blood flow in mood disorders. I. Comparison of major depressives and normal controls at rest. *Arch. Gen. Psychiatry* **47**:60–70.

Sahyoun, C., Floyer-Lea, A., Johansen-Berg, H., and Matthews, P. M. 2003. Towards an understanding of gait control: brain activation during the anticipation, preparation and execution of foot movements. *Neuroimage* **21**:568–575.

Sandson, J., and Albert, M. L. 1987. Perseveration in behavioral neurology. *Neurology* **37**:1736–1741.

Seeman, M. V. 1997. Psychopathology in women and men: focus on female hormones. *Am. J. Psychiatry* **154**:1641–1647.

Selemon, L. D., Rajkowska, G., and Goldman-Rakic, P. S. 1995. Abnormally high neuronal density in the schizophrenic cortex. A morphometric analysis of prefrontal area 9 and occipital area 17. *Arch. Gen. Psychiatry* **52**:805–818.

Sirigu, A., Cohen, L., Zalla, T., Pradat-Diehl, P., Van Eeckhout, P., Grafman, J., and Agid, Y. 1998. Distinct frontal regions for processing sentence syntax and story grammar. *Cortex* **34**:771–778.

Smiley, J. F., and Goldman-Rakic, P. S. 1996. Serotonergic axons in monkey prefrontal cerebral cortex synapse predominately on interneurons as demonstrated by serial section electron microscopy. *J. Comp. Neurol.* **467**:431–443.

Smith, E. E., and Jonides, J. 1999. Storage and executive processes in the frontal lobes. *Science* **283**:1657–1661.

Smith, J. D., Reisberg, D., and Wilson. M. 1992. Subvocalization and auditory imagery: interactions between the inner ear and inner voice. In: D. Reisberg (ed.) *Auditory Imagery*. New Jersey: Lawrence Erlbaum, pp. 95–119.

Sonnby-Borgström, M. 2002. Automatic mimicry reactions as related to differences in emotional empathy. *Scand. J. Psychol.* **43**:433–443.

Sowell, E. R., Thompson, P. M., Tessner, K. D., and Toga, A. W. 2001. Mapping continued brain growth and gray matter density reduction in dorsal frontal cortex: inverse relationships during post adolescent brain maturation. *J. Neurosci.* **21**:8819–8829.

Starkstein, S. E., and Robinson, R. G. 1993. Depression in cerebrovascular disease. In: S. E. Starkstein and R. G. Robinson (eds.) *Depression in Neurologic Disease*. Baltimore, Md.: Johns Hopkins Press, pp. 28–49.

Starkstein, S. E., Robinson, R. G., and Price, T. R. 1987. Comparison of cortical and subcortical lesions in the production of post-stroke mood disorders. *Brain* **110**:1045–1059.

Sukhwinder, S. S., Bullmore, E., Simmons, A., Murray, R., and McGuire, P. 2000. Functional anatomy of auditory verbal imagery in schizophrenic patients with auditory hallucinations. *Am. J. Psychiatry* **157**:1691–1693.

Swedo, S. E., Pietrini, P., Leonard, H. L., Schapiro, M. B., Rettew, D. C., Goldberger, E. L., Rapoport, S. I., Rapoport, J. L., and Grady, C. L. 1992. Cerebral glucose metabolism in childhood-onset obsessive-compulsive disorder. Revisualization during pharmacotherapy. *Arch. Gen. Psychiatry* **49**:690–694.

Tamminga, C. A. 1999. Pruning during development. *Am. J. Psychiatry* **156**:168.

Tamminga, C. A., Thaker, G. K., Buchanan, R., Kirkpatrick, B., Alphs, L. D., Chase, T. N., and Carpenter, W. T. 1992. Limbic system abnormalities identified in schizophrenia using positron emission tomography with fluorodeoxyglucose and neocortical alterations with deficit syndrome. *Arch. Gen. Psychiatry* **49**:522–530.

Teasdale, J. D., Howard, R. J., Cox, S. F., Ha, Y., Brammer, M. J., Williams, S. C. R., and Checkley, S. A. 1999. Functional MRI study of the cognitive generation of affect. *Am. J. Psychiatry* **156**:209–215.

Volkow, N. D., Hitzemann, R., Wang, G. -J., Fowler, J. S., Wolf, A. P., Dewey, S. L., and Handlessman, L. 1992. Long-term frontal brain metabolic changes in cocaine abusers. *Synapse* **11**:184–190.

Wager, T. D., and Smith, E. E. 2003. Neuroimaging studies of working memory: a meta-analysis. *Cognit. Affect. Behav. Neurosci.* **3**(4):255–274.

Weinberger, D. R., Berman, K. F., and Chase, T. N. 1986. Prefrontal cortex physiological activation in Parkinson disease: effect of l-dopa. *Neurology* **36**(Suppl.):170.

Wicker, B., Perrett, D. I., Baron-Cohen, S., and Decety, J. 2003. Being the target of another's emotion: a PET study. *Neuropsychologia* **41**(2):139–146.

Williams, M. S., and Goldman-Rakic, P. S. 1993. Characterization of the dopaminergic innervation of the primate frontal cortex using a dopamine-specific antibody. *Cerebr. Cortex* **3**:199–222.

Wise, S. P., Fried, I., Olivier, A., Paus, T., Rizzolatti, G., and Zilles, K. J. 1996. Workshop on the anatomic definition and boundaries of the supplementary sensorimotor area. In: H. O. Lunders (ed.) *Supplementary Sensorimotor Area.* Philadelphia, Pa.: Lippincott–Raven, pp. 489–496.

Wise, S. P., Boussaloud, D., Johnson, P. B., and Caminiti, R. 1997. Premotor and parietal cortex: corticocortical connectivity and combinatorial computations. *Annu. Rev. Neurosci.* **20**:25–42.

Yingling, C. D., and Skinner, J. E. 1977. Gating of thalamic input to cerebral cortex by nucleus reticularis thalami. In: J. Desmedt (ed.) *Attention, Voluntary Contraction and Event Related Cerebral Potential.* Basel: Karger, pp. 70–96.

Zald, D. H., and Kim, S. W. 1996. Anatomy and function of the orbital frontal cortex: II. Function and relevance to obsessive-compulsive disorder. *J. Neuropsychiatry Clin. Neurosci.* **8**(3):249–261.

Zametkin, A. J., Nordahl, T. E., Gross, M., King, A. L., Semple, W. E., Rumsey, J., Hamberger, S., and Cohen, R. M. 1990. Cerebral glucose metabolism in adults with hyperactivity of childhood onset. *N. Engl. J. Med.* **323**:1361–1366.

7 Basal ganglia

The basal ganglia (basal nuclei) have been regarded traditionally as a motor control system. Lesions in the basal ganglia almost always result in movement disorders. Recently, these structures have been found to influence other emotionally related behaviors. Research on the behavioral influence of the basal ganglia was prompted by the repeated observation that emotional and cognitive dysfunctions frequently accompany movement disorders of basal ganglia origin. In some cases, psychiatric manifestations precede the onset of motor symptoms. With the advent of neuroimaging techniques, investigation into the anatomy and metabolic physiology of these structures in the awake behaving human has revealed intriguing behavioral relationships.

Motor activity is controlled by the intricate interaction of three major systems: the cerebral cortex, the cerebellum, and the basal ganglia. The few milliseconds that intervene between thought and action are crucial for our adjustment in modern society. Understanding the structures that influence those few milliseconds, such as the basal ganglia, will help unravel some of the mysteries of human behavior. It is interesting that the main input to the basal ganglia comes from the cerebral cortex and that its output returns (via the thalamus) to the frontal cortex (motor, premotor, and prefrontal cortex). The frontal cortex, including the prefrontal areas, thus mediates and plays a significant role in the various functions of the basal ganglia.

Originally the basal ganglia were described as a group of cerebral (telencephalic) nuclei. These classical basal ganglia included the caudate nucleus, putamen, globus pallidus, claustrum, and amygdala. Since that time the amygdala has been reassigned to the limbic system. Little is known of the function of the claustrum, and it is not considered here. A diencephalic nucleus, the subthalamic nucleus, has been added to the group since it is closely tied to the caudate/putamen–globus pallidus. The substantia nigra and ventral tegmental area (mesencephalic nuclei) and the pedunculopontine tegmental nucleus (a midbrain–pontine nucleus; see Chapter 10) have been added for the same reason (Figure 7.1). Some authors describe the nigral complex as consisting of the substantia nigra proper and the ventral tegmental area, which lies just medial to it.

The basal ganglia are divided into dorsal and ventral divisions (Figure 7.2; see Haber and Fudge (1997a) for a detailed review). The dorsal division consists of the neostriatum (caudate nucleus and putamen) and the paleostriatum (globus pallidus). The striatal complex is recognized as a functional unit that includes the dorsal division of the

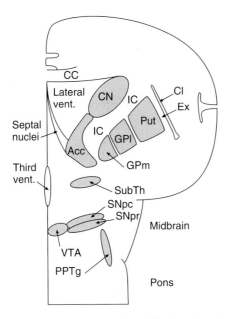

Figure 7.1.   A schematic representation of the basal ganglia and nearby structures. Clinically significant basal ganglia are highlighted in red. Acc, nucleus accumbens; CC, corpus callosum; Cl, claustrum; CN, caudate nucleus (head); IC, internal capsule; Ex, external capsule; GPl, lateral segment of globus pallidus; GPm, medial segment of globus pallidus; PPTg, pedunculopontine tegmental nucleus; Put, putamen; SNpc, substantia nigra pars compacta; SNpr, substantia nigra pars reticulata; SubTh, subthalamic nucleus; VTA, ventral tegmental nucleus.

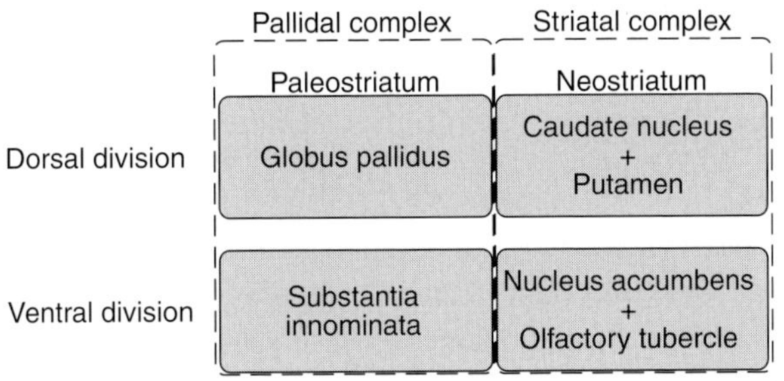

	Pallidal complex	Striatal complex
	Paleostriatum	Neostriatum
Dorsal division	Globus pallidus	Caudate nucleus + Putamen
Ventral division	Substantia innominata	Nucleus accumbens + Olfactory tubercle

Figure 7.2.   The basal ganglia consist of a dorsal division and a ventral division. The dorsal division contains the globus pallidus (paleostriatum) and the caudate nucleus and putamen (neostriatum). The paleostriatum is continuous ventrally with the substantia innominata. The neostriatum is continuous ventrally with the nucleus accumbens and the olfactory tubercle.

neostriatum (i.e., caudate nucleus and putamen) and the ventral striatum (nucleus accumbens and olfactory tubercle as well as ventromedial extensions of the caudate and putamen). The pallidal complex consists of the globus pallidus (dorsal division) and the substantia innominata (ventral division). Included as part of the substantia innominata is the basal nucleus (of Meynert).

The basal ganglia receive signals from the cerebral cortex and route integrated responses to these signals back to the cerebral cortex (Figure 7.3). The cortical information is

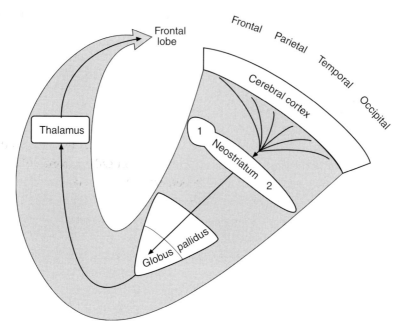

Figure 7.3.   The generalized pattern of connections involving the basal ganglia form a loop from the cortex to the basal ganglia and back to the cortex by way of the thalamus. 1, Caudate nucleus; 2, putamen. Compare with Figure 7.1 and the direct pathway of Figure 7.4.

processed through a series of multiple parallel channels as the signals pass through the basal ganglia: the basic mechanism of operation of the basal ganglia is through a process of disinhibition. Consequently, damage to the basal ganglia often results in the release of behavior, usually in the form of uncontrollable motor activity (e.g., the tremor seen in Parkinson's disease).

The basal ganglia are viewed as part of a planning mechanism that drives motor pattern generators. They work closely with executive levels of the frontal lobe to help select the motor response appropriate to the current situation. The basal ganglia also operate in close harmony with the frontal lobes in the acquisition, retention, and expression of cognitive behavior (Graybiel, 1997). Regions of the caudate nucleus (dorsal striatum) as well as the ventral striatum seem to be important in cognitive function.

Anatomy and behavioral considerations

Dorsal striatopallidum and associated nuclei

Dorsal striatum (neostriatum)

The neostriatum is made up of the putamen and the caudate nucleus (see Figure 7.2). The putamen and caudate are separated anatomically by fibers of the internal capsule (see Figure 7.1). The caudate nucleus occupies a position in the floor of the lateral ventricle dorsolateral to the thalamus. It consists of a head, body, and tail. The body continues caudally, lateral to the thalamus, and tapers gradually to form the tail, which curves ventrally into the temporal lobe to end near the amygdaloid nucleus. The putamen lies behind the anterior limb of the internal capsule and medial to the external capsule (see Figure 9.1).

The neostriatum is the gateway to the basal ganglia (see Figure 7.3). It receives fibers from all portions of the cerebral cortex and from the intralaminar nuclei of the thalamus. The neurotransmitter from the cortex is glutamate. Afferent fibers from regions of the frontal and parietal lobes may have preferential targets within the neostriatum. Fibers from the motor area of the frontal lobe (BA 4 and 6) and from the primary somesthetic cortex (BA 1, 2, and 3) end predominantly on cells in the putamen. Fibers from the dorsolateral prefrontal cortex and from the somesthetic association cortex (BA 5 and 7) terminate on cells in the caudate nucleus. These differences in cortical projection fibers support the concept of differences in function between the caudate nucleus and putamen. Neurons located within the neostriatum (interneurons) use acetylcholine as a neurotransmitter. Efferent fibers from both components of the neostriatum are GABAergic. Gamma-aminobutyric acid (GABA) is one of the major inhibitory neurotransmitters of the central nervous system. Efferent fibers from the neostriatum terminate in the substantia nigra and in both the lateral and the medial segments of the globus pallidus (Figure 7.4).

It has been theorized that the neostriatum is a repository of common motor programs and acts as a comparator that serves gating and screening functions. It can act in response to external sensory signals or to commands from various regions of the cortex. Normally the neostriatum works in conjunction with the frontal cortex to inhibit motor and thought impulses that are inappropriate to the task at hand. For example, it is normal to generate a waving action of the arm in response to the sight of a person leaving the house. However, it is inappropriate to generate the same arm-waving motor response to the sight of a spouse leaving the house to carry the trash out to the curb. It is suggested that the putamen deals with motor behaviors whereas portions of the caudate nucleus deal with thoughts and sensations (Baxter *et al.*, 1990).

The caudate nucleus plays a key role in the serial order of movements and behavior (Aldridge and Berridge, 1998). Dopaminergic input from the substanta nigra correlates with learning-related activation of the left dorsolateral prefrontal cortex and anterior cingulate area. This correlation was found to be lost in early stage Parkinson patients (Carbon et al., 2004). An increase in cortical activation was seen in Parkinson patients suggesting cortical compensation for loss in striatal function in sequential learning (Nakamura *et al.*, 2001).

Continuous administration of d-amphetamine over 3 days produces degeneration of axons in the neostriatum as well as in the motor frontal cortex of rats. The damage to dopamine axon terminals appears much like that seen in the neostriatum after administration of 1-methyl-4-phenyl-1,2,3,6-tetrahydropyridine (MPTP) (Ryan *et al.*, 1990).

In the motor sphere, lesions in the rostroventral caudate nucleus can produce choreoathetosis on the contralateral side. In the behavioral sphere, abulia is the most common disturbance reported with lesions of the caudate nucleus. Abulia includes apathy, loss of initiative, and loss of spontaneous thoughts and emotional responses (Bhatia and Marsden, 1994).

A suggestion of reduced caudate nucleus volume has been reported in schizophrenic patients by DeLisi and associates (1991). More recently a significant (14%) reduction was seen in the volume of

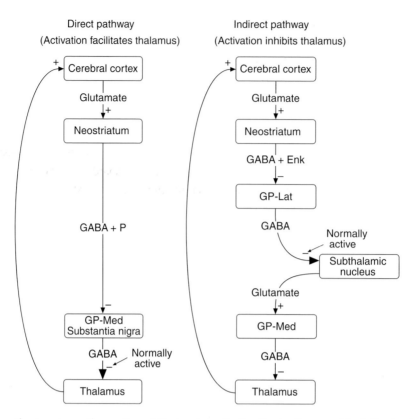

Figure 7.4.   There are two pathways through the basal ganglia: the direct pathway and the indirect pathway. When the body is at rest, the thalamus is inhibited. When muscular activity is called for, the thalamus is disinhibited. When activated by the cerebral cortex, the direct pathway increases the output of the thalamus. The indirect pathway decreases the output of the thalamus. Substantia nigra identified in this illustration represents only substantia pars reticulata. GABA in the neostriatal direct pathway is accompanied by the cotransmitter substance P (P). GABA in the neostriatal indirect pathway is accompanied by the cotransmitter enkephalin (Enk). GP, globus pallidus; Med, medial; Lat, lateral.

the caudate nucleus in neuroleptic-naive schizophrenic patients (Keshavan *et al.*, 1998). This reduction does not appear to be diagnostically specific since reductions in caudate nucleus volume have been reported in nonschizophrenic psychotic patients and in patients with depression (Krishnan *et al.*, 1992). These reductions were not accompanied by volume reductions of the putamen.

Striatal binding sites have been reported to be significantly more abundant in cocaine users. The severity of cocaine use is correlated with the number of binding sites (Little *et al.*, 1999).

Huntington's disease

Atrophy of the caudate has been reported in patients with Huntington's disease (Luxenberg *et al.*, 1988). Cell loss is seen first in the dorsomedial caudate nucleus. The greatest neuron loss is in the caudate, then the putamen, with more subtle cell loss in the ventral tegmental area (Peyser and Folstein, 1993). Both the motor disturbances and mood disorder seen in Huntington's disease correlate with cell loss in the caudate nucleus. Depression, seen in 41% of 186 Huntington's patients, preceded other symptoms by an average of 5 years. In many cases patients suffer episodes of depression before they are even aware that they are at risk for Huntington's disease (Folstein *et al.*, 1990).

Obsessive-compulsive disorder

Obsessive-compulsive disorder (OCD) is a multidimensional disorder that includes obsessions, checking, symmetry and ordering, cleanliness and washing, and hoarding (Leckman *et al.*, 1997). A response bias exists toward stimuli related to socioterritorial concerns about danger, violence, hygiene, order, and sex. These behaviors are mediated by orbitofrontal-subcortical circuits. In healthy individuals socioterritorial concerns and responses to stimuli perceived as dangerous are processed through the orbitofrontal-caudate circuit and inhibited when appropriate by the indirect pathway. Patients with OCD are particularly sensitive to socioterritorial stimuli and related concerns of danger, violence, hygiene, order, etc., and have an imbalance in the direct/indirect pathway that prevents them from inhibiting behaviors related to these stimuli and switching to alternative behaviors (Saxena *et al.*, 1998). Luxenberg and associates (1988) and Robinson and colleagues (1995) reported atrophy of the caudate in patients with OCD. An increase in metabolism over control subjects has been reported in the whole cerebral hemispheres, the orbital gyri, and the heads of the caudate nuclei in patients with OCD (see Figure 12.7; Baxter, 1992; Saxena *et al.*, 1998). It is theorized that small, restricted caudate lesions may be responsible for OCD, whereas larger lesions of the caudate nuclei result in more global symptoms such as those seen in Huntington's disease (*Baxter et al.*, 1990). Baxter and coworkers (1990) have proposed that chronic motor tics are due to small lesions in the putamen. Baxter (1992) theorized that a deficit in caudate function leads to inadequate repression (i.e., filtering) of input from the orbital cortex ("worry"). This deficit allows input from other cortical areas to continue on to the globus pallidus, where it frees the thalamus to drive the cortex to carry out a behavior (Figure 7.5). For example, sensations that signal dirty hands may normally match with an appropriate response: hand washing. However, in the case of OCD, the screening capability of the neostriatum is decreased, and the slightest sensory input from the hands may trigger hand washing. In this scenario even sensory input unrelated to the hands may cross over and produce hand washing. Motivation and the initiation of the activity may originate in the anterior cingulate gyrus (see Chapter 12). According to Houck and Wise (1995) the basal ganglia make use of old rules when presented with familiar environmental and contextual stimuli. It is up to the frontal cortex to alter a learned response pattern when old rules need to be rejected and new rules applied (Rapoport and Fiske, 1998). The presence of dopamine in the frontal cortex may be important both in activating old rules and in learning new rules (Houck and Wise, 1995).

Effective therapy allows the patient to enhance the filtering effect of the caudate to limit behavioral responses from signals from the orbital cortex. PET scans of OCD patients revealed that the metabolic rates in the basal ganglia and in the orbital cortex are higher in OCD patients than in controls (Baxter *et al.*, 1990). The increase in metabolism may reflect attempts by the patient to control the disorder. Similar changes seen in caudate metabolism following successful therapy reflect the role played by the caudate in learning new habits and skills (Schwartz *et al.*, 1996).

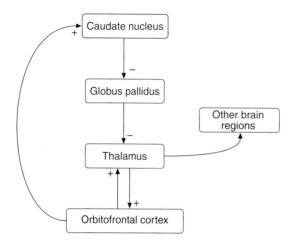

Figure 7.5.   It is proposed that overactivity in the orbital prefrontal cortex ("worry") drives the caudate nucleus. The resulting increase in the output of the caudate nucleus reduces inhibition on the thalamus. The thalamus becomes overactive and further drives the orbital prefrontal cortex. In the model, the orbital prefrontal cortex also drives the thalamus directly. Successful treatment may reduce the input to the caudate nucleus and/or it may reduce the facilitation of the thalamus by direct input from the prefrontal orbital cortex (after Baxter, 1992).

Stereotaxic lesions of the bifrontal pathways located beneath and in front of the head of the caudate nucleus (subcaudate tractotomy or capsulotomy; see Chapter 12) have been used as a surgical treatment for intractable affective disorder (Kartsounis *et al.*, 1991). Capsulotomy has been found to benefit intractable cases of OCD. The effect is believed to result from interrupting the connections between the caudate and frontal and anterior cingulate cortex (Rapoport, 1991).

Tourette's syndrome

Neuroimaging studies provide evidence that the head of the caudate is involved in Tourette's syndrome (Hyde *et al.*, 1995). The caudate nucleus is smaller in volume in both children and adults with Tourette's but there is no correlation between size and severity of symptoms (Peterson *et al.*, 2003). It is speculated that the dysfunction of the caudate seen in patients with Tourette's syndrome is responsible for the compulsive component of tics (Wolf *et al.*, 1996). It is suggested that patients with Tourette's syndrome exhibit supersensitivity of the D_2 dopamine receptor or have an excess of dopamine in the caudate nucleus (Singer, 1997). The similarity in caudate nucleus abnormalities seen both in patients with OCD and in those with Tourette's, along with the fact that OCD is frequently a comorbid condition with Tourette's syndrome, suggests that the caudate may be involved in both conditions. These two disorders may represent overlapping neurobehavioral conditions, although OCD involves, in addition, orbitofrontal and cingulate areas (Wolf *et al.*, 1996).

The right putamen is normally larger than the left in control subjects. Of 37 Tourette's syndrome patients, 13 demonstrated the reverse asymmetry with the right larger than the left putamen (Singer *et al.*, 1993). The abnormal anatomical asymmetry is paralleled by abnormal asymmetry in behavioral tests performed by these patients (Yank *et al.*, 1994).

Other

Trichotillomania (repetitive hair-pulling) has been referred to as compulsive and contains elements similar to the compulsions of OCD (Swedo and Leonard, 1992). Patients with trichotillomania exhibit significantly smaller left putamen volume (13.2%) than control subjects. These differences more closely parallel those seen in Tourette's syndrome than those in OCD (O'Sullivan *et al.*, 1997).

The density of D_2-like dopamine receptors is increased in the caudate nucleus of patients with bipolar disorder and psychotic symptoms compared with normal control subjects and with nonpsychotic patients with bipolar disorder (Pearlson *et al.*, 1995). It has been suggested that changes in the dopamine system are secondary to primary abnormalities in the serotonergic and noradrenergic systems.

Peyser and Folstein (1993) propose that when the caudate is damaged or caudate function is disrupted by lesions elsewhere in the brain, depression is often produced. This fits with the "subcortical triad" of depression, movement disorder, and dementia that often results from damage to the caudate and nearby structures (Folstein *et al.*, 1990; McHugh, 1990; Folstein *et al.*, 1991). Stroke patients who are identified to have mood disorders and are found to have unilateral lesions restricted to the head of the caudate, with or without extension into the internal capsule, exhibit depression if the lesion is on the left, and mania if it is on the right (Mayberg, 1993).

There is some evidence that the basal ganglia may be involved in schizophrenia (Buchsbaum, 1990; Liddle *et al.*, 1992). Catatonia in schizophrenia may be related to cell loss and gliosis found in the globus pallidus (Falkai and Bogerts, 1993). In contrast other investigators have found an increase in size in the striatum and pallidum (Heckers *et al.*, 1991), although more recent findings suggest that the increased size is due to the use of neuroleptics (Heckers, 1998).

Dorsal pallidum (paleostriatum)

The globus pallidus is the dorsal division of the paleostriatum (see Figure 7.2). It lies medial to the putamen (see Figures 7.1, 7.3, and 9.1). The globus pallidus consists of a lateral segment and a medial segment separated by a band of fibers. Cell bodies in the lateral segment project fibers that terminate in the medial segment. The medial segment is a major output nucleus of the basal ganglia. The putamen and the globus pallidus lie directly adjacent to one another and collectively are called the *lentiform nucleus*.

Depression is a common finding in diseases that affect the globus pallidus. A neuroanatomical model of depression after pallidal lesions focuses on enhanced inhibition of the prefrontal cortex (Lauterbach *et al.*, 1997, Lauterbach, 1999).

Of 46 patients with frontal lobe degeneration, 78% demonstrated repetitive behaviors ranging from motor stereotypies to complex obsessive-compulsive behavior. These patients had additional damage in the basal ganglia, caudate, and pallidal regions. It is postulated that the combined damage to the frontal lobe, caudate nucleus, and globus pallidus may account for the repetitive behavior seen in the frontal lobe degeneration and possibly in idiopathic OCD (Ames *et al.*, 1994). Anoxic injury, such as that produced by carbon monoxide poisoning, can result in bilateral infarctions of the globus pallidus and can cause obsessions, compulsions, and a Tourette-like syndrome (Salloway and Cummings, 1994).

Subthalamic nucleus (subthalamus)

The subthalamic nucleus lies below the thalamus and is contiguous with the substantia nigra at its caudal end. Cell bodies located in the lateral segment of the globus pallidus project to the subthalamus (see Figure 7.4). Efferent fibers from the subthalamus project to the medial segment of the globus pallidus and to the substantia nigra pars reticulata. The subthalamus is a key component of the indirect pathway through the basal ganglia. Strokes or tumors that affect the subthalamus produce contralateral hemiballismus. The affected extremities often exhibit a decrease in muscle tone.

Substantia nigra

The substantia nigra is one of the basal ganglia and is located in the midbrain (see Figures 7.1 and 7.5). Neuromelanin found in the substantia nigra pars compacta is a by-product of dopamine metabolism and gives the "nigra" its dark appearance as seen at autopsy. The substantia nigra consists of two distinct divisions, the pars reticulata and pars compacta.

The substantia nigra pars compacta contains cells that produce dopamine and give rise to fibers that project to the caudate nucleus and to the putamen. These fibers make up the nigrostriatal (mesostriatal) tract. The axons that make up the nigrostriatal projection are believed to interact with dopamine receptor sites where neuroleptics cause movement disorders. The substantia nigra pars compacta sends dopaminergic fibers to the neostriatum, involving both the direct pathway and the indirect pathway.

Dopaminergic fibers that act on D_1 dopamine receptors activate the direct pathway and increase motor activity. In contrast, dopaminergic fibers that act on D_2 receptors activate the indirect pathway and decrease motor activity. D_2 receptors tend to be concentrated in the lateral segment of the globus pallidus. Overall it appears that an increase in the level of dopamine in the neostriatum shifts the balance toward the direct pathway and an increase in activity (Figure 7.6).

Dopamine is a relatively slow-acting neurotransmitter, and, because of this slow action, some authors describe it as a neuromodulator. Release of dopamine precedes motor activity. Dopamine is inhibitory on neurons of the striatum; when released, it decreases the spontaneous firing rate of these neurons. The suppression of spontaneous firing makes individual striatal neurons more sensitive to excitatory signals from the cerebral cortex. In this manner, the release of dopamine primes the striatum for motor activity under the direction of the cerebral cortex.

Evidence from mouse studies supports the hypothesis that midbrain stem cells result in neurogenesis in the substantia nigra. The rate of turnover is less than that of the dentate gyrus (Chapter 11). Lesions result in an increase in neuronal replacement (Zhao *et al.*, 2003).

The substantia nigra pars reticulata is an output nucleus of the basal ganglia much like the medial segment of the globus pallidus. This division of the substantia nigra gives rise to the nigrothalamic fibers. The substantia nigra pars reticulata and the medial segment of the globus pallidus are the two major output nuclei of the basal ganglia. Both project to the thalamus.

Extrapyramidal side-effects of antipsychotic drugs are due to their ability to block D_2 receptor sites. These side-effects include dystonia, akathisia, pseudoparkinsonism, and tardive dyskinesia. Akathisia is motor restlessness and may be mistaken for psychotic restlessness and agitation. Tardive dyskinesia is the worst of the side-effects and is associated with long-term therapy. It

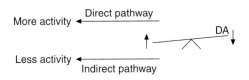

Figure 7.6.   The indirect system is the normally active pathway. The action of an increase in the level of dopamine is to facilitate motor activity. DA, dopamine.

is seen in up to 50% of patients who are receiving long-term treatment and may not disappear even when the drug is discontinued. Although dopamine or dopamine receptors or both may be involved in schizophrenia, there is no difference in the density of D_2 receptors in the neostriatum of drug-free schizophrenic patients compared to control subjects (Okubo *et al.*, 1997).

Atrophy of neuron cell bodies in the substantia nigra pars compacta leads to dopamine loss and Parkinson's disease. Side-effects of dopamine replacement therapy (levodopa, l-dopa) include dyskinesias and hallucinations. Intracerebral transplantation of dopaminergic fetal mesencephalic tissue has few reported psychiatric sequelae; however, transplantation of adrenal medullary tissue often causes psychosis or delirium (Price *et al.*, 1995). Patients with Parkinson's disease have been shown to exhibit cognitive impairment. Impairments in visuospatial function, executive function, and memory have been described (Savage, 1997).

Neuroimaging revealed that metabolism in the caudate nuclei and orbitofrontal cortex of depressed patients with Parkinson's disease is lower than that of nondepressed patients with Parkinson's disease (Mayberg *et al.*, 1990). Left anterior lesions involving the caudate nucleus have the greatest risk of depression regardless of the level of disability caused by the stroke (Starkstein *et al.*, 1987). These and other results (George *et al.*, 1993) suggest that depression associated with Parkinson's disease may involve the caudate nucleus (Lafer *et al.*, 1997).

Patients with Parkinson's disease are diagnosed with depression significantly more frequently than are patients with other disabilities (Ehmann *et al.*, 1990; Menza and Mark, 1994). The mean frequency of depression in parkinsonian patients is 40%, and the depression is accompanied by a high rate of anxiety symptoms (Cummings, 1992; Starkstein and Mayberg, 1993). Parkinson's patients with depression show significant cell loss in the ventral tegmental area (Torack and Morris, 1988). This area lies just medial to the substantia nigra and supplies dopamine to the limbic system and cortex (see later in text). It has been suggested that depression in Parkinson's disease is seen more commonly in patients with more prominent dopamine-responsive signs such as gait disturbance and rigidity. Parkinson's patients with left brain dysfunction have a higher incidence of depression than do patients with right brain dysfunction (Cummings, 1992; Starkstein and Mayberg, 1993). Depression correlates with lowered metabolism in the head of the caudate and the orbitofrontal cortex (Mayberg *et al.*, 1990).

Connections of the dorsal striatopallidal system (skeletomotor circuit)

Parallel circuits

Four distinct circuits are recognized involving the basal ganglia. These circuits run parallel to each other, but each serves a separate behavior. The best known circuit is associated with the movement disorders of basal ganglia disease. It is called the *skeletomotor circuit* and consists of both a direct and an indirect circuit (see Figure 7.4). The oculomotor circuit controls the action of the extraocular muscles. Two additional circuits are recognized but are less well known. These are the association circuit, which is believed to subserve cognition, and the limbic circuit, which is thought to subserve emotions. All four circuits have certain elements in common. First, each receives input from many areas of the cortex. Second, each sends signals through the basal ganglia, but the specific regions used by each of the circuits may differ. Third, all four circuits relay in the thalamus before sending signals back to the cortex. Fourth, all four circuits send signals back to the frontal lobe, but the exact portion of the frontal lobe targeted by each circuit differs. Although each of the circuits is separate, it is thought that each of their actions is influenced by actions of the others by way of interneurons located within the basal ganglia. Three of the circuits are associated with the dorsal striatopallidal system. The fourth, the limbic circuit, is associated with the ventral striatopallidal system.

Skeletomotor circuit

Direct pathway

The connections of the classical basal ganglia are relatively well known even though their exact mode of operation remains unclear (Graybiel, 1995). The direct pathway is a loop that has its origin in the cerebral cortex (see Figures 7.3 and 7.4). The pathway loops down into the basal ganglia and then returns to the cortex by way of the thalamus. Fibers from many areas of the cortex project into the neostriatum (caudate nucleus and putamen), effectively funneling many fibers onto relatively few cells. Fibers from the neostriatum course to the medial segment of the globus pallidus. Efferents from the globus pallidus terminate in the anterior division of the ventrolateral nucleus of the thalamus, which projects back to the frontal lobe. Cortical neurons that receive input from the basal ganglia seem to have common properties. They receive significant sensory input, they are commonly involved in premovement activities, and they respond to stimuli that have motivational significance. Lesions in these cortical areas result in attentional deficits and defective movements.

The direct (basic) pathway functions on the principle of disinhibition. The cells of the ventrolateral thalamus project to the supplementary motor cortex and facilitate motor activity. These cells would fire constantly if it were not for the fact that the output cells of the medial segment of the globus pallidus are tonically active. These tonically active cells contain GABA, which inhibits activity in the ventrolateral nucleus of the thalamus.

Efferents from the cortex contain glutamate, an excitatory neurotransmitter. When a signal arrives in the neostriatum from the cortex requesting a particular motor response, glutamate causes selected cells in the neostriatum to fire. The cells of the neostriatum contain GABA, which inhibits the tonically active GABA cells of the medial segment of the globus pallidus. The action of the neostriatal GABA inhibits the action of the GABAergic cells of the globus pallidus, which normally inhibit the action of the thalamus. By inhibiting the action of inhibitory globus pallidus neurons, the neurons of the ventrolateral nucleus of the thalamus are released (disinhibited); the thalamus fires and activates motor regions of the frontal lobe.

Indirect pathway

The components of the indirect pathway are similar to those of the direct pathway but with the addition of a detour through the lateral segment of the globus pallidus and the subthalamic nucleus (see Figure 7.5). In the case of the indirect pathway, the ventrolateral nucleus of the thalamus is inhibited by the activity of GABAergic neurons of the medial segment of the globus pallidus – just the same as with the direct pathway. However, these GABAergic neurons are encouraged to fire more rapidly only when the normally active GABAergic neurons of the lateral segment of the globus pallidus are inhibited.

The overall effect of activation of the direct pathway is to increase cortical activity. The overall effect of activation of the indirect pathway is to decrease cortical activity. During a normal resting state the two pathways are in balance with a slight edge given to the indirect pathway. Note that the neostriatal GABAergic neurons serving the two pathways each carry a different cotransmitter (see Figure 7.4).

There are a number of parallel circuits, probably thousands, that run from the prefrontal cortex to the basal ganglia and then to the thalamus and back to the cortex. Each of these circuits contains a direct and an indirect pathway. The striatum plays a role in supporting movement and thought, and is active in procedural learning.

Oculomotor circuit

The oculomotor circuit is involved with the control of eye movements and arises from more restricted areas of the cortex than the other circuits. The input to the oculomotor circuit arises from cell bodies located in the frontal eye field and the posterior parietal cortex. The oculomotor circuit targets oculomotor control areas in the frontal cortex.

Association circuit

The association circuit receives input from many areas of the cortex. It is hypothesized that this circuit is responsible for relating motor activity to targets in the extrapersonal space and may play a special role in eye–hand coordination. The association circuit projects to the frontal association area. This area, especially the dorsolateral prefrontal cortex, is important in organizing behavior in space and in time.

Hyperkinetic movement disorders

Chorea and athetosis are common hyperkinetic movement disorders. Choreoathetoid movements are typical of Huntington's disease. These movement disorders correlate with loss of striatal neurons. Ballism is seen rarely and usually as a result of an infarction of the subthalamic nucleus. The violent movements of ballism may represent extreme choreoathetoid movements. Tics are also a form of hyperkinetic movement disorder. The forced vocalizations of Tourette's syndrome may represent a form of complex tic. Hyperkinetic movements may be suppressed with D_2 receptor antagonists. Cholinergic agonists are sometimes used for control of chorea in Huntington's disease.

Hypokinetic movement disorders

Akinesia, bradykinesia, and rigidity are examples of hypokinesis, which are seen in Parkinson's disease. A loss of dopamine-producing cells in the substantia nigra pars compacta occurs in Parkinson's disease. Tardive dyskinesia may appear after long-term treatment with antipsychotic agents (phenothiazines and the butyrophenones). These drugs appear to block dopaminergic transmission and may eventually cause dopaminergic receptors in the basal ganglia to become hypersensitive to dopamine.

Pallidotomy and subthalamic deep brain stimulation for Parkinson's disease have demonstrated positive effects for motor function. Decreased semantic verbal fluency has been reported but was unaccompanied by cognitive defects (Gironell *et al.*, 2003). Hypersexuality (Roane *et al.*, 2002; Mendez *et al.*, 2004), transient manic behavior (Okun *et al.*, 2003), and confusion have been reported (Higuchi and Iacono, 2003; Hua *et al.*, 2003).

Ventral striatopallidum and associated nuclei

Ventral striatum (limbic striatum)

The ventral striatum is also known as the limbic striatum and includes a number of structures found in the basal forebrain, including the nucleus accumbens, the olfactory tubercle, and the ventral extensions of the caudate nucleus and putamen. Much of the ventral pallidum appears to be a ventral extension of the globus pallidus and includes the substantia innominata and basal nucleus (of Meynert).

Nucleus accumbens

The nucleus accumbens is a small nucleus near the midline just rostral to the diencephalon. It lies at the base of the septum pellucidum (see Figure 7.1). The nucleus accumbens is continuous above with the caudate/putamen and extends ventrally as the olfactory tubercle.

Clinical vignette

The appearance of the movement abnormality and the psychiatric symptoms may be separated by many years. Casanova and associates (1995) reported the case of a woman who was diagnosed with Sydenham's chorea at age 5. The abnormal movements abated spontaneously after a few months and never returned. At age 28, she developed auditory and visual hallucinations, delusions of persecution, and antagonistic behavior. Her affect was inappropriate, and she had no insight. She did not respond to treatment with typical neuroleptics. She died at the age of 60. Results of microscopic examination revealed basophilic concretions tracking the vessel walls of the basal ganglia. Moderate amounts of mineral deposits were seen lying free in the basal ganglia tissue, including at least iron and calcium.

Two major subdivisions of the nucleus are recognized: the core and the shell. The core represents a ventromedial extension of the caudate/putamen. There is no distinguishable border between the caudate/putamen and the core. The shell of the nucleus accumbens surrounds the core on its medial and ventral borders. The shell extends caudomedially to blend with the central division of the extended amygdala, providing evidence of the close relationship between the nucleus accumbens and the limbic system. Distinctive cell clusters throughout the nucleus suggest that different regions of the nucleus may operate selectively under different functional conditions (de Olmos and Heimer, 1999).

Projections from the prefrontal cortex, from the midline nuclei of the thalamus, and from the hippocampus and basal amygdala terminate in both the core and the shell of the nucleus accumbens. Projections from the shell terminate in the nucleus basalis (of Meynert), which is the source of cholinergic fibers to the cortex.

These connections through the nucleus basalis may allow the shell of the nucleus accumbens to influence arousal, attention, and cognitive function (Heimer *et al.*, 1997).

The shell is different from the core in that it has fibers that project directly to the central nucleus of the extended amygdala and to the lateral hypothalamus.

The connections of the shell to the amygdala suggest that the nucleus accumbens may facilitate autonomic and goal-directed behavior (Alheid and Heimer, 1996).

The nucleus accumbens has been described as a limbic–motor interface. It is in a position to bring together input from limbic "motivational" structures, and its output goes to structures associated with motor processes, including the globus pallidus, substantia nigra, and pedunculopontine tegmental nucleus (Winn *et al.*, 1997).

The nucleus accumbens and dopamine have been closely associated with the rewarding effects of carbohydrates as well as abusive drugs including alcohol, cocaine, amphetamine, and morphine (Blum *et al.*, 1996a). The nucleus accumbens also is involved with both withdrawal effects related to these drugs and effects of antipsychotic drugs (Alheid and Heimer, 1996). One model of schizophrenia proposes that an increase in the quantity of dopamine released in the nucleus accumbens by the mesolimbic pathway from the ventral tegmental area is responsible for positive psychotic symptoms (Gray *et al.*, 1991; Gray, 1998). Another model of the pathophysiology of schizophrenia suggests that abnormalities in the projection from the hippocampus to the nucleus accumbens may be responsible for the psychosis and thought disorganization of schizophrenia (Csernansky and Bardgett, 1998).

Ventral pallidum

Several nuclei within the substantia innominata along with the lateral preoptic area make up the ventral pallidum. The ventral pallidum is continuous with the globus pallidus (dorsal pallidum), which lies above it.

Basal nucleus (of Meynert)

The basal nucleus makes up a large portion of the substantia innominata. The majority of acetylcholine found in the brain arises from the neurons of the basal nucleus. It projects fibers to the neocortex, hippocampus, amygdala, thalamus, and brainstem. It receives fibers from the amygdala, hypothalamus (see Chapter 8), pedunculopontine nucleus, and midbrain (see Chapter 10).

The basal nucleus is believed to be important in integrating subcortical functions. Drugs such as scopolamine that block acetylcholine can cause confusion and memory disorders.

Loss of the acetylcholinergic neurons of the basal nucleus has been described in Alzheimer's disease (Price *et al.*, 1982). However, acetylcholine disappears from the axon terminals before it is reduced in the cell bodies in the basal nucleus. This suggests that nerve cell loss in the basal nucleus is secondary to a dying back of the axons (Sofroniew *et al.*, 1983; Herholz *et al.*, 2004).

Ventral tegmental area

The ventral tegmental area has recently been included as one of the basal ganglia (see Figures 7.1, 10.3, and 10.4). It is located in the midbrain and appears as a ventromedial extension of the substantia nigra pars compacta. In addition to their close proximity, the ventral tegmental area and substantia nigra pars compacta serve similar functions and they have a similar histochemical makeup. For this reason they have been identified as the two components of the "nigral complex" (Ma, 1997). Like substantia nigra pars compacta, the ventral tegmental area contains a large population of dopaminergic neurons.

Similarity between cells found in the substantia nigra and the ventral tegmental area has suggested the existence of a dorsal tier and a ventral tier of dopaminergic neurons. The dorsal tier includes a band of neurons stretching across the dorsal substantia nigra pars compacta and contiguous ventral tegmental area. The ventral tier consists of cells of the ventral substantia nigra pars compacta and a corresponding ventral group of ventral tegmental area neurons. Evidence suggests that the dorsal tier neurons are tightly linked with the limbic system. The ventral tier dopaminergic neurons are influenced by limbic regions but are more closely linked with areas of the striatum that are important in sensorimotor control (Haber and Fudge, 1997b).

Descending projections to the ventral tegmental area include indirect connections from the hippocampus by way of septal nuclei and the hypothalamus. These close connections with limbic system structures led Nauta (1958) to include the ventral tegmental area as part of the "midbrain limbic area."

The ventral tegmental area projects through the medial forebrain bundle to limbic areas (mesolimbic system) and to cortical areas (mesocortical system). Targets of the dopaminergic fibers from the ventral tegmental area include the dorsolateral and medial prefrontal cortex, the anterior cingulate gyrus (mesocortical system) and nucleus accumbens, the hippocampus, and the amygdala (mesolimbic system). The midline and medial thalamic nuclei are considered part of the limbic thalamus and are also targets of ascending dopaminergic fibers (see Chapter 9).

There is evidence that many of the fibers that make up the mesocortical projection arise from neurons from both the ventral tegmental area and adjacent areas of the midbrain. The adjacent areas include widespread regions of the substantia nigra and the retrorubral field. A few fibers even originate from within the parabrachial nucleus. Although this is described as a dopaminergic system, a surprising number of the fibers are not from dopamine-producing neurons. It appears that the mesocortical projections to the dorsal prefrontal cortex, to the ventromedial prefrontal cortex, and to the anterior cingulate cortex are served by midbrain neurons from three different regions of the midbrain (Williams and Goldman-Rakic, 1998).

The ventral tegmental area dopaminergic system is postulated to be involved in reward associated with newly learned behaviors in contrast to the maintenance of previously learned behaviors (Schultz *et al.*, 1995). This system responds to the novelty of an unexpected stimulus, to primary rewards, and to the conditioned stimulus associated with that reward (Haber and Fudge, 1997a). Systemic injection of cocaine in rats produced an increase in extracellular glutamate in the ventral tegmental area and may underlie behavioral sensitization to cocaine (Kalivas and Duffy, 1998).

The size of neuromelanin-containing neurons in the ventral tegmental area was decreased and the volume of the substantia nigra area was reduced in the brains of six schizophrenic patients. There was no change in the number of neurons or glia cells (Bogerts *et al.*, 1983). An increase in activity in the mesolimbic system has been reported in schizophrenia. This is accompanied by a decrease in activity in the prefrontal area. It has been suggested that the positive symptoms of schizophrenia may reflect mesolimbic hyperactivity, and the negative symptoms may reflect mesocortical hypoactivity (Weinberger, 1987).

Pedunculopontine tegmental nucleus

The pedunculopontine tegmental nucleus extends caudally from the substantia nigra just medial to the lateral lemniscus (see Figures 7.1 and 10.3). It is usually considered as one of the reticular formation nuclei (see Chapter 10); however, its connections with the basal ganglia and importance in motor control have motivated some authors to include it among the basal ganglia (Winn *et al.*, 1997). Like the nucleus basalis, the pedunculopontine tegmental nucleus is an important source of acetylcholine; however, it also contains noncholinergic neurons, much the same as the substantia nigra contains dopaminergic and nondopaminergic neurons. Fibers from the pedunculopontine nucleus project to the frontal cortex, septum, amygdala, globus pallidus, substantia nigra, hypothalamus, and thalamus. The largest and most studied are those projections to the thalamus. The pedunculopontine tegmental nucleus receives fibers from: (1) the dorsal striatum (putamen, globus pallidus, substantia nigra pars reticulata, subthalamic nucleus), (2) ventral striatum (nucleus accumbens), (3) amygdala, and (4) brainstem reticular formation (raphe nuclei and locus ceruleus) (Jones, 1990; Wainer and Mesulam, 1990).

Clinical vignette

A 52-year-old hypertensive man developed a delirium which slowly cleared leaving a profoundly apathetic state. He remained detached and disinterested and would not initiate any activity. When spoken to he would reply in a few words, but he never initiated conversation. There was a recent infarct in the head of the right caudate on CT scan, clearly delineated 2 months later on MRI (Figure 7.7). One year following the event he was distractible, irritable, and easily frustrated. There was decreased initiative, disengagement from prior activities, and decreased attention to his appearance and weight. He eventually lost his job as school principal.

Clinical vignette

A 59-year-old, right-handed man underwent a right pallidotomy for long-standing Parkinson's disease. Immediately after the pallidotomy, the patient began demanding sex up to 12–13 times a day. He masturbated frequently and propositioned his wife's female friends for sex. He began hiring strippers and driving

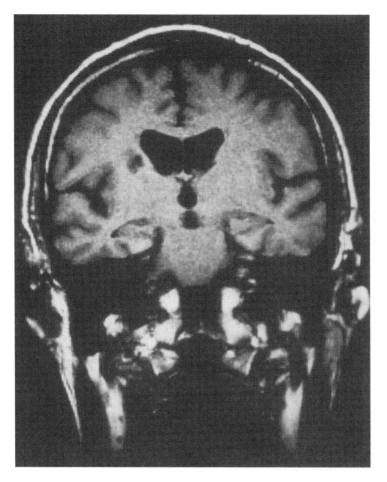

Figure 7.7.   A magnetic resonance image (T1-weighted), coronal view, taken 2 months after his acute event showed predominant dorsolateral involvement of the right caudate nucleus. (Reprinted with permission from Mendez *et al.*, 1989.)

around town searching for prostitutes. He spent hours on the internet looking for sex and buying pornographic materials. The patient also had increased irritability and energy suggesting hypomanic behavior.

The variation in placement of the pallidotomy (Figure 7.8), or its extension beyond the appropriate site, could have caused hypersexuality, and possible manic-type behavior. His pallidotomy could have affected the patient's ventral striatopallidal system.

Limbic connections of the pedunculopontine nucleus (septum, amygdala, ventral pallidum, prefrontal cortex), along with behavioral studies, underscore its importance in working memory and cognition. It plays a role in the regulation of the basal nucleus (Decker and McGaugh, 1991). Connections with other basal ganglia nuclei suggest its importance in motor activity. It is known to be important in locomotion and possibly may be involved in the pill-rolling tremor of Parkinson's disease. It appears to be critical in the reward effects of opiates and other stimulants and plays a role in attention and arousal (Steckler *et al.*, 1994).

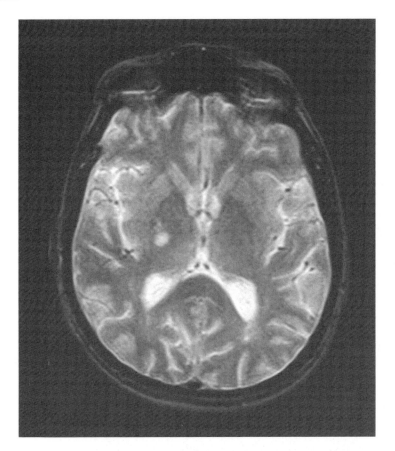

Figure 7.8.   A magnetic resonance image (T2-weighted) demonstrated increased signal intensity in the ventrolateral globus pallidus on the right. (Reprinted with permission from Mendez *et al.*, 2004.)

Like the nucleus accumbens, the pedunculopontine tegmental nucleus is considered a limbic–motor interface and may be involved with response switching and perseveration. It is speculated to be in a position to respond to signals from the ventral striatum in order to inhibit an ongoing response maintained by the dorsal striatum (Winn *et al.*, 1997).

Neuron cell loss in the pedunculopontine tegmental nucleus has been reported in Parkinson's disease (Jellinger, 1991), Alzheimer's disease (Mufson *et al.*, 1988), and progressive supranuclear palsy (Jellinger, 1988). Impairment of attentional processes is a common denominator of all of these disorders.

Connections of the ventral striatopallidal system (limbic circuit)

In addition to the other circuits of the basal ganglia, the ventral striatopallidal system forms yet another circuit called the *limbic circuit* (Figure 7.9). It is the least known of the circuits. It is believed to provide an interface between the limbic system and the motor systems. From what is known of the connections of the ventral striatopallidal system, there appear to be many similarities between the general pattern of connectivity of this system and the

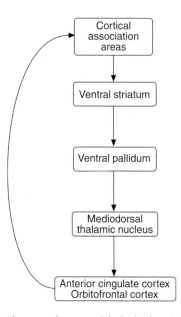

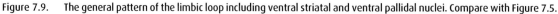

Figure 7.9.   The general pattern of the limbic loop including ventral striatal and ventral pallidal nuclei. Compare with Figure 7.5.

dorsal striatopallidal system (see Figures 7.3 and 7.6). Limbic fibers to the ventral stria-topallidal system arise from the hippocampus and the amygdala (Burns *et al.*, 1996). Fibers from many cortical areas and from several brainstem nuclei, including the raphe nuclei and locus ceruleus, funnel together and converge on the ventral striatum. A large contingent of fibers is from the ventral tegmental area. The bulk of the efferents from the nucleus accumbens project to the ventral pallidum. The ventral pallidum projects back to both cortical and brainstem targets. The primary cortical target is the prefrontal cortex directly, and via the mediodorsal nucleus of the thalamus indirectly. Brainstem targets include the pedunculopontine tegmental nucleus.

Evidence indicates that the ventral striatal system is involved in emotional behavior and with motivational aspects of motor behavior (Graybiel, 1995).

Serotonin is much less studied than dopamine but also plays a role in the function of the basal ganglia and is found throughout the caudate nucleus and putamen (Pazos and Palacios, 1985; Pazos *et al.*, 1985). Clomipramine, which acts on the serotonergic system, has been useful in treating symptoms of obsessive-compulsive disorder. It has been questioned whether serotonin may play a role in this disorder (Insel and Winslow, 1992).

Further behavioral notes

Wilson's disease is a neurodegenerative disorder that results from an abnormality in copper metabolism and manifests mainly through a movement disorder, psychiatric symptoms, and liver disease. The abnormal movements include rigidity, coarse proximal tremor, and choreoathetosis. Patients may have a facial expression of silliness or indifference, but their emotions are usually not affected. The disorder may start at an early age (7–15) or at a late age (after 30). Psychiatric symptoms may include impulsiveness, irritability, and affective changes. The late form has been more closely associated with psychosis, usually of a paranoid type. In approximately 20% of patients, psychiatric symptoms precede other signs or symptoms of the disease (Lohr and Wisniewski, 1987).

The A1 allele of the D_2 dopamine receptor gene is dysfunctional in some cases of alcoholism. Variants of the D_2 dopamine receptor gene have been correlated with crack/cocaine dependency, obesity, carbohydrate binge eating, attention-deficit hyperactivity disorder, Tourette's syndrome, pathological gambling, and smoking. The association of these various behavioral disorders with a single genetic anomaly supports the concept of a "reward deficiency syndrome"(Blum *et al.*, 1996a, 1996b).

Lesions in the striatum on the dominant side can cause atypical aphasias. This indicates a possible role of the basal ganglia in language. Neurological conditions that commonly accompany psychotic episodes suggest basal ganglia involvement.

In summary, evidence from several different sources suggests that the basal ganglia may be partially involved in the regulation of attentional and cognitive functions by correlating and integrating motor and sensory information. Both operate by way of a simple loop from the cortex down into the basal ganglia and back to the cortex (see Figure 7.3). The motor loops are concerned with motor functions, whereas the limbic circuit is concerned with emotions. The filtering and gating functions of the basal ganglia appear to be used by both the motor and the limbic circuits.

SELECT BIBLIOGRAPHY

G. W. Arbuthnott and P. C. Emson, eds. Chemical signalling in the basal ganglia. *Progress in Brain Research*, **99** (1993).

P. F. Buckley, ed. Schizophrenia. *Psychiatric Clinics of North America*, **21** (1998).

B. J. Carroll, and J. E. Barrett, *Psychopathology and the Brain*. (New York: Raven Press, 1991.)

E. R. Kandel, J. H. Schwartz, and T. M. Jessell, *Principles of Neural Science*, 3rd edn. (Norwalk, Conn.: Appleton and Lange, 1991.)

K. Kultas-Ilinsky, and I. A. Ilinsky, eds. *Basal Ganglia and Thalamus in Health and Movement Disorders*. (New York: Kluwer Academic / Plenum Publishers, 2000.)

T. P. Ma, The basal ganglia. In *Fundamental Neuroscience*, ed. D. E. Haines. (New York: Churchill Livingstone, 1997), pp. 363–378.

E. C. Miguel, S. L. Rauch and J. F. Leckman, *Psychiatric Clinics of North America: Neuropsychiatry of the Basal Ganglia*, **20** (1997).

M. Sandler, C. Feuerstein, and B. Scatton, eds. *Neurotransmitter Interactions in the Basal Ganglia*. (New York: Raven Press, 1985.)

J. S. Schneider, and T. I. Lidsky, eds. *Basal Ganglia and Behavior: Sensory Aspects of Motor Functioning*. (Toronto: Hans Huber, 1985.)

P. B. Strange, *Brain Biochemistry and Brain Disorders*. (New York: Oxford University Press, 1992.)

W. J. Weiner, and A. E. Lang, eds. Behavioral Neurology of Movement Disorders. *Advances in Neurology*, **65**, (1995).

REFERENCES

Aldridge, J.W., and Berridge, K.C. 1998. Coding of serial order by neostriatal neurons: a "natural action" approach to movement sequence. *J. Neurosci.* **18(7)**:2777–2787.

Alheid, G. F., and Heimer, L. 1996. Theories of basal forebrain organization and the "emotional motor system." *Prog. Brain Res.* **107**: pp. 461–484.

Ames, D., Cummings, J. L., Wirshing, W. C., Quinn, B., and Mahler, M., 1994. Respective and compulsive behavior in frontal lobe degenerations. *J. Neuropsychiatry Clin. Neurosci.* **6(2)**: 100–113.

Baxter, L. R. Jr. 1992. Neuroimaging studies of obsessive compulsive disorder. *Psychiatr. Clin. North Am.* **15**:871–884.

Baxter, L. R., Schwartz, J. M., Guze, B. H., Bergman, K., and Szuba, M. P. 1990. Neuroimaging in obsessive-compulsive disorder: seeking the mediating neuroanatomy. In: M. A. Jenike, L. Baer, and W. E. Minichiello (eds.) *Obsessive-Compulsive Disorders: Theory and Management.* Littleton, Mass.: Year Book Medical Publishers.

Bhatia, K. P., and Marsden, C. D. 1994. The behavioural and motor consequences of local lesions of the basal ganglia in man. *Brain* **117**:859–876.

Blum, K., Cull, J. G., Braverman, E. R., and Comings, D. E. 1996a. Reward deficiency syndrome. *Am. Sci.* **84**:132–145.

Blum, K., Sheridan, P. J., Wood, R. C., Braverman, E. R., Chen, T. J. H., Cull, J. G., and Comings, D. E. 1996b. The D2 dopamine receptor gene as a determinant of reward deficiency syndrome. *J. R. Soc. Med.* **89**:396–400.

Bogerts, B., Hantsch, J., and Herzer, M. 1983. A morphometric study of the dopamine-containing cell groups in the mesencephalon of normals, Parkinson patients, and schizophrenics. *Biol. Psychiatry* **18**:951–969.

Buchsbaum, M. S. 1990. The frontal lobes, basal ganglia, and temporal lobes as sites for schizophrenia. *Schizophr. Bull.* **16**:379–389.

Burns, L. H., Annett, L., Kelley, A. E., Everitt, B. J., and Robbins, T. W. 1996. Effects of lesions to amygdala, ventral subiculum, medial prefrontal cortex, and nucleus accumbens on the reaction to novelty: implication for limbic-striatal interactions. *Behav. Neurosci.* **110**:60–73.

Carbon, M., Ma, Y., Barnes, A., Dhawan, V., Chaly, T., Ghilardi, M. F., and Eidelberg, D. 2004. Caudate nucleus: influence of dopaminergic input on sequence learning and brain activation in Parkinsonism. *Neuroimage* **21**:1497–1507.

Casanova, M. F., Crapanzano, K. A., Mannheim, G., and Kruesi, M. 1995. Sydenham's chorea and schizophrenia: a case report. *Schizophr. Res.* **16**:73–76.

Csernansky, J. G., and Bardgett, M. E. 1998. Limbic-cortical neuronal damage and the pathophysiology of schizophrenia. *Schizophr. Bull.* **24**:231–248.

Cummings, J. L. 1992. Depression and Parkinson's disease: a review. *Am. J. Psychiatry* **149**:443–454.

Decker, M. W., and McGaugh, J. L. 1991. The role of interactions between the cholinergic system and other neuromodulatory systems in learning and memory. *Synapse* **7**:151–168.

DeLisi, L. E., Hoff, A. L., Schwartz, J. E., Shields, G. W., Halthore, S. N., Gupta, S. M., Henn, F. A., and Anand, A. K. 1991. Brain morphology in first-episode schizophrenic-like psychotic patients: a quantitative magnetic resonance imaging study. *Biol. Psychiatry* **29**:159–175.

deOlmos, J. S., and Heimer, L. 1999. The concepts of the ventral striatopallidal system and the extended amygdala. *Ann. N.Y. Acad. Sci.* **877**:1–32.

Ehmann, T. S., Beninger, R. J., Gawel, M. J., and Riopelle, R. J. 1990. Depressive symptoms in Parkinson's disease: a comparison with disabled control subjects. *J. Geriatr. Psychiatry Neurol.* **1**:3–9.

Falkai, P., and Bogerts, B. 1993. Cytoarchitectonic and developmental studies in schizophrenia. In: R. W. Kerwin (ed.) *Cambridge Medical Reviews. Neurobiology and Psychiatry*, vol. **2**. Cambridge, UK: Cambridge University Press, pp. 43–52.

Folstein, S. E., Folstein, M. F., and Starkstein, S. E. 1990. Diseases of the caudate as a model for a manic depressive disorder. In: A. J. Franks (ed.) *Function and Dysfunction in the Basal Ganglia.* Manchester: Manchester University Press, pp. 239–246.

Folstein, S. E., Peyser, C. E., Starkstein, S. E., and Folstein, M. F. 1991. The subcortical triad of Huntington's disease: a model for a neuropathology of depression, dementia and dyskinesia. In: B. J. Carroll and J. E. Barrett, (eds.) *Psychopathology and the brain.* New York: Raven Press, pp. 65–75.

George, M. S., Ketter, T. A., and Post, R. M. 1993. SPECT and PET imaging in mood disorders. *J. Clin. Psychiatry* **54** (Suppl. 11):6–13.

Gironell, A., Kulisevsky, J., Rami, L., Fortuny, N., Garcia-Sanchez, C., and Pascual-Sedano, B. 2003. Effects of pallidotomy and bilateral subthalamic stimulation on cognitive function in Parkinson disease. A controlled comparative study. *J. Neurol.* **250 (8)**:917–923.

Gray, J. A. 1998. Integrating schizophrenia. *Schizophr. Bull.* **24**:249–266.

Gray, J. A., Feldon, J., Rawlins, J. N. R., Hemsley, D. R., and Smith, A. D. 1991. The neuropsychology of schizophrenia. *Behav. Brain Res.* **14**:1–20.

Graybiel, A. M. 1995. The basal ganglia. *Trends Neurosci.* **18**:60–62.

1997. The basal ganglia and cognitive pattern generators. *Schizophr. Bull.* **23**:459–469.

Haber, S. N., and Fudge, J. L. 1997a. The primate substantia nigra and VTA: integrative circuitry and function. *Crit. Rev. Neurobiol.* **11**:323–342.

1997b. The interface between dopamine neurons and the amygdala: implications for schizophrenia. *Schizophr. Bull.* **23**:471–482.

Heckers, S. 1998. Neuropathology of schizophrenia: cortex, thalamus, basal ganglia, and neurotransmitter-specific projection systems. *Schizophr. Bull.* **23**:403–421.

Heckers, S., Heinsen, H., Heinsen Y. C., and Beckmann, H. 1991. Cortex, white matter, and basal ganglia in schizophrenia: a volumetric postmortem study. *Biol. Psychiatry* **29**:556–566.

Heimer, L., Alheid, G. F., de Olmos, J. S., Groenewegen, H. J., Haber, S. N., Harlan, R. E., and Zahm, D. S. 1997. The accumbens: beyond the core-shell dichotomy. *J. Neuropsychiatry Clin. Neurosci.* **9**:354–381.

Herholz, K., Weisenbach, S., Zündorf, G., Lenz, O., Schröder, H., Bauer, B., Kalbe, E., and Heiss, W.-D. 2004. In vivo study of acetylcholine esterase in basal forebrain, amygdala, and cortex in mild to moderate Alzheimer disease. *Neuroimage* **21**:136–143.

Higuchi, Y., and Iacono, R. P. 2003. Surgical complications in patients with Parkinson's disease after posterioventral pallidotomy. *Neurosurgery* **52(3)**:568–571.

Houck, J., and Wise, S. P. 1995. Distributed modular architectures linking basal ganglia, cerebellum, and cerebral cortex: their role in planning and controlling action. *Cereb. Cortex* **5**:95–110.

Hua, Z., Guodong, G., Qinchuan, L., Yaqun, A., Qinfen, W., and Xuelian, W. 2003. Analysis of complications of radiofrequency pallidotomy. *Neurosurgery* **52(1)**:99–101.

Hyde, T. M., Stacey, M. E., Coppola, R. C., Handel, S. F., Rickler, K. C., and Weinberger, D. R. 1995. Cerebral morphometric abnormalities in Tourette's syndrome: a quantitative MRI study in monozygotic twins. *Neurology* **45**:1176–1182.

Insel, T. R., and Winslow, J. T. 1992. Neurobiology of obsessive compulsive disorder. *Psychiatr. Clin. North Am.* **15**:813–824.

Jellinger, K. 1988. The pedunculopontine nucleus in Parkinson's disease, progressive supranuclear palsy and Alzheimer's disease. *J. Neurol. Neurosurg. Psychiatry* **51**:540–543.

——— 1991. Pathology of Parkinson's disease: changes other than the nigrostriatal pathway. *Mol. Chem. Neuropathol.* **14**:153–197.

Jones, B. E. 1990. Immunohistochemical study of choline acetyltransferase-immunoreactive processes and cells innervating the pontomedullary reticular formation in the rat. *J. Comp. Neurol.* **295**:485–491.

Kalivas, P. W., and Duffy, P. 1998. Repeated cocaine administration alters extracellular glutamate in the ventral tegmental area. *J. Neurochem.* **70(4)**:1497–1502.

Kartsounis, L. D., Poynton, A., Bridges, P. K., and Bartlett, J. R. 1991. Neuro-psychological correlates of stereotactic subcaudate tractotomy. *Brain* **114**:2657–2673.

Keshavan, M. S., Rosenberg, D., Sweeney, J. A., and Pettegrew, J. W. 1998. Decreased caudate volume in neuroleptic-naive psychotic patients. *Am. J. Psychiatry* **155**:774–778.

Krishnan, K. R. R., McDonald, W. M., Escalona, P. R., Doraiswamy, P. M., Na, C., Husain, M. M., Figiel, G. S., Boyko, O. B., Ellinwood, E. H., and Nemeroff, C. B. 1992. Magnetic resonance imaging of the caudate nuclei in depression: preliminary observations. *Arch. Gen. Psychiatry* **49**:553–557.

Lafer, B., Renshaw, P. F., and Sachs, G. S. 1997. Major depression and the basal ganglia. *Psychiatr. Clin. North Am.* **20**:885–896.

Lauterbach, E. C. 1999. The external globus pallidus in depression. *J. Neuropsychiatry Clin. Neurosci.* **11(4)**:515–516.

Lauterbach, E. C., Jackson, J. G., Price, S. T., Wilson, A. N., Kirsh, A. D., and Dever, G. E. A. 1997. Clinical, motor, and biological correlates of depressive disorders after focal subcortical lesions. *J. Neuropsychiatry Clin. Neurosci.* **9(2)**:259–266.

Leckman, J. F., Grice, D. E., Boardman, J., Zhang, H., Vitale, A., Bondi, C., Alsobrook, J., Peterson, B. S., Cohen, D. J., Rasmussen, S. A., Goodman, W. K., McDougle, C. J., and Pauls, D. L. 1997. Symptoms of obsessive-compulsive disorder. *Am. J. Psychiatry* **154**:911–917.

Liddle, P. F., Friston, K. J., Frith, C. D., Hirsch, S. R., Jones, T., and Frackowiak, R. S. 1992. Patterns of cerebral blood flow in schizophrenia. *Br. J. Psychiatry* **160**:179–186.

Little, K. Y., Zhang, L., Desmond, T., Frey, K. A., Dalach, G. W., and Cassin, B. J. 1999. Striatal dopaminergic abnormalities in human cocaine users. *Am. J. Psychiatry* **156**:238–245.

Lohr, J. B., and Wisniewski, A. A. 1987. *Movement Disorders; A Neuropsychiatric Approach.* New York: Guilford.

Luxenberg, J. S., Swedo, S. E., Flament, M. F., Friedland, R. P., Rapoport, J., and Rapoport, S. I. 1988. Neuroanatomical abnormalities in obsessive-compulsive disorder determined with quantitative x-ray computed tomography. *Am. J. Psychiatry* **145**:1089–1093.

Ma, T. P. 1997. The basal ganglia. In: D. E. Haines (ed.) *Fundamental Neuroscience.* New York: Churchill Livingstone, pp. 363–378.

Mayberg, H. S. 1993. Neuroimaging studies of depression in neurologic disease. In: S. E. Starkstein and R. G. Robinson (eds.) *Depression in Neurologic Disease.* Baltimore, Md.: Johns Hopkins Press, pp. 186–216.

Mayberg, H. S., Starkstein, S. E., Sadzot, B., Preziosi, T., Andrezejewski, P. L., Dannals, R. F., Wagner, H. N. Jr., and Robinson, R. G. 1990. Selective hypometabolism in the inferior frontal lobe in depressed patients with Parkinson's disease. *Ann. Neurol.* **28**:57–64.

McHugh, P. R. 1990. The basal ganglia: the region, the integration of its systems and implications for psychiatry and neurology. In: A. J. Franks (ed.) *Function and Dysfunction in the Basal Ganglia.* Manchester, UK: Manchester University Press, pp. 259–269.

Mendez, M. F., Adams, N. L., and Skoog, K. M. 1989. Neurobehavioral changes associated with caudate lesions. *Neurology* **39**:349–354.

Mendez, M. F., O'Connor, S. M., and Gerald, T. H. 2004. Hypersexuality after right pallidotomy for Parkinson's disease. *J. Neuropsychiatry Clin. Neurosci.* **16(1)**:37–40.

Menza, M. A., and Mark, M. H. 1994. Parkinson's disease and depression: the relationship to disability and personality. *J. Neuropsychiatry Clin. Neurosci.* **6**:165–169.

Mufson, E. J., Mash, D. C., and Hersh, L. B. 1988. Neurofibrillary tangles in cholinergic pedunculopontine neurons in Alzheimer's disease. *Ann. Neurol.* **24**:623–629.

Nakamura, T., Ghilardi, M. F., Mentis, M., Dhawan, V., Fukuda, M., Hacking, A., Moeller, J. R., Ghez, C., and Eidelberg, D. 2001. Functional networks in motor sequence learning: abnormal topographies in Parkinson's disease. *Hum. Brain Mapp.* **12**:42–60.

Nauta, W. J. H. 1958. Hippocampal projections and related neural pathways to the midbrain in the cat. *Brain* **81**:319–340.

Okubo, Y., Suhara, T., Suzuki, K., Kobayashi, K., Inoue, O., Terasaki, O., Someya, Y., Sassa, T., Sudo, Y., Matsushima, E., Iyo, M., Tateno, Y., and Toru, M. 1997. Decreased prefrontal dopamine D1 receptors in schizophrenia revealed by PET. *Nature* **385**:634–636.

Okun, M. S., Bakay, R. A. E., DeLong, M. R., and Vitek, J. L. 2003. Transient manic behavior after pallidotomy. *Brain Cogn.* **52(2)**:281–283.

O'Sullivan, R. L., Rauch, S. L., Breitr, H. C., Grachev, I. D., Baer, L., Kennedy, D. N., Keuthen, N. J., Savage, C. R., Manzo, P. W., Caviness, V. S., and Jenike, M. A. 1997. Reduced basal ganglia volumes in trichotillomania measured via morphometric magnetic resonance imaging. *Biol. Psychiatry* **42**:39–45.

Pazos, A., and Palacios, J. M. 1985. Quantitative autoradiographic mapping of serotonin receptors in the rat brain. I: Serotonin-1 receptors. *Brain Res.* **346**:205–230.

Pazos, A., Cortes, R., and Palacios, J. M. 1985. Quantitative autoradiographic mapping of serotonin receptors in the rat brain. II: Serotonin-2 receptors. *Brain Res.* **346**:231–249.

Pearlson, G. D., Wong, D. F., Tune, L. E., Ross, C. A., Chase, G. A., Links, J. M., Dannals, R. F., Wilson, A. A., Ravert, H. T., Wagner, H. N., and DePaulo, J. R. 1995. In vivo D2 dopamine receptor density in psychotic and nonpsychotic patients with bipolar disorder. *Arch. Gen. Psychiatry* **52**:471–477.

Peterson, B. S., Thomas, P., Kane, M. J., Scahill, L., Zhang, H., Bronen, R., King, R. A., Leckman, J. F., and Staib, L. 2003. Basal ganglia volumes in patients with Gilles de la Tourette syndrome. *Arch. Gen. Psychiatry* **60(4)**:15–24.

Peyser, C. E., and Folstein, S. E. 1993. Depression in Huntington disease. In: S. E. Starkstein and R. G. Robinson (eds.) *Depression in Neurologic Disease.* Baltimore, Md.: Johns Hopkins Press, pp. 117–138.

Price, D. L., Whitehouse, P. J., Struble, R. G., Clark, A. W., Coyle, J. T., DeLong, M. R., and Hedreen, J. C. 1982. Basal forebrain cholinergic systems in Alzheimer's disease and related dementia. *Neurosciences* **1**:84–92.

Price, L. H., Spencer, D. D., Marek, K. L., Robbins, R. J., Leranth, C., Farhi, A., Naftolin, F., Roth, R. H., Bunney, B. S., Hoffer, P. B., Makuch, R., and Redmond, D. E. Jr. 1995. Psychiatric status after human fetal mesencephalic tissue transplantation in Parkinson's disease. *Biol. Psychiatry* **38**:498–505.

Rapoport, J. L. 1991. Basal ganglia dysfunction as a proposed cause of obsessive-compulsive disorder. In: B. J. Carroll and J. E. Barrett (eds.) *Psychopathology and the Brain.* New York: Raven Press, pp. 77–95.

Rapoport, J. L., and Fiske, A. 1998. The new biology of obsessive-compulsive disorder: implications for evolutionary psychology. *Perspect Biol. Med.* **41**:159–175.

Roane, D. M., Yu, M., Feinberg, T. E., and Rogers, J. D. 2002. Hypersexuality after pallidal surgery in Parkinson disease. *Neuropsychiatry Neuropsychol. Behav. Neurol.* **15**(4):247–251.

Robinson, D., Wu, H., Munne, R. A., Ashtari, M., Alvir, J., Ma, J., Lerner, G., Koreen, A., Cole, K., and Bogerts, B. 1995. Reduced caudate nucleus volume in obsessive-compulsive disorder. *Arch. Gen. Psychiatry* **52**:393–398.

Ryan, L., Martone, M., Linder, J., and Groves, P. 1990. Histological and ultrastructural evidence that d-amphetamine causes degeneration in neostriatum and frontal cortex of man. *Brain Res.* **518**:67–77.

Salloway, S., and Cummings, J. 1994. Subcortical disease and neuro-psychiatric illness. *J. Neuropsychiatry Clin. Neurosci.* **6**:93–97.

Savage, C. 1997. Neuropsychology of subcortical dementias. *Psychiatr. Clin. North Am.* **20**:911–933.

Saxena, S., Brody, A. L., Schwartz, J. M., and Baxter, L. R. 1998. Neuroimaging and frontal-subcortical circuitry in obsessive-compulsive disorder. *Br. J. Psychiatry* **173**(Suppl. 35):26–37.

Schultz, S. K., Miller, D. D., Arndt, S., Ziebell, S., Gupta, S., and Andreasen, N. C. 1995. Withdrawal-emergent dyskinesia in patients with schizophrenia during antipsychotic discontinuation. *Biol. Psychiatry* **38**:713–719.

Schwartz, J. M., Stoessel, P. W., Baxter, L. R. Jr., Martin, K. M., and Phelps, M. E. 1996. Systematic changes in cerebral glucose metabolic rate after successful behavior modification treatment of obsessive-compulsive disorder. *Arch. Gen. Psychiatry* **53**:109–113.

Singer, H. S. 1997. Neurobiology of Tourette syndrome. *Neurol. Clin.* **15**:357–379.

Singer, H. S., Reiss, A. L., Brown, J. E., Aylwar, E. H., Shih, B., Chee, B., Harris, E. L., Reader, M., Chase, G. A., and Bryan, R. N. 1993. Volumetric MRI changes in basal ganglia of children with Tourette's syndrome. *Neurology* **43**:950–956.

Sofroniew, M. V., Pearson, R. C., Eckenstein, F., Cuello, A. C., and Powell, T. P. 1983. Retrograde changes in cholinergic neurons in the basal forebrain of the rat following cortical damage. *Brain Res.* **289**:370–374.

Starkstein, S. E., and Mayberg, H. S. 1993. Depression in Parkinson disease. In: S. E. Starkstein and R. G. Robinson (eds.) *Depression in Neurologic Disease.* Baltimore, Md.: Johns Hopkins Press, pp. 97–116.

Starkstein, S. E., Robinson, R. G., and Price, T. R. 1987. Comparison of cortical and subcortical lesions in the production of post-stroke mood disorders. *Brain* **110**:1045–1059.

Steckler, T., Inglis, W., Winn, P., and Sahgal, A. 1994. The pedunculopontine tegmental nucleus: a role in cognitive processes? *Brain Res. Brain Res. Rev.* **19**:298–318.

Swedo, S. E., and Leonard, H. L. 1992. Trichotillomania: an obsessive compulsive spectrum disorder? *Psychiatr. Clin. North Am.* **151**:777–790.

Torack, R. M., and Morris, J. C. 1988. The association of ventral tegmental area histopathology with adult dementia. *Arch. Neurol.* **45**:497–501.

Wainer, B. H., and Mesulam, M. M. 1990. Ascending cholinergic pathways in the rat brain. In: M. Steriade and D. Biesold (eds.) *Brain Cholinergic Systems.* Oxford, UK: Oxford University Press, pp. 65–199.

Weinberger, D. R. 1987. Implications of normal brain development for the pathogenesis of schizophrenia. *Arch. Gen. Psychiatry* **44**:660–669.

Williams, S. M., and Goldman-Rakic, P. S. 1998. Widespread origin of primate mesofrontal dopamine system. *Cerebr. Cortex* **8**:321–345.

Winn, P., Brown, V. J., and Inglis, W. L. 1997. On the relationships between the striatum and the pedunculopontine nucleus. *Crit. Rev. Neurobiol.* **11**:241–261.

Wolf, S. S., Jones, D. W., Knable, M. B., Gorey, J. G., Lee, K. S., Hyde, T. M., Coppola, R., and Weinberger, D. R. 1996. Tourette syndrome: prediction of phenotypic variation in monozygotic twins by caudate nucleus D2 receptor binding. *Science* **273**:1225–1227.

Yank, M., Yazgan, B. P., Wexler, B. E., and Leckman, J. F. 1994. Behavioral laterality in individual with Gilles de la Tourette's syndrome and basal ganglia alterations: a preliminary report. *Biol. Psychiatry* **38**:386–390.

Zhao, M., Momma, S., Delfani, K., Carlén, M., Cassidy, R. M., Johansson, C. B., Brismar, H., Shupliakov, O., Frisén, J., and Janson, A. M. 2003. Evidence for neurogenesis in the adult mammalian substantia nigra. *Proc. Natl. Acad. Sci. U.S.A.* **100(13)**:7925–7930.

8 Diencephalon: hypothalamus and epithalamus

Hypothalamus

The hypothalamus is the region of the mammalian brain that is most important in the coordination of behaviors essential for the maintenance and continuation of the species. Although the hypothalamus occupies only about 0.15% of the volume of the human brain, it plays a major role in the regulation and release of hormones from the pituitary gland, maintenance of body temperature, and organization of goal-seeking behaviors such as feeding, drinking, mating, and aggression. It is the primary center for the control of autonomic function. It is also the region of the brain that is essential for behavioral adjustments to changes in the internal or external environment (Figure 8.1). The hypothalamus is a very old structure with striking similarity between humans and lower animals. It is made up of a number of nuclei and scattered cell groups. Some hypothalamic cell groups control specific functions (e.g., blood pressure, heart rate, etc.) through the coordinated action of short intrahypothalamic connections. Other nuclei operate by projections to structures outside the confines of the hypothalamus.

Anatomical and behavioral considerations

The hypothalamus lies on either side of the walls of the third ventricle below the level of the hypothalamic sulcus (Figure 8.2, see Figures 9.2, 9.3, and 14.6). It is bounded in front (rostrally) by the lamina terminalis and optic chiasm, laterally by the optic tracts, and behind by the mamillary bodies. Some hypothalamic nuclei are continuous across the floor of the third ventricle. On the bottom (ventral surface) of the hypothalamus is the infundibulum, to which the pituitary (hypophysis) is attached. The median eminence forms the floor of the third ventricle and is the staging area from which the hypothalamic releasing factors leave to enter the hypothalamohypophyseal portal system (Figure 8.2). The borders of the individual hypothalamic nuclei are often indistinct and the location of some borders varies from author to author. Some hypothalamic subdivisions are referred to as areas or zones because of the difficulty in establishing distinct borders.

The hypothalamus and amygdala bilaterally were more activated in men than women when viewing identical sexual stimuli even when the females reported greater arousal (Hamann *et al.*, 2004).

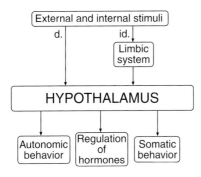

Figure 8.1.   The hypothalamus is positioned between incoming sensory signals and the body's response to those signals. Some sensory signals arrive directly (d.) from the sensory receptor. Other sensory signals are processed through higher centers and are considered indirect (id.). Output may involve only internal controls (e.g., change in heart rate) or may be more complex (e.g., eating behavior).

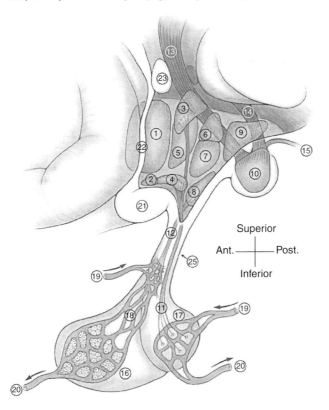

Hypothalamic nuclei:
1. Preoptic
2. Suprachiasmatic
3. Paraventricular
4. Supraoptic
5. Anterior
6. Dorsomedial
7. Ventromedial
8. Arcuate
9. Posterior
10. Mamillary

Tracts:
11. Hypothalamohypophyseal
12. Tuberohypophyseal
13. Column of fornix
14. Mamillothalamic

Other structures:
15. Mamillotegmental tr.
16. Anterior pituitary
17. Posterior pituitary
18. Hypophyseal portal system
19. Hypophyseal arteries
20. Hypophyseal veins
21. Optic chiasm
22. Lamina terminalis
23. Anterior commissure
25. Infundibulum

Figure 8.2.   A three-dimensional view of the medial zone of the hypothalamus showing principal nuclei and surrounding structures. (Reproduced by permission from Young, P.A., and Young, P.H. 1997. *Basic Clinical Anatomy.* Baltimore, Md.: Williams and Wilkins.)

   The organization of the hypothalamus can be simplified by viewing it as made up of one area and three zones (Figure 8.3). The *preoptic area* makes up the rostral (anterior) portion of the hypothalamus. Its major components are the medial and lateral preoptic nuclei (Figure 8.4). The thin *periventricular zone* lies just inside the walls of the third ventricle and

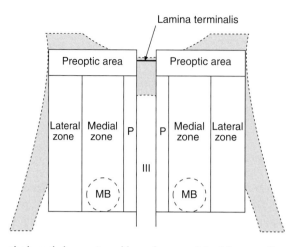

Figure 8.3.   The hypothalamus viewed from above consists of the preoptic area in front and three parallel zones behind. From the cavity of the third ventricle (III) moving laterally are the periventricular zone (P), the medial zone, and the lateral zone. The medial zone can be further subdivided and includes the mamillary bodies (MB). The optic nerve, chiasm, and optic tract are shown as *dotted lines*.

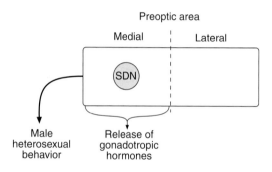

Figure 8.4.   The preoptic area contains the medial and lateral preoptic nuclei. The medial preoptic nucleus produces luteinizing hormone-releasing hormone and influences motor behaviors. SDN, Sexually dimorphic nucleus.

makes up the most medial of the three zones. The *medial zone* contains the majority of the hypothalamic nuclei (see Figure 8.5). The separation between the medial and lateral zones is formed by the fibers of the fornix. The lateral zone contains incoming axons from limbic and other structures. The *lateral zone* also contains the nerve cell bodies that give rise to many of the axons that leave the hypothalamus. The medial forebrain bundle is a diffuse fiber system that passes through the lateral zone interconnecting structures above and below with the hypothalamus.

The pituitary is made up of the posterior lobe and the anterior lobe (nos. 17 and 16, Figure 8.2). The posterior lobe of the pituitary is innervated directly by neurons whose cell bodies lie in the hypothalamus. The axons from these neurons make up the hypothalamohypophyseal tract (no. 11, Figure 8.2). Neurotransmitters (vasopressin and oxytocin) from these neurons are released directly into capillaries located in the posterior lobe

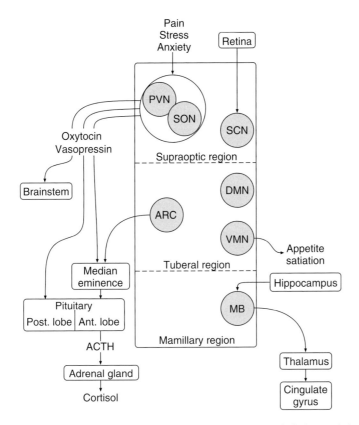

Figure 8.5.   The medial hypothalamic zone is rich in nuclei. Efferents link the medial zone of the hypothalamus with the pituitary and with other brain centers. Oxytocin/vasopressin from the PVN/SON follow three separate pathways. ACTH, adrenocorticotropic hormone; ARC, arcuate nucleus; DMN, dorsomedial nucleus; MB, mamillary body; PVN, paraventricular nucleus; SCN, suprachiasmatic nucleus; SON, supraoptic nucleus; VMN, ventromedial nucleus.

of the pituitary. The anterior lobe is controlled indirectly via "releasing substances." Neurotransmitters (releasing substances) from many of the hypothalamic nuclei enter into the hypophyseal portal system to be passed downstream to the anterior lobe of the pituitary, where they control the release of many anterior pituitary lobe hormones (Table 8.1).

There are both monosynaptic (direct) and polysynaptic (indirect) inputs to the hypothalamus (see Figure 8.1). Both inputs reflect sensory signals from internal (visceral) and external (somatosensory) domains (Figure 8.6). Several monosynaptic pathways arise from within the dorsal horn of the spinal cord and from within the trigeminal spinal nucleus. These fibers project directly to many areas of the hypothalamus.

The monosynaptic pathways provide a route for reflex autonomic and endocrine behaviors (Katter *et al.*, 1991). These behaviors include heart rate change in response to pain, shivering in response to cold, milk letdown in response to suckling, and so forth.

Polysynaptic pathways receive sensory signals that are relayed from spinal cord and brainstem autonomic nuclei (e.g., solitary and parabrachial nuclei). These afferent signals

Table 8.1. *Hypothalamic releasing hormones and their actions on the anterior pituitary.*

Releasing hormone	Action on anterior pituitary
Corticotropin-releasing hormone (CRH)	Stimulates secretion of adrenocorticotropic hormone (ACTH)
Thyrotropin-releasing hormone (TRH)	Stimulates secretion of thyroid-stimulating hormone (TSH)
Gonadotropin-releasing hormone (GnRH), luteinizing hormone-releasing hormone (LHRH)	Stimulates secretion of follicle-stimulating hormone (FSH) and luteinizing hormone (LH)
Growth hormone-releasing hormone (GHRH)	Stimulates secretion of growth hormone (GH)
Somatostatin, somatotropin release-inhibiting hormone (SRIH)	Inhibits secretion of GH
Dopamine	Inhibits biosynthesis and secretion of prolactin (PRL)

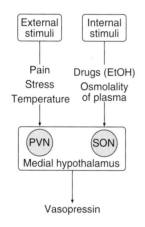

Figure 8.6.   Both external and internal stimuli can affect the release of hormones controlled by the hypothalamus. In this example the output of vasopressin (antidiuretic hormone) is increased by heat and dehydration and decreased by pain, stress, and alcohol. EtOH, Ethyl alcohol; PVN, paraventricular nucleus; SON, supraoptic nucleus.

are processed through structures such as the amygdala, nucleus accumbens, and limbic association cortex before being relayed to the hypothalamus.

Polysynaptic pathways are responsible for behaviors such as sleep, food intake, freezing and flight, and affects such as depression, rage, and fear (Burstein, 1996).

Preoptic hypothalamic area

The preoptic area (no. 1, Figure 8.2) includes the medial and lateral preoptic nuclei (see Figure 8.4). Many neurons in the preoptic area and nearby anterior hypothalamus contain both androgen and estrogen receptors. Stimulation of these areas has been shown to initiate sexual behavior in animals. Lesions of the preoptic area reduce or abolish copulatory behavior in many species (Van de Poll and Van Goozen, 1992).

Fibers that project to the medial preoptic area arise in the cingulate cortex, hippocampus, septum, and lateral habenular nucleus. These are all limbic structures

(Corodimas *et al.*, 1993). The medial preoptic area receives input from the olfactory system by way of the amygdala and the stria terminalis and projects heavily to the periaqueductal gray of the midbrain and to the rostral ventral medulla. Both of these brainstem areas have been implicated in the control of incoming pain signals, in sexual behavior, and in the initiation of maternal and defensive/aggressive behaviors (Shipley *et al.*, 1996). It is hypothesized that this pathway is important in the olfactory cues related to these behaviors.

One or more nuclei found within the medial preoptic area are sexually dimorphic in animals; however, the concept remains controversial for humans (Martin, 1996). One cluster of neurons is called the *sexually dimorphic nucleus (SDN)*. It is also known as INAH1 (interstitial nucleus of the anterior hypothalamus, number 1). It contains at birth only about 20% of the number of neurons that are seen at 2–4 years of age. After age 4 years the cell number decreases in girls but remains constant in boys. No difference in cell number in the SDN is seen between homosexual and heterosexual men (Swaab *et al.*, 1995). The anterior nucleus (see Figure 8.2), sometimes described as INAH3, is also sexually dimorphic (LeVay, 1991; LeVay and Hamer, 1994). It is larger in the male and contains approximately twice the number of neurons in adult male than in adult female humans. However, its size is reported to be similar on average when the brains of male homosexuals and female heterosexuals are compared (Friedman and Downey, 1993). Before birth the anterior nucleus is similar in size in both male and female rats. It is smaller in male offspring of rats that were stressed while pregnant. It is larger in sexually active male rats. Many of the cells of INAH3 die in the female shortly after birth. However, testosterone present from 4 days before until 10 days following birth protects these neurons from cell death in the male rat. Differential cell death accounts for the sexual dimorphism of this nucleus. These same neurons in human females begin to undergo programmed death at about 4 years of age.

The medial preoptic area contains neurons that produce luteinizing hormone-releasing hormone. In the pituitary, this releasing hormone regulates the level of gonadotropins. The medial preoptic area plays an important role in maternal behavior (Numan and Sheenan, 1997). Surgical or chemical lesions of the medial preoptic area severely disrupt the induction as well as the maintenance of maternal behavior (DeVries and Villalba, 1997). The ventral tegmental area (see Chapter 7) may be the target of fibers that arise from the medial preoptic area (Numan and Smith, 1984; Hansen and Ferreira, 1986).

The medial preoptic area is also critical in the expression of male-typical heterosexual behavior. Activity in the medial preoptic area increases in the male monkey during sexual arousal but decreases during copulation and ceases after ejaculation. A lesion of the medial preoptic area produces a dramatic reduction in female-directed sexual behavior, although masturbation continues. Electrical stimulation of the medial preoptic area initiates sexual behavior but only if a receptive female is available. The medial preoptic area shows the greatest testosterone uptake of any region of the brain. Efferent connections from the medial preoptic area include projections to the dorsomedial hypothalamic nucleus and to brainstem areas linked with penile erection. Stimulation of the medial preoptic area in the female rat inhibits lordosis. In contrast, stimulation in the male rat induces copulation (Marson and McKenna, 1994).

The periventricular hypothalamic zone

The periventricular zone is a thin layer that lies just lateral to the ependymal cells that form the lining of the third ventricle. This zone is important in regulating the release of hormones from the anterior pituitary.

The medial hypothalamic zone

The medial hypothalamic zone includes the majority of the well-defined nuclei of the hypothalamus (see Figures 8.2 and 8.5). Several important regions in this zone include, from front to back, the *supraoptic region*, the *tuberal region*, and the *mamillary region*. In addition to containing important nuclei, the tuberal region is continuous below with the infundibular stalk of the pituitary gland.

Supraoptic region

The supraoptic region is located directly above the optic chiasm and includes the supraoptic, the paraventricular, and the suprachiasmatic nuclei (see Figures 8.2 and 8.5). Clusters of magnocellular neurons within the supraoptic and paraventricular nuclei produce oxytocin and vasopressin. The paraventricular nucleus consists of one subdivision that projects to the median eminence and a second subdivision that projects to the posterior pituitary. A third subdivision, which also produces oxytocin and vasopressin, projects to brainstem and to spinal cord autonomic nuclei. The axons from the third subdivision enter the medial forebrain bundle and descend in the dorsolateral brainstem. Axons of some neurons pass through the infundibular stalk to terminate on capillaries in the posterior lobe of the pituitary. When these neurons depolarize, their neurotransmitter (oxytocin or vasopressin) is released directly into the blood stream. These neurons receive input from brainstem autonomic nuclei (solitary nucleus) and from circumventricular organs. The latter are vascular neural structures that lack the blood–brain barrier. One of these, the subfornical region located in the wall of the third ventricle, sends axons that terminate in the hypothalamus. It is presumed that the circumventricular organs sense osmolality and blood-borne chemicals. Many areas of the hypothalamus are sensitive to hormones. Some hormones cross the blood–brain barrier, and others bind to intracellular receptors.

Other neurons in the paraventricular nucleus that also produce oxytocin and vasopressin project to limbic structures, including the amygdala and hippocampus. Descending fibers project to the brainstem to terminate in the locus ceruleus and in the raphe nuclei (see Chapter 10). Some oxytocin axons extend to the spinal cord where they terminate on presynaptic neurons of the sympathetic nervous system (Sofroniew, 1983).

Oxytocin release causes contraction of the smooth muscles of the uterus during childbirth as well as contraction of the myoepithelial cells of the mammary gland during nursing. Surprisingly, the number of oxytocin-producing cells is about the same in the female and male. Intraventricular injection of oxytocin in the female rat rapidly stimulates maternal behavior (Pedersen and Prange, 1979). In contrast, oxytocin infusion in males results in an increase in nonsexual social interaction (Witt, 1997). Receptors for oxytocin in both the medial preoptic area of the hypothalamus and the ventral tegmental area of the midbrain are critical for the postpartum onset of maternal behavior in the rat. The oxytocin-producing neurons are located in the lateral preoptic area and in the paraventricular nucleus. Proximal separation of rat pups from their mothers (i.e., the pups remain in olfactory and auditory contact) markedly depletes oxytocin levels in the mothers. It is speculated that stimuli that reactivate the mechanisms of attachment between mother and offspring may contribute to the sense of longing and other strong emotions that accompany the loss of a close relationship in humans (Pedersen, 1997). These emotions may be related to a reduction in the level of oxytocin. Oxytocin released by the paraventricular nucleus may play a role in the sedation, relaxation, and decreased sympathoadrenal activity at the hypothalamic level that occurs during friendly social interaction (Uvnas-Moberg, 1997).

There appears to be a central dysregulation of vasopressin secretion in patients with anorexia nervosa (Demitrack and Gold, 1988). The number of vasopressin- and oxytocin-expressing neurons in the paraventricular nucleus of patients with mood disorder is significantly increased (Purba *et al.*, 1996). An increase in both vasopressin and oxytocin was reported in bulimic patients (Demitrack *et al.*, 1990). The levels of vasopressin and oxytocin are altered in the cerebrospinal fluid of depressed patients (Legros *et al.*, 1993). No correlation was found between the extent of the depressive symptomatology and the level to which vasopressin levels were reduced (Gjerris, 1990).

The suprachiasmatic nucleus (see Figures 8.2 and 8.5) is found in the supraoptic region of the medial zone. It lies just above the optic chiasm and just below and lateral to the supraoptic nucleus. The suprachiasmatic nucleus is critical in controlling the day–night circadian rhythm of the body and functions as the "master clock." It receives primary visual afferents from the retina and secondary afferents from the lateral geniculate body of the visual system. The suprachiasmatic nucleus has intimate connections with the pineal gland and plays a key role in circadian functions as well as in seasonal function (Pevet *et al.*, 1996; Reuss, 1996).

The suprachiasmatic nucleus may be related to seasonal fluctuations in mood (seasonal affective disorder or SAD), and the number of vasopressin-expressing neurons is greatest in October and November in the northern hemisphere, when the incidence of depression is greatest (Hofman *et al.*, 1993). Exposure to prolonged periods of light following transportation to a distant time zone can facilitate recovery from jet lag. More specifically, exposure to bright light in the morning delays the light–dark cycle (phase advance), whereas exposure to bright light in the evening advances this cycle (phase delay). Most SAD patients with winter depression are abnormally phase delayed and therefore respond positively to bright morning light. The bright light itself is not an antidepressant, but the reversal of the abnormal phase delay acts as an antidepressant (Lewy and Sack, 1996).

Tuberal region

The arcuate nucleus (see Figures 8.2 and 8.5) as well as other hypothalamic nuclei contain neurons that produce various release and release-inhibiting hormones. These include gonadotropin-releasing hormone, luteinizing hormone-releasing hormone, and corticotropin-releasing hormone (CRH). The close connections between the hypothalamus, the pituitary, and the adrenal gland are recognized as the hypothalamic–pituitary–adrenal (HPA) axis. CRH is responsible for triggering the release of adrenocorticotropic hormone (ACTH) from the anterior lobe of the pituitary gland. Abnormalities in the HPA axis have been linked to several disorders.

The neurons of the paraventricular nucleus that control the HPA are strongly activated in depression (Raadsheer *et al.,* 1994). Excessive ACTH secretion and a concomitant increase in cortisol release by the adrenal cortex are seen in 40 – 60% of depressed patients, primarily during afternoon and evening hours. The hypersecretion of cortisol is not dependent on stress. The synthetic corticosteroid dexamethasone, when administered to normal subjects, suppresses CRH. HPA activity can be assessed by measures of cortisol in the blood, urine, saliva, and in cerebrospinal fluid (DeMoranville and Jackson, 1996). When synthetic corticosteroid dexamethasone is administered to depressed patients during the evening, approximately 40% show no decline in cortisol levels. Improvement in the dexamethasone suppression test is seen in successful antidepressant treatment (Holsboer-Trachsler *et al.,* 1991).

Subtle alterations in HPA function have been observed in patients with panic disorder (Abelson and Curtis, 1996). Weinstock (1997) hypothesized that prenatal stress impairs the ability of the child's HPA to cope in novel situations.

The periventricular hypothalamus, the arcuate nucleus, and other hypothalamic regions that produce CRH represent the origin of the hypothalamic–pituitary–adrenocortical axis. The regulation of the HPA is dependent on three major factors. First, the pulsatile release of CRH is under the control of the suprachiasmatic nucleus. Second, psychological and physical stresses are mediated by way of pathways from the brainstem and limbic system to the hypothalamus. Third, circulating levels of glucocorticoids are sensed by the hypothalamus in a negative feedback mechanism that regulates the output of CRH. The hippocampus also has many glucocorticoid receptors and appears to play an important role in monitoring stress and regulating the production and release of CRH by the hypothalamus. Exposure to stress down-regulates glucocorticoid receptors in both the hippocampus and hypothalamus. Therefore, the feedback receptors are less sensitive to circulating glucocorticoids and the hypothalamus secretes inordinately high levels of CRH (Herman *et al.,* 1995). The separation of partners that show signs of emotional attachment activates the HPA axis, whereas separation of partners that show little emotional attachment has little or no effect on the HPA (Hennessy, 1997). Significantly decreased bone density in women with depression is consistent with dysfunction of the HPA axis (Michelson *et al.,* 1996).

Many neurons in the arcuate nucleus produce beta-endorphin. This peptide is known to play an important role in the control of pain. In addition, some of these same neurons project to the periaqueductal gray, which is a midbrain region known to function in the suppression of incoming pain signals (see Chapter 10). The arcuate nucleus and its connections with the paraventricular nucleus also are a hypothalamic pathway involved in the control of body weight. This pathway may be the target of the hormone leptin, which is secreted by fat cells (Schwartz and Seeley, 1997). A nucleus adjacent to the arcuate nucleus (the periventricular nucleus) produces dopamine, which inhibits prolactin release.

Abnormal levels of endorphins have been reported in the hypothalamic tissue of schizophrenic patients. Both "endorphin excess" and "endorphin deficiency" hypotheses of schizophrenia have been proposed (Wiegant *et al.,* 1992).

Neurons located in the arcuate (infundibular) nucleus of the medial zone are hypertrophied in postmenopausal women. Some cells of the arcuate nucleus are sensitive to circulating levels of estrogen and regulate the activity of substance-P-producing neurons found there. Substance P production in neurons in the arcuate nucleus varies with the sexual cycle and may regulate the release of gonadotropin-releasing hormone from the hypothalamus into the hypophyseal portal system. It has been hypothesized that an increase in the pulsatile release of substance P may coincide with menopausal flushes (Rance, 1992).

The dorsomedial nucleus (see Figures 8.2 and 8.5) lies immediately above the ventromedial nucleus. Stimulation of the dorsomedial nucleus in laboratory animals produces unusually aggressive behavior that lasts only as long as the stimulus is present. This aggressive behavior is known as sham rage and can be produced by stimulation in other regions of the hypothalamus.

The ventromedial nucleus (see Figures 8.2 and 8.5) lies near the midline just rostral to the mamillary bodies. It receives input from the amygdala. It projects heavily to the magnocellular nuclei of the basal forebrain including the basal nucleus (of Meynert). These nuclei in turn project to all areas of the cerebral cortex. The ventromedial nucleus has been described in the past as the satiety center. It regulates the amount of food consumed in order to maintain a normal body weight. The ventromedial nucleus is interconnected with the lateral hypothalamic zone (see the following section), which has been described in the past as the hunger center. The concept of hunger and satiety centers is a convenient concept. Feeding control is probably more complex than this comparison would imply, however, and involves a number of additional structures (Kupfermann, 1991).

Clinical vignette

A 36-year-old male was found to have an anterior hypothalamic tumor when he was evaluated for a 65-pound weight gain, hallucinations, paranoid delusions, and confusion. After surgical removal of the tumor, he became apathetic and akinetic mutism developed. He responded well to treatment with dopamine agonists (bromocriptine) (Ross and Stewart, 1981). The case suggests that akinesia may be related to loss of dopaminergic input to anterior cingulate or other frontal lobe regions. The postsurgical clinical picture may have been produced by damage to the mesolimbic/mesocortical dopamine fibers. These fibers are found within the medial forebrain bundle, which courses from the ventral tegmental area to the cingulate cortex and passes through the lateral hypothalamic zone.

A lesion of the ventromedial nucleus results in appetite disorders and dramatic increase in body weight. Stereotactic lesions of the ventromedial nucleus have been used in an attempt to treat alcoholism, drug addiction, and hypersexuality. Increase in body weight was a common side-effect of these lesions (Nadvornik *et al.*, 1975).

The ventrolateral portion of the ventromedial nucleus is responsible for typical female sexual behavior. Stimulation of this area produces lordosis in rats. The ventromedial nucleus is a site of action of estrogen and progesterone hormones. Projections from the ventromedial nucleus to the periaqueductal gray may be the route by which this region of the hypothalamus induces sexual behavior (Pfaff *et al.*, 1994).

A number of nuclei in the hypothalamus have receptor sites for estrogen. Under experimental conditions food intake is increased when estrogen levels decrease. There is evidence that during the second half of the menstrual cycle when estrogen levels drop there is also an increase in food intake and preference for carbohydrates (Bray, 1992).

The mamillary bodies and the cells of the posterior hypothalamic nucleus that lie dorsal to the mamillary bodies mark the caudal extent of the medial hypothalamus. The largest number of afferents to the mamillary bodies come from the hippocampus by way of the fornix (nos. 20 and 2, Figure 13.5). This connection with the hippocampus suggests that the mamillary bodies are also involved in emotion as well as memory. For example, the mamillary bodies have been implicated in penile erection (Segraves, 1996). Fibers from the mamillary bodies ascend to the anterior nucleus of the thalamus and make up the mamillothalamic tract (no. 8, Figure 13.5). The anterior nucleus of the thalamus is a major component of the limbic thalamus (see Figure 9.2). **Cell loss is seen in the mamillary bodies as well as in the mediodorsal nucleus of the thalamus in alcoholic Korsakoff's syndrome (Delis and Lucas, 1996).**

Lateral hypothalamic zone and medial forebrain bundle

The lateral zone contains several groups of cells, the largest of which is the tuberomamillary nucleus, which extends in a posterior direction lateral to and below the mamillary body. The lateral tuberal nuclei consist of two or three sharply delineated cell groups that often produce small visible bumps on the basal surface of the hypothalamus. The medial forebrain bundle courses through the lateral zone and makes delineation of specific nuclei difficult. Axons from the limbic system terminate in the lateral zone, which, in turn, integrates and relays the signals to other parts of the hypothalamus as well as to the midbrain. Of particular significance are projections from the infralimbic area of the cingulate cortex (see Chapter 12). This is a key route by which the visceral motor cortex (infralimbic area) influences autonomic tone, and the lateral zone is believed to be important as an integrative center for ingestive behavior (Bernardis and Bellinger, 1996; Saper, 1996).

The lateral zone has been described as the hunger center. A lesion placed in this zone will eliminate an animal's motivation to seek food, and the animal will lose weight and will eventually die. Electrical stimulation of the medial forebrain bundle seems to induce pleasure in the animal. The rate of self-stimulation (and thus the amount of pleasure induced) is maximal when the stimuli are delivered directly to the lateral hypothalamus. Indeed, if the lateral region is destroyed, the experience of pleasure and emotional responsiveness is almost completely attenuated (Saver *et al.*, 1996). Electrical stimulation or the infusion of acetylcholine into the posterior lateral hypothalamus produces aggressive attack behavior in animals (Kruck, 1991). The lateral hypothalamic zone is important in the cardiovascular response to fearful stimuli. Neurons in the lateral zone project to the lower brainstem, which directly controls alterations in blood pressure (LeDoux, 1996). Signals arrive in the lateral zone of the hypothalamus from the amygdala and from other regions.

The medial forebrain bundle (fasciculus telencephalicus medialis) is a complex collection of fibers that resembles a freeway with many on and off ramps (no. 18, Figure 13.5). It extends from the midbrain to the frontal cortex and passes through the lateral hypothalamus. Fibers representing many different functions enter the medial forebrain bundle, course through it for a short or long distance, and then exit. Mesolimbic and mesocortical fibers are part of the medial forebrain bundle (see Chapter 7). Descending fibers from the hypothalamus extend caudally to the brainstem. Raphe serotonergic nuclei (see Chapter 10) and basal forebrain acetylcholinergic nuclei (see Chapter 13) both project through the medial forebrain bundle.

Lesions of the lateral hypothalamus have been found to be responsible for anorexia in humans (Martin and Riskind, 1992). Significant neuronal loss is reported in the lateral tuberal nucleus in Huntington's disease, adult-onset dementia (Braak and Braak, 1989), and in a patient with severe depressive illness (Horn *et al.,* 1988). It is hypothesized that loss of neurons in the lateral hypothalamus may be responsible for the weight loss that commonly accompanies these disorders (Kremer, 1992).

Connections of the hypothalamus

Neural signals reach the hypothalamus over many pathways. A major pathway that carries ascending signals from the brainstem reticular formation is the medial forebrain bundle, which courses through the lateral hypothalamus. The lateral hypothalamus, in turn, is richly interconnected with the periventricular, medial, and hypothalamic zones and the preoptic area.

Incoming

Ascending input to the hypothalamus includes fibers from the locus ceruleus and raphe nuclei (see Chapter 10). These inputs provide signals that have a general alerting effect on the hypothalamus. In particular, fibers to the lateral hypothalamus from the locus ceruleus as well as from the amygdala have been implicated in the sympathetic activation and hormonal release associated with fear and anxiety (Charney *et al.,* 1996). Fibers from the brainstem solitary nucleus provide specific information from visceral afferents, including taste as well as signals from the thoracic and abdominal viscera.

Descending influences to the hypothalamus include signals from the limbic system, especially from the hippocampus and amygdala (see Figures 11.2 and 11.5). The prefrontal cortex projects directly to the hypothalamus via the medial forebrain bundle. The cingulate gyrus influences the hypothalamus by way of the septal nuclei and hippocampus (see Figure 12.4).

Clinical vignette

A 19-year-old man sustained a fall with head injury and underwent neurosurgical evacuation of a right-sided epidural hematoma. Two months after the head trauma and surgery, he began eating excessively, particularly a great many sweets, and gained about 176 lb (80 kg). During the following 18 months, he had periodic episodes of 6–10 weeks where he would sleep up to 16 h a night with continued drowsiness during the rest of the day. He was periodically irritable and aggressive, with mood alterations and increased interest in pornographic material.

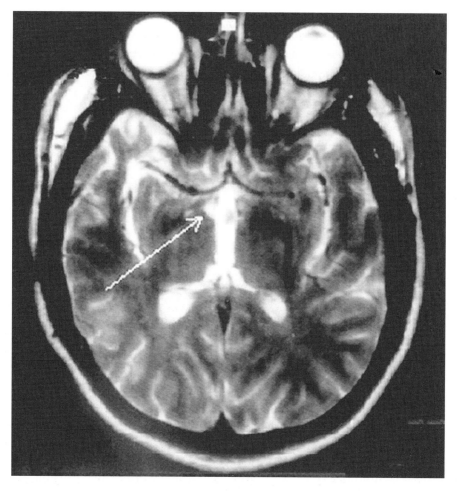

Figure 8.7.   A magnetic resonance image (T2-weighted) demonstrated a high-intensity lesion in the right hypothalamus (arrow). (Reprinted with permission from Kostic *et al.,* 1998.)

The patient developed the Kleine–Levin syndrome probably consequent to hypothalamic injury. His magnetic resonance imaging showed a post-traumatic lesion in the right hypothalamus (Figure 8.7). The Kleine–Levin syndrome includes hypersomnolence, hyperphagia, and sexual disinhibition or other behavioral disorders.

Outgoing

Efferent signals from the hypothalamus tend to leave by way of long axons that arise from cell bodies located in the medial and lateral hypothalamic zones. The hypothalamus has reciprocal (back-and-forth) connections with most of the structures that provide afferents, including the periaqueductal gray, the locus ceruleus, and the raphe nuclei in the brainstem. Descending fibers to the brainstem are responsible for the direct control of the sympathetic and parasympathetic systems. Efferent fibers to the limbic system include connections with the septal nuclei, amygdala, and hippocampus. Some fibers project directly from the hypothalamus to the prefrontal cortex via the medial forebrain bundle. The hypothalamus influences the cingulate cortex indirectly by way of signals relayed in the anterior thalamic nucleus. Other efferents terminate in the mediodorsal thalamic nucleus, which relays information to the prefrontal lobe.

Further behavioral considerations

The hypothalamus lies in a position between the "thinking brain" (neocortex) and the "emotional brain" (limbic system) on the one hand and the body systems that are controlled by the autonomic and endocrine systems on the other. Mental state can operate through the hypothalamus to alter endocrine function and autonomic tone.

Clinical vignette

Tonkonogy and Geller (1992) reported two cases of craniopharyngioma presenting with and meeting Diagnostic and Statistical Manual of Mental Disorders-III-R criteria for intermittent explosive disorder. The first case is that of a 21-year-old man who presented with frequent episodes of explosive behavior and threats to cut himself or to kill his mother. He complained of insomnia, depressed mood, periodic hypnagogic visual and auditory hallucinations, and periods of 15–20 min of spacing out. He had a family history of alcoholism and personality disorder, and he grew up in foster homes. A decline in his IQ, progressive weight loss, dizziness, and fatigue prompted a medical examination. Polydipsia, polyuria, lack of pigmentation, and diabetes insipidus eventually developed. Removal of the tumor did not lead to behavioral improvement.

The second case is that of a 24-year-old woman who presented with episodes of explosive behavior, including threats to start fires and a history of assaults on staff. She complained of depressed mood and attempted suicide a number of times. She was markedly obese. At age 11, the patient had developed growth retardation, weight loss, and other signs of hypopituitarism. A craniopharyngioma was removed at that time. After surgery, her assaultive and self-threatening behavior manifested itself. She did not respond to neuroleptics, antidepressants, or substitute hormonal therapy. An abnormal encephalogram led to treatment with carbamazepine, to which the patient responded with a marked improvement in behavior.

Emotional stress can induce ulcers. In women stress can block the menstrual cycle. Normally the milk ejection reflex is induced by the infant suckling at the nipple. An experienced, nursing mother can sometimes cause milk to trickle from her nipples by forming a mental image of her infant. There is some evidence that mental processes can operate through the hypothalamus to influence the immune system.

The hypothalamus is in a position to control the outward manifestations of emotion. Heart rate, blood pressure, pupil size, and vasoconstriction are all controlled by the hypothalamus. Other behaviors that involve striated muscles are also controlled by the hypothalamus. Shivering for heat conservation, piloerection during rage and facial expression reflecting emotion are all under hypothalamic influence. It is thought that much of the autonomic and somatic expression of emotion is controlled by the hypothalamus. It is believed that emotional expression is controlled by the hypothalamus, whereas the feelings of emotion lie elsewhere, particularly within the limbic system. Sham rage in experimental animals can be seen when the hypothalamus is electrically stimulated. The animal's rage is nondirected and dies out quickly. For example, cats exhibiting sham rage may alternately growl and purr when lapping warm milk (DeMoranville and Jackson, 1996).

Social subjugation of hamsters during puberty resulted in males that were more aggressive toward intruders and were significantly more likely to bite smaller males than were control males. This behavior is not unlike that of schoolyard bullies. Analysis revealed a 50% decrease in the level of vasopressin in the anterior hypothalamus of the subjugated hamsters but an increase in the number of serotonin-containing fibers. The number of vasopressin fibers suggested that less vasopressin is produced and released in the subjugated hamsters. The increase in serotonin fibers suggested to the authors that the capacity to release serotonin was increased. An increase in serotonin is consistent with reduced aggression and may account for the fact that the subjected hamsters were less aggressive than controls when in the presence of males of equal or greater size (Delville *et al.*, 1998).

Many case reports of intermittent explosive disorders associated with hypothalamic lesions appear in the literature. A number of these are remarkable since the patients were diagnosed with behavioral disorders, sometimes years before the underlying tumor was discovered. Visual hallucinations have been reported by these patients (Tonkonogy and Geller, 1992). An association between precocious puberty and hypothalamic lesions (particularly hamartomas) has been repeatedly noted (Takeuchi *et al.*, 1979). An even more interesting association is between hypothalamic hamartomas, precocious puberty, and gelastic (laughing) seizures (Breningstall, 1985). It is suggested that the area of the hypothalamus that is critical for the expression of intermittent explosive disorder is the posterior lateral hypothalamic region. This region was at one time surgically destroyed for the treatment of aggressive behavior (Tonkonogy and Geller, 1992).

In summary, at the hypothalamic level, the emotional states elicited are primitive, undirected, and unrefined. Higher-level emotions such as love or hate require the involvement of other limbic, as well as neocortical, regions.

Epithalamus

Pineal (epiphysis)

The pineal is found in the midline, above the third ventricle, and in front of the superior colliculus (see P in Figure 13.5). It is glandular in appearance and contains a unique cell called the *pinealocyte*. It is richly vascular with its rate of blood flow second only to that of the kidney. In lower forms the pineal forms the parietal eye, a photosensitive organ important in circadian rhythms.

The pineal has been called a "tranquilizing organ" due to the hypnotic properties of melatonin (Romijn, 1978) and is described as a neuroendocrine transducer that transforms a neural signal into an endocrine signal (Reuss, 1996). The prominent pinealocytes synthesize serotonin and melatonin, both of which are released into the extracellular space. Exposure to light blocks the transmission of neural signals to the pineal gland from the hypothalamus and therefore blocks the production of melatonin. The synthesis of melatonin and release into the bloodstream are normally observed to take place only during the

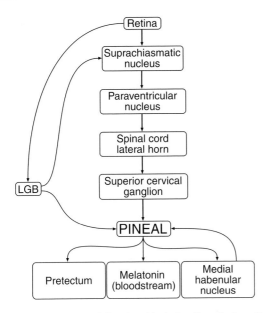

Figure 8.8.   The connections of the pineal include afferents from the retina and lateral geniculate body (LGB). Exposure to light inhibits melatonin production by the pinealocytes. The lines leaving the pineal represent cytoplasmic extensions of the pinealocytes. Feedback from the pineal to the suprachiasmatic nucleus is by way of melatonin in the bloodstream.

night-time hours. Blinded animals continue to produce melatonin in rhythm with the day–night cycle. However, a lesion of the suprachiasmatic nucleus of the hypothalamus abolishes the rhythm. Pinealocytes found in the deep portion of the pineal give rise to long, beaded processes that terminate in the pretectum and in the medial nucleus of the habenula (see the following section). (The pretectum is part of the visual system and is found in the midbrain in front of the superior colliculus.) The ends of these processes form neuron-like connections with neurons located in these two sites (Figure 8.8). The pineal is usually considered an endocrine organ; however, the axon-like processes and point-to-point organization suggest that it may have neuronal connections as well (Korf *et al.,* 1990).

The pineal is the most influential component of the melatonin system. However, melatonin is also synthesized in photoreceptors of the retina. Retinal melatonin is secreted locally, whereas pineal melatonin is released into the bloodstream. A well-recognized pathway to the pineal originates with the retinohypothalamic tract to the suprachiasmatic nucleus, paraventricular nucleus of the hypothalamus, medial forebrain bundle, lateral horn of the upper thoracic spinal cord, superior cervical ganglion, and sympathetic pre- and postganglionic nerves to the pineal (Figure 8.8). This route includes the sympathetic innervation of the pineal from the superior cervical ganglion. A second pathway involves the lateral geniculate nucleus, which sends efferent fibers to both the suprachiasmatic nucleus and to the pineal (Reuss, 1996).

The suprachiasmatic nucleus and the anterior pituitary are two regions where melatonin exerts its major effects. Melatonin feedback to the suprachiasmatic nucleus regulates the output of melatonin by the pineal. The effect of melatonin in the anterior pituitary is to regulate neuroendocrine and gonadal function (Morgan *et al.*, 1994). Melatonin synchronizes daily activity/inactivity with daily changes in light/dark. It also synchronizes other body functions and is responsible for maternal entrainment of fetus activity (Reppert *et al.*, 1989). The pain threshold is raised by melatonin. Since this effect is blocked by naloxone, it appears that melatonin acts through opiate mechanisms (Golombek *et al.*, 1991). Melatonin has also been demonstrated to have anticonvulsant properties and has anxiolytic effects in laboratory animals (Golombek *et al.*, 1996). It increases the turnover of the inhibitory neurotransmitter gamma-aminobutyric acid (GABA) in the hypothalamus, cerebral cortex, and cerebellum, suggesting that a melatonin–GABA interaction is responsible for some of its behavioral effects (Golombek *et al.*, 1996).

Parenchymatous pinealomas are associated with depression of gonadal function and delayed pubescence. Destruction of the pineal is associated with precocious puberty. The pineal is frequently calcified in schizophrenics, and the melatonin system may be involved in seasonal affective disorder (SAD) (Sandyk, 1992).

The level of melatonin normally rises at night. Melatonin given during the day, when levels are normally low, induces fatigue. Exposure to bright light at night suppresses the normal nocturnal elevation of circulating melatonin (Dollins *et al.*, 1993). It has been suggested that melatonin or melatonin analogues may be therapeutic for the control of circadian clock dysfunctions such as jet lag, shift-work syndrome, and sleep disorders. Melatonin has been used effectively for treatment of insomnia to correct the sleep/wake cycle (Tzichinsky *et al.*, 1992). However, it has not always proved effective in the treatment of SAD (Wehr, 1991). Sleep patterns are often affected by depression, although it is believed that there is no primary disturbance of the circadian rhythm system in this disease (Moore, 1997).

Habenula

The habenula (habenular nuclei) is located in the wall of the third ventricle rostral to the pineal (see Figure 9.3, and nos. 9 and 23, Figure 13.3). It consists of a smaller medial nucleus, which contains small cells, and a larger lateral nucleus, which contains larger cells. The stria medullaris is the major afferent bundle serving the habenula and brings signals from the medial forebrain and septum, limbic lobe hypothalamus, and ventral striatum. The fasciculus retroflexus (habenulointerpeduncular tract; no.11, Figure 13.5) is the major efferent pathway that projects primarily to the nigral complex (ventral tegmental area and substantia nigra; see Chapter 7) and to brainstem nuclei, including the raphe nuclei and locus ceruleus (see Chapter 10). The habenula is positioned to link limbic structures with nuclei in the upper brainstem (Figure 8.9).

Lateral habenular nucleus

The lateral habenular nucleus receives fibers from the frontal cortex, the septal nuclei (limbic system), the lateral preoptic area, and the lateral hypothalamus as well as the ventral tegmental area. It has reciprocal connections (back-and-forth) with the raphe nuclei, an important source of serotonin (see Chapter 10). The lateral habenula contains

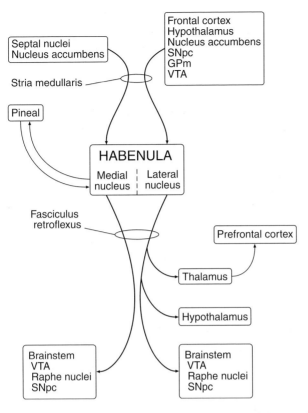

Figure 8.9. The medial habenula links the septal nuclei with the thalamus. The lateral habenula links the frontal cortex, hypothalamus, and dopaminergic nuclei to the brainstem and allows for feedback to the medial preoptic area of the hypothalamus and to the frontal cortex. GPm, medial segment of globus pallidus; SNpc, substantia nigra pars compacta (dopamine); VTA, ventral tegmental area (dopamine).

a high concentration of D_2 dopamine receptors (Dawson *et al.*, 1986). The incoming dopaminergic fibers terminate in the medial portion of the lateral habenular nucleus. These fibers arise from cell bodies in the medial preoptic area, ventral tegmental area, midbrain periaqueductal gray, substantia nigra pars compacta, and dorsal raphe nucleus. Dopamine may regulate the endocrine-specific proteins expressed in the habenula that are involved in endocrine-related reproductive function (Darlington *et al.*, 1996).

A large number of efferent fibers from the lateral habenular nucleus terminate in the dorsal raphe nucleus. The lateral habenula is an estrogen-concentrating region that correlates with its importance in female sexual and maternal behavior (Pfaus *et al.*, 1993). Other fibers project to the substantia nigra, the ventral tegmental area, and various brainstem nuclei.

Stimulation of the lateral habenular nucleus is reported to facilitate the release of norepinephrine in the medial frontal cortex, nucleus accumbens, and neostriatum (caudate nucleus and putamen) of the rat. Stimulation also causes inhibition of more than 85% of the dopamine neurons in the nigral complex (ventral tegmental area and substantia nigra). In addition, electrical stimulation of the lateral habenular nucleus inhibits release of serotonin by the neurons of the dorsal raphe (Reisine *et al.*, 1982). The lateral habenular nucleus is also involved in the initiation and propagation of limbic seizures induced by pilocarpine in the rat. Lesions of the lateral habenula produce severe deficits in maternal behavior in the rat (Matthews-Felton *et al.*, 1995).

Fibers from nucleus accumbens to the lateral habenular nucleus are believed to be part of a unidirectional loop that terminates in the periaqueductal gray of the midbrain. Electrical stimulation or microinjection of morphine into the habenula has reduced pain in several pain tests. However, lesions of the habenula do not affect pain levels or morphine analgesia, indicating that the habenula plays a role in pain control but is not a critical link (Ma *et al.*, 1992). The lateral habenular nucleus appears to be part of a negative feedback loop connecting the limbic cortex with brainstem nuclei that are responsible for providing serotonin, norepinephrine, and dopamine to rostral brain areas. This places the lateral habenular nucleus in a unique position to regulate the levels of these critical neurotransmitters.

Lesions in the lateral habenular nucleus result in an activation of the mesocortical, mesolimbic, and mesostriatal systems. These lesions result in an increase in dopamine turnover in the prefrontal cortex, nucleus accumbens, and striatum (Nishikawa *et al.*, 1986). Continuous amphetamine and cocaine administration has been shown to induce a strong pattern of degeneration that is highly confined to the lateral habenula and its principal output pathway, the fasciculus retroflexus. These findings suggest that habenular abnormalities may play a role in the genesis of psychotic conditions, particularly psychostimulant-induced psychosis (Ellison, 1994).

Medial habenular nucleus

The medial habenular nucleus shares many of the same incoming afferent fibers with its lateral counterpart. It also receives melatonin-containing axons from the pinealocytes of the pineal. The septum is an especially rich source of incoming fibers to the medial habenular nucleus. Outgoing fibers from the medial habenular nucleus, which course in the lateral forebrain bundle, terminate as acetylcholine endings in the intralaminar, reticular, and medial mediodorsal nuclei of the thalamus. These three thalamic nuclei are also the target of fibers from the ascending brainstem reticular formation and are believed to be involved with alerting the cortex.

The habenular nuclei have been observed to be significantly more calcified in schizophrenics than in normal control subjects. It is hypothesized that the calcification may be correlated with the enlargement of the third ventricle. Calcification of the habenula may disrupt the role played by the habenula in providing a link between the limbic system and the upper brainstem (Ellison, 1994).

SELECT BIBLIOGRAPHY

J. Arendt, *Melatonin and the Mammalian Pineal Gland.* (New York: Chapman and Hall, 1995).

R. M. Buijs, A. Kalsbeek, H. J. Romijn, C. M. A. Pennartz, and M. Mirmiran, Hypothalamic integration of circadian rhythms. *Progress in Brain Research*, **111** (1996).

C. S. Carter, I. I. Lederhendler, and B. Kirkpatrick, The integrative neurobiology of affiliation. *Annals of the New York Academy of Sciences*, **807** (1997).

R. Joseph, *Neuropsychology, Neuropsychiatry, and Behavioral Neurology*. (New York: Plenum Press, 1989.)

D. F. Swaab, M. A. Hofman, M. Mirmiran, R. Ravid, and F. W. van Leeuwen, The human hypothalamus in health and disease. *Progress in Brain Research*, **93** (1992).

REFERENCES

Abelson, J. L., and Curtis, G. C 1996. Hypothalamic-pituitary-adrenal axis activity in panic disorder. *Arch. Gen. Psychiatry* **53**:323–331.

Bernardis, L. L., and Bellinger, L. L. 1996. The lateral hypothalamic area revisited: ingestive behavior. *Neurosci. Biobehav. Rev.* **20**:189–287.

Braak, H., and Braak, E. 1989. Cortical and subcortical argyrophilic grains characterize a disease associated with adult onset dementia. *Neuropathol. Appl. Neurobiol.* **15**:13–26.

Bray, G. A. 1992. Genetic, hypothalamic and endocrine features of clinical and experimental obesity. In: D. F. Swabb, M. A. Hofman, M. Mirmiran, R. Ravid, and F. W. van Leeuwen (eds.) The human hypothalamus in health and disease. *Prog. Brain Res.* **93**:333–341.

Breningstall, G. N. 1985. Gelastic seizures, precocious puberty, and hypothalamic hamartomas. *Neurology* **35**:1180–1183.

Burstein, R. 1996. Somatosensory and visceral input to the hypothalamus and limbic system. In: G. Holstege, R. Bandler, and C. B. Saper (eds.) The emotional motor system. *Prog. Brain Res.* **107**: 257–267.

Charney, D. S., Nagy, L. M., Bremner, J. D., Goddard, A. W., Yehuda, R., and Southwick, S. M. 1996. Neurobiological mechanisms of human anxiety. In: B. S. Fogel, R. B. Schiffer, and S. M. Rao (eds.) *Neuropsychiatry*. Baltimore, Md.: Williams and Wilkins, pp. 257–286.

Corodimas, K. P., Rosenblatt, J. S., Canfield, M. E., and Morrell, J. I. 1993. Neurons in the lateral subdivision of the habenular complex mediate the hormonal onset of maternal behavior in rats. *Behav. Neurosci.* **107**:827–843.

Darlington, D. N., Mains, R. E., and Eipper, B. A. 1996. Location of neurons that express regulated endocrine-specific protein-18 in the rat diencephalon. *Neuroscience* **71**:477–488.

Dawson, T. M., Gehlert, D. R., McCabe, R. T., Barnett, A., and Wamsley, J. K. 1986. D-1 dopamine receptors in the rat brain: a quantitative autoradiographic analysis. *J. Neurosci.* **6**:2352–2365.

Delis, D. C., and Lucas, J. A. 1996. Memory. In: B. S. Fogel, R. B. Schiffer, and S. M. Rao (eds.) *Neuropsychiatry*. Baltimore, Md.: Williams and Wilkins, pp. 365–399.

Delville, Y. U., Melloni, R. H. Jr., and Ferris, C. F. 1998. Behavioral and neurobiological consequences of social subjugation during puberty in golden hamsters. *J. Neurosci.* **18**:2667–2672.

Demitrack, M. A., and Gold, P. W. 1988. Oxytocin: neurobiologic considerations and their implications for affective illness. *Prog. Neuropsychopharmacol.* **12**:S23–S51.

Demitrack, M. A., Lesem, M. D., Listwak, S. J., Brandt, H. A., Jimerson, D. C., and Gold, P. W. 1990. Cerebrospinal fluid oxytocin in anorexia nervosa and bulimia nervosa: clinical and pathophysiological considerations. *Am. J. Psychiatry* **147**:882–886.

DeMoranville, B. M., and Jackson, I. M. D. 1996. Psychoneuroendocrinology. In: B. S. Fogel, R. B. Schiffer, and S. M. Rao (eds.) *Neuropsychiatry*. Baltimore, Md.: Williams and Wilkins, pp. 173–192.

DeVries, G. J., and Villalba, C. 1997. Brain sexual dimorphism and sex differences in parental and other social behaviors. In: C. S. Carter, I. I. Lederhendler, and B. Kirkpatrick (eds.) The integrative neurobiology of affiliation. *Ann. N.Y. Acad. Sci. U.S.A.* **807**:273–286.

Dollins, A. B., Lynch, H. J., Wurtman, R. J., Deng, M. H., and Lieberman, H. R. 1993. Effects of illumination on human nocturnal serum melatonin levels and performance. *Physiol. Behav.* **53**:153–160.

Ellison, G. 1994. Stimulant-induced psychosis, the dopamine theory of schizophrenia and the habenula. *Brain Res. Brain Res. Rev.* **19**:223–239.

Friedman, R. C., and Downey, J. 1993. Neurobiology and sexual orientation. *J. Neuropsychiatry Clin. Neurosci.* **5**:147–148.

Gjerris, A. 1990. Studies on cerebrospinal fluid in affective disorders. *Pharmacol. Toxicol.* **66** (Suppl.3): 133–138.

Golombek, D. A., Escolar, E., Burin, L., Brito Sanchez, M. G., and Cardinali, D. P. 1991. Time-dependent melatonin analgesia in mice: inhibition by opiate or benzodiazepine antagonism. *Eur. J. Pharmacol.* **194**:25–30.

Golombek, D. A., Pevet, P., and Cardinali, D. P. 1996. Melatonin effects on behavior: possible mediation by the central GABAergic system. *Neurosci. Biobehav. Rev.* **20**:403–412.

Hamann, S., Herman, R. A., Nolan, C. L., and Wallen, K. 2004. Men and women differ in amygdala response to visual sexual stimuli. *Nature Neurosci.* **7**:411–416.

Hansen, S., and Ferreira, A. 1986. Food intake, aggression, and fear behavior in the mother rat: control by neural systems concerned with milk ejection and maternal behavior. *Behav. Neurosci.* **100**:64–70.

Hennessy, M. B. 1997. Hypothalamic-pituitary-adrenal responses to brief social separation. *Neurosci. Biobehav. Rev.* **21**:11–29.

Herman, J. P., Adams, D., and Prewitt, C. 1995. Regulatory changes in neuroendocrine stress-integrative circuitry produced by a variable stress paradigm. *Neuroendocrinology* **61**:180–190.

Hofman, M. A., Puirba, J. S., and Swaab, D. F. 1993. Annual variation in the vasopressin neuron population of the human suprachiasmatic nucleus. *Neuroscience* **53**:1103–1112.

Holsboer-Trachsler, E., Stohler, R., and Hatzinger, M. 1991. Repeated administration of the combined dexamethasone–human corticotropin releasing hormone stimulation test during treatment of depression. *Psychiatry Res.* **38**:163–171.

Horn, E., Lach, B., Lapierre, Y., and Hrdina, P. 1988. Hypothalamic pathology in the neuroleptic malignant syndrome. *Am. J. Psychiatry* **145**:617–620.

Katter, J. T., Burstein, R., and Giesler, G. J. 1991. The cells of origin of the spinohypothalamic tract in cats. *J. Comp. Neurol.* **303**:101–112.

Korf, H. W., Sato, T., and Oksche, A. 1990. Complex relationship between the pineal organ and the medial habenular nucleus–pretectal region of the mouse as revealed by S-antigen immunocytochemistry. *Cell* **261**:493–500.

Kostic, V. S., Stefanova, E., Svetel, M., and Kovic, D. 1998. A variant of the Kleine–Levin syndrome following head trauma. *Behav. Neurol.* **11**:105–108.

Kremer, H. P. H. 1992. The hypothalamic lateral tuberal nucleus: normal anatomy and changes in neurological diseases. In: R. M. Buijs, A. Kalsbeek, H. J. Romijn, C. M. A. Pennartz, and M. Mirmiran (eds.) Hypothalamic integration of circadian rhythms. *Prog. Brain Res.* **111**:249–261.

Kruck, M. R. 1991. Ethology and pharmacology of hypothalamic aggression in the rat. *Neurosci. Biobehav. Rev.* **15**:527–538.

Kupfermann, I. 1991. Hypothalamus and limbic system: peptidergic neurons, homeostasis, and emotional behavior. In: E. R. Kandel, J. H. Schwartz, and T. M. Jessell (eds.) *Principles of neural science*, 3rd edn. New York: Elsevier, pp. 735–749.

LeDoux, J. 1996. Emotional networks and motor control: a fearful view. In: G. Holstege, R. Bandler, and C. B. Saper (eds.) The emotional motor system. *Prog. Brain Res.* **107**: 437–446.

Legros, J. J., Ansseau, M., and Timsit-Berthier, M. 1993. Neurohypophyseal peptides and psychopathology. *Prog. Brain Res.* **93**:455–461.

LeVay, S. 1991. A difference in hypothalamic structure between heterosexual and homosexual men. *Science* **253**:1034–1037.

LeVay, S., and Hamer, D. H. 1994. Evidence for a biological influence in male homosexuality. *Sci. Am.* **270**:44–49.

Lewy, A. J., and Sack, R. L. 1996. The role of melatonin and light in the human circadian system. In: R. M. Buijs, A. Kalsbeek, H. J. Romijn, C. M. A. Pennartz, and M. Mirmiran (eds.) Hypothalamic integration of circadian rhythms. *Prog. Brain Res.* **111**:205–216.

Ma, Q. P., Shi, Y. S., and Han, J. S. 1992. Further studies on interactions between periaqueductal gray, nucleus accumbens and habenula in antinociception. *Brain Res.* **583**:292–295.

Marson, L., and McKenna, K. E. 1994. Stimulation of the hypothalamus initiates the urethrogenital reflex in male rats. *Brain Res.* **638**:103–108.

Martin, J. B., and Riskind, P. N. 1992. Neurologic manifestations of hypothalamic disease. In: D. F. Swabb, M. A. Hofman, M. Mirmiran, R. Ravid, and F. W. van Leeuwen (eds.) The human hypothalamus in health and disease. *Prog. Brain Res.* **93**:31–42.

Martin, J. H. 1996. *Neuroanatomy: Text and Atlas.* Stamford, Conn.: Appleton and Lange, p. 434.

Matthews-Felton, T., Corodimas, K. P., Rosenblatt, J. S., and Morrell, J. I. 1995. Lateral habenula neurons are necessary for the hormonal onset of maternal behavior and for the display of post-partum estrus in naturally parturient female rats. *Behav. Neurosci.* **109(6)**:1172–1188.

Michelson, D., Stratakis, C., Hill, L., Reynolds, J., Galliven, E., Chrousos, G., and Gold, P. 1996. Bone mineral density in women with depression. *N. Engl. J. Med.* **335**:1176–1181.

Moore, R. Y. 1997. Circadian rhythms: basic neurobiology and clinical applications. *Annu. Rev. Med.* **48**:253–266.

Morgan, P. J., Barrett, P., Howell, H. E., and Helliwell, R. 1994. Melatonin receptors: localization, molecular pharmacology and physiological significance. *Neurochem. Int.* **24**:101–146.

Nadvornik, P., Sramka, M., and Patoprsta, G. 1975. Transventricular anterior hypothalamotomy in stereotactic treatment of hedonia. In: W. H. Sweet, S. Obrador, and J. G. Martin-Rodriguez (eds.) *Neurosurgical Treatment in Psychiatry, Pain and Epilepsy.* Baltimore, Md.: University Park Press, pp. 445–450.

Nishikawa, T., Fage, D., and Scatton, B. 1986. Evidence for and nature of the tonic inhibitory influence of the habenulointerpeduncular pathways upon cerebral dopaminergic transmission in the rat. *Brain Res.* **373**:324–336.

Numan, M., and Sheenan, T. P. 1997. Neuroanatomical circuitry for mammalian maternal behavior. In: C. S. Carter, I. I. Lederhendler, and B. Kirkpatrick (eds.) The integrative neurobiology of affiliation. *Ann. N.Y. Acad. Sci.* **807**:101–125.

Numan, M., and Smith, H. G. 1984. Maternal behavior in rats: evidence for the involvement of preoptic projections to the ventral tegmental area. *Behav. Neurosci.* **98**:712–727.

Pedersen, C. A. 1997. Oxytocin control of maternal behavior: regulation by sex steroids and offspring stimuli. *Ann. N. Y. Acad. Sci.* **807**:126–145.

Pedersen, C. A., and Prange, A. J. Jr. 1979. Induction of maternal behavior in virgin rats after intracerebroventricular administration of oxytocin. *Proc. Natl. Acad. Sci. U.S.A.* **76**:6661–6665.

Pevet, P., Pitrosky, B., Vuillez, P., Jacob, N., Teclemariam-Mesbah, R., Kirsch, R., Vivien-Roels, B., Lakhdar-Ghazal, N., Canguilhem, B., and Masson-Pevet, M. 1996. The suprachiasmatic nucleus: the biological clock of all seasons. In: R. M. Buijs, A. Kalsbeek, H. J Romijn, C. M. A. Pennartz, and M. Mirmiran (eds.) Hypothalamic integration of circadian rhythms. *Prog. Brain Res.* **111**: 369–384.

Pfaff, D. W., Schwartz-Giblin, S., McCarthy, M. M., and Kow, L.-M. 1994. Cellular mechanisms of female reproductive behavior. In: E. Knobil, and J. Neill (eds.) *The Physiology of Reproduction*, 2nd edn. New York: Raven Press, pp. 107–220.

Pfaus, J. G., Kleopoulos, S. P., Mobbs, C. V., Gibbs, R. B., and Pfaff, D. W. 1993. Sexual stimulation activates c-fos within estrogen-concentrating regions of the female rat forebrain. *Brain Res.* **624**:253–267.

Purba, J. S., Hoogendijk, W. J. G., Hofman, M. A., and Swaab, D. F. 1996. Increased number of vasopressin- and oxytocin-expressing neurons in the paraventricular nucleus of the hypothalamus in depression. *Arch. Gen. Psychiatry* **53**:137–143.

Raadsheer, F. C., Hoogendijk, W. J. G., Stam, F. C., Tilders, F. J. H., and Swaab, D. F. 1994. Increased number of corticotropin-releasing hormone neurons in the hypothalamic paraventricular nuclei of depressed patients. *Neuroendocrinology* **60**:436–444.

Rance, N. E. 1992. Hormonal influences on morphology and neuropeptide gene expression in the infundibular nucleus of post-menopausal women. In: D. F. Swabb, M. A. Hofman, M. Mirmiran, R. Ravid, and F. W. van Leeuwen (eds.) The human hypothalamus in health and disease. *Prog. Brain Res.* **93**:221–236.

Reisine, T. D., Soubrie, P., Artaud, F., and Glowinski, J. 1982. Involvement of lateral habenula-dorsal raphe neurons in the differential regulation of striatal and nigral serotonergic transmission in cats. *J. Neurosci.* **2**: 1062–1071.

Reppert, S. M., Rivkees, S. A., and Weaver, D. R. 1989. Prenatal entrainment of a circadian clock. In: S. M. Reppert (ed.) *The Development of Circadian Rhythmicity and Photoperiodism in Mammals.* New York: Perinatology Press, pp. 25–44.

Reuss, S. 1996. Components and connections of the circadian timing system in mammals. *Cell Tissue Res.* **285**:353–378.

Romijn, H. 1978. The pineal: a tranquilizing organ? *Life Sci.* **3**:2257–2274.

Ross, E. D., and Stewart, R. M. 1981. Akinetic mutism from hypothalamic damage: successful treatment with dopamine agonists. *Neurology* **31**:1435–1439.

Sandyk, R. 1992. Pineal and habenula calcification in schizophrenia. *Int. J. Neurosci.* **67**: 19–30.

Saper, C. B. 1996. Role of the cerebral cortex and striatum in emotional motor response. In: G. Holstege, R. Bandler, and C. B. Saper (eds.) The emotional motor system. *Prog. Brain Res.* **107**: 537–550.

Saver, J. L., Salloway, S. P., Devinsky, O., and Bear, D. M. 1996. Neuropsychiatry of aggression. In: B. S. Fogel, R. B. Schiffer, and S. M. Rao (eds.) *Neuropsychiatry.* Baltimore, Md.: Williams and Wilkins, pp. 523–548.

Schwartz, M. W., and Seeley, R. J. 1997. The new biology of body weight regulation. *J. Am. Diet. Assoc.* **97**:558.

Segraves, R. T. 1996. Neuropsychiatric aspects of sexual dysfunction. In: B. S. Fogel, R. B. Schiffer, and S. M. Rao (eds.) *Neuropsychiatry.* Baltimore, MD.: Williams and Wilkins, pp. 757–770.

Shipley, M. T., Murphy, A. Z., Rizvi, T. A., Ennis, M., and Behbehani, M. M. 1996. Olfaction and brainstem circuits of reproductive behavior in the rat. In: G. Holstege, R. Bandler, and C. B. Saper (eds.) The emotional motor system. *Prog. Brain Res.* **107**:353–377.

Sofroniew, M. W. 1983. Vasopressin and oxytocin in the mammalian brain and spinal cord. *Trends Neurosci.* **6**:467–472.

Swaab, D. F., Gooren, L. J., and Hofman, M. A. 1995. Brain research, gender and sexual orientation. *J. Homosex.* **28**:283–301.

Takeuchi, J., Handa, H., and Miki, Y. 1979. Precocious puberty due to hypothalamic hamartoma. *Surg. Neurol.* **11**:456–460.

Tonkonogy, J. M., and Geller, J. L. 1992. Hypothalamic lesions and intermittent explosive disorder. *J. Neuropsychiatry Clin. Neurosci.* **4**:45–50.

Tzichinsky, O., Pal, I., Epstein, R., Dagan, Y., and Lavie, P. 1992. The importance of timing in melatonin administration in a blind man. *J. Pineal Res.* **12**:105–108.

Uvnas-Moberg, K. 1997. Physiological and endocrine effects of social contact. *Ann. N. Y. Acad. Sci.* **807**:146–163.

Van de Poll, N. E., and Van Goozen, S. H. M. 1992. Hypothalamic involvement in sexuality and hostility: comparative psychological aspects. In: D. F. Swabb, M. A. Hofman, M. Mirmiran, R. Ravid, and F. W. van Leeuwen (eds.) The human hypothalamus in health and disease. *Prog. Brain Res.* **93**:343–361.

Wehr, T. A. 1991. The duration of human melatonin secretion and sleep respond to changes in daylength (photoperiod). *J. Clin. Enocrinol. Metab.* **73**:1276–1280.

Weinstock, M. 1997. Does prenatal stress impair coping and regulation of hypothalamic-pituitary-adrenal axis? *Neurosci. Biobehav. Rev.* **21**:1–10.

Wiegant, V. M., Ronken, E., Kovacs, G., and DeWied, D. 1992. Endorphins and schizophrenia. In: D. F. Swabb, M. A. Hofman, M. Mirmiran, R. Ravid, and F. W. van Leeuwen (eds.) The human hypothalamus in health and disease. *Prog. Brain Res.* **93**:433–453.

Witt, D. W. 1997. Regulatory mechanisms of oxytocin-mediated sociosexual behavior. *Ann. N. Y. Acad. Sci.* **807**:287–301.

Young, P. A., and Young, P. H. 1997. *Basic Clinical Anatomy*. Baltimore, Md.: Williams and Wilkins.

9 Diencephalon: thalamus

The thalamus functions as the principal relay station for sensory information destined for the cerebral cortex. It is made up of a number of nuclei, which can be grouped into relay nuclei and diffuse-projection nuclei (Table 9.1). Each relay nucleus is associated with a single sensory modality or motor system and projects to a specific region of the cerebral cortex with which it has reciprocal connections. The diffuse-projection group of nuclei have more widespread connections with the cortex and also interact with other thalamic nuclei. It is believed that this group of nuclei is involved with regulating the level of arousal of the brain. The limbic thalamus consists of a number of the thalamic nuclei that project to the limbic cortex and includes both relay and diffuse-projection nuclei.

Anatomy and behavioral considerations

The thalamus consists of a symmetrical pair of ovoid structures located above (dorsal to) the hypothalamus. The left thalamus and right thalamus are separated medially by the third ventricle and bounded laterally by the posterior limb of the internal capsule (Figures 9.1–9.3). The massa intermedia (interthalamic adhesion) is a bridge of cells that spans the third ventricle and joins the left with the right thalamus. The thalamus is bounded in front (anteriorly) by the head of the caudate nucleus and the genu of the internal capsule and behind (posteriorly) by the midbrain. The subthalamic nucleus (subthalamus) lies immediately below (ventral to) the thalamus and is sandwiched between the thalamus, internal capsule, and pretectal area (Figures 9.2 and 9.3).

The internal medullary lamina is a sheet of fibers that runs through the center of the thalamus, dividing it into three subdivisions (Figures 9.2 and 9.3). The anterior subdivision is embraced within the split anterior leaves of the internal medullary lamina. The anterior subdivision consists of the anterior group of thalamic nuclei. The medial subdivision lies medial to the internal medullary lamina and consists of the midline and medial nuclear groups. The lateral subdivision lies lateral to the internal medullary lamina and consists of the lateral, ventral, and reticular nuclei as well as the medial and lateral geniculate bodies. The intralaminar nuclei represent a fourth subdivision, and these nuclei are found encapsulated within the fibers of the internal medullary lamina. The most prominent of the intralaminar nuclei is the centromedian nucleus (CM in Figure 9.3).

Table 9.1. *Major connections of thalamic nuclei that make up the four nuclear groups found in the human thalamus.*

Nucleus	Functional class	Major inputs	Major outputs	Function
Anterior group				
Anterior*	Relay	Hypothalamus (mamillary body)	Cingulate gyrus	Learning, emotion, memory
Medial group				
Midline*	Diffuse-projecting	Reticular formation, hypothalamus	Cerebral cortex including cingulate gyrus, amygdala	Regulation of forebrain excitability
Mediodorsal*	Relay	Basal ganglia, amygdala, hypothalamus, nucleus accumbens, olfactory system	Prefrontal cortex, cingulate gyrus, nucleus basalis	Emotion, cognition, learning, memory
Lateral group				
Ventral anterior*	Relay	Basal ganglia	Supplementary motor cortex, cingulate gyrus	Movement planning
Ventral lateral	Relay	Cerebellum	Premotor and primary motor cortex	Movement planning and control
Ventral posterior	Relay	Spinal cord, brainstem, ascending discriminative touch systems	Parietal cortex	Touch, limb position sense
Lateral dorsal*	Relay	Hippocampus	Cingulate gyrus, parietal cortex	?
Lateral posterior	Relay	Superior colliculus pretectum, occipital lobe	Posterior parietal cortex	Sensory integration
Pulvinar	Relay	Superior colliculus; parietal, temporal, occipital lobes	Parietal, temporal, occipital association cortices; cingulate gyrus	Sensory integration, perception, eye movement control, language
Lateral geniculate	Relay	Retina	Primary visual cortex	Vision
Medial geniculate	Relay	Inferior colliculus	Primary auditory cortex	Hearing
Reticular		Thalamus, cortex	Thalamus	Regulation of thalamic activity
Intralaminar*	Diffuse-projecting	Brainstem, spinal cord, basal ganglia	Cerebral cortex, basal ganglia	Regulation of cortical activity

* Nuclei that are considered to be part of the limbic thalamus.

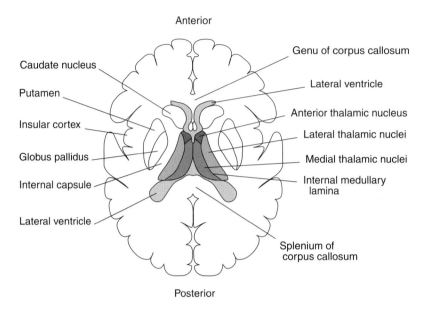

Figure 9.1.   The brain section in this view is cut perpendicular to the long axis of the body and parallel to the horizontal limb of the neuraxis (see Figure 1.1). It is as if we are standing at the foot of the bed and looking at the patient. This diagram is identical to that of the insert on the left-hand side of Figure 9.2. Anterior refers to the front of the head, posterior to the back of the head.

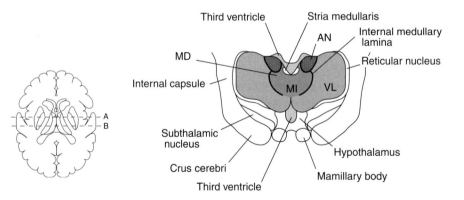

Figure 9.2.   The level of this cross-section is indicated by A in the inset. The massa intermedia (MI) contains the midline nuclei. AN, anterior group of nuclei; MD, mediodorsal nucleus; VL, ventrolateral nuclei.

Thalamic nuclei

Anterior thalamic nuclei

The anterior group of thalamic nuclei consists of the anterodorsal, the anteroventral, and the anteromedial nuclei. The anterior thalamic nuclei receive input from the mamillary body of the hypothalamus by way of the mamillothalamic tract. The anterior group projects to the cingulate gyrus. The anterior thalamic nuclear group is part of the limbic

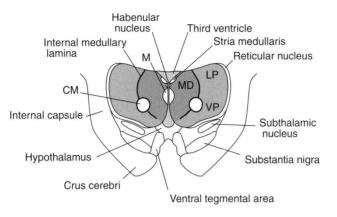

Figure 9.3.   The level of this cross-section is indicated by B in the inset of Figure 9.2. The centromedian nucleus (CM) lies within the internal medullary lamina. LP, lateral posterior nucleus; M, midline nuclei; MD, mediodorsal nucleus; VP, ventral posterior nuclei.

circuitry and constitutes the original "limbic thalamus." It is part of the circuit of Papez (see Figures 9.2 and 13.8). Disorientation has been seen following lesions of the anterior thalamic nuclei (Graff-Radford *et al.*, 1984). The anterior thalamus is activated during pain processing more so in men than in women (Zubieta *et al.*, 2002).

Midline and medial nuclei

Two groups of thalamic nuclei lie medial to the internal medullary lamina. These are the medial nuclei and the midline nuclei (see Figures 9.2 and 9.3). The midline nuclei are continuous with the periaqueductal gray of the midbrain reticular formation (see Chapter 10). They are the target of dopaminergic fibers and express dopamine receptors. These are two criteria that qualify them as part of the ascending dopaminergic system (see Chapter 7). Fibers from the midline nuclei project diffusely, and targets include the amygdala and the anterior cingulate gyrus. The midline nuclei provide an indirect link from the brainstem to these limbic structures.

Clinical vignette

A lesion of the ventral lateral nucleus along with the intralaminar nuclei and the dorsomedial nucleus on the right side was postulated to be the cause of a disinhibition syndrome that appeared in a 72-year-old woman (Bogousslavsky *et al.*, 1988b). The patient, who had no prior psychiatric history, developed a syndrome of increased speech, jokes, laughing, inappropriate comments, and confabulations. The authors suggest that this behavioral syndrome was produced by interrupting the link provided by the mediodorsal nucleus between the limbic system and the prefrontal lobe. Mania following thalamic lesions is associated with damage to the right side (Cummings and Mendez, 1984).

A bilateral surgical lesion placed in the anterior portion of the internal capsule (anterior capsulotomy) disconnects the orbital frontal cortex from the midline thalamic nuclei and is thought to decrease symptoms of obsessive-compulsive disorder (OCD) (see Chapter 12; Martuza *et al.*, 1990).

The medial nuclear group is dominated by the mediodorsal nucleus. It is a very large nucleus that occupies most of the space between the midline nuclei and the internal medullary lamina. The mediodorsal nucleus is described as the thalamic relay nucleus for association areas in the frontal lobe. It receives input from the amygdala, the nucleus accumbens, the olfactory region, the hypothalamus, and the basal ganglia. It projects to the nucleus basalis (of Meynert), the frontal eye fields, the prefrontal cortex, and the cingulate gyrus (Baleydier and Mauguiere, 1987). The mediodorsal nucleus relays limbic system information to the prefrontal cortex and to the cingulate cortex. It has been subdivided into several regions. The magnocellular portion of the mediodorsal nucleus, which lies medially, has close connections with the pyriform cortex, the amygdala, and the neocortex of the temporal lobe, as well as with the cingulate cortex. The parvicellular portion is much larger and lies laterally; it projects heavily to the prefrontal cortex.

Thalamic dementia presents with amnesia, speech disturbances, confusion, apathy, flattened affect, and aspontaneity of motor acts. It often results from bilateral paramedian infarction of the thalamus (Clarke *et al.*, 1994). The lesion apparently interrupts reciprocal connections between the thalamus and areas of the frontal cortex. In contrast, some patients with bilateral paramedian thalamic infarction exhibit thalamic pseudodementia (robot syndrome) in which they act in a manner similar to patients with thalamic dementia but can act normally if they are constantly stimulated by other people who show them what to do. It is suggested that both syndromes result from damage to the mediodorsal nucleus but that only the nonmagnocellular portions are involved in robot syndrome. The magnocellular portion of the mediodorsal nucleus appears to be important in memory (Graff-Radford *et al.*, 1990; Bogousslavsky, 1991; Bogousslavsky *et al.*, 1991).

Eight patients with bilateral thalamic tumors exhibited personality change, memory loss, inattention, confusion, and hallucinations. In each case, the tumor involved the medial aspect of the left and right thalamus (Partlow *et al.*, 1992). Personality changes often are severe enough to result in institutional care. Most symptoms seen following an infarct improve over time with the exception of amnesia.

It has been hypothesized that the magnocellular portion of the mediodorsal nucleus may be released (disinhibited) in obsessive-compulsive disorder. The release in behavior is similar to that seen in the involuntary motor activity following lesions in other parts of the basal ganglia responsible for Parkinson's and Huntington's disease (Baxter, 1990).

The mediodorsal nucleus has been implicated in schizophrenia. It has been reported to be reduced in size in early-onset schizophrenia (Pakkenberg, 1992). However, a study of late-onset schizophrenia demonstrated that the thalamus was increased in size (Corey-Bloom *et al.*, 1995), leading to the speculation that the thalamus may compensate for abnormalities and delay the onset of symptoms in some individuals (Jeste *et al.*, 1996).

Ventral thalamic nuclei

The ventral thalamic group contains three major nuclei: the ventral anterior nucleus, the ventral lateral nucleus, and the ventral posterior nucleus. The border between the ventral anterior and the ventral lateral nuclei is indistinct and makes it difficult to clearly separate the function of these two nuclei, which relay signals from the cerebellum and basal ganglia to the cortex. A small number of cells in the ventral anterior nucleus project to the cingulate cortex. These cells are located in the region of the nucleus that receives input from the globus pallidus and substantia nigra.

The ventral anterior nucleus is the most common lesion site in the thalamus associated with aphasia (Nadeau *et al.*, 1994). Mild transient hemiparesis and hemiataxia may be present following damage to the ventral lateral nucleus (Bogousslavsky *et al.*, 1986; Melo and Bogousslavsky, 1992). Hemineglect may be observed in right-sided lesions (Graff-Radford *et al.*, 1985).

Touch (somesthetic) signals are relayed from the head and body to the somesthetic (parietal) cortex through the ventral posterior nucleus. This nucleus is frequently sub-divided into the ventral posterolateral nucleus (VPL), which mediates touch from the body to the parietal cortex, and the ventral posteromedial nucleus (VPM), which mediates touch from the head region to the parietal cortex (see Chapter 4).

A lesion of the ventral posterior nucleus produces sensory loss on the contralateral side without major cognitive deficits. Paresthesias, including pain, may be the first symptoms. The patient may exhibit contralateral neglect. In some cases pain may develop only after several weeks. The thalamic pain syndrome is now more accurately called the *central poststroke pain syndrome.* It can occur after thalamic lesions as well as lesions in the spinal cord, brainstem, or cerebral hemispheres (Bovie *et al.*, 1989).

Neuropathic pain has been treated with varying degrees of success with electrical stimulation of VPM/VPL. It is theorized that the pain results from lack of proprioceptive stimuli reaching the thalamus (Head and Holmes, 1911). Stimulation correlates with increased blood flow to the region including VPM/VPL contralateral to the painful body site. Increased blood flow was also seen in the rostral insula ipsilateral to the thalamic stimulation (Duncan *et al.*, 1998).

Clinical vignette

A 61-year-old right-handed carpet salesman became acutely unable to perform the calculations needed to determine the amount of carpet for a floor area. He underwent tests of his calculation ability. On 16 written problems, he made the following errors: $5+6 = 36$, $26+17 = 53$, $621-72 = 541$, $5 \times 13 = 75$, $78/13 = 5.5$. On a word problem ("18 books on 2 shelves, put twice as many on top shelf"), he stated, "18 on the top and none on the bottom." Further testing revealed difficulties related to working memory, a frontal-executive function.

This patient had cognitive difficulties from a thalamic stroke (Figure 9.4). On magnetic resonance imaging, he had a new lacunar infarct in the left thalamus. Infarction in the territory of the left tuberothalamic artery, with injury to the medial group of thalamic nuclei and their prefrontal connections, can produce difficulty in the working memory necessary to perform calculations.

Lateral thalamic nuclei

The lateral thalamic nuclear group makes up the largest of the thalamic nuclear groups. It consists of three nuclei. The lateral dorsal nucleus, the most rostral of the group, is functionally related to the anterior thalamic nuclear group and lies immediately behind the anterior nuclei.

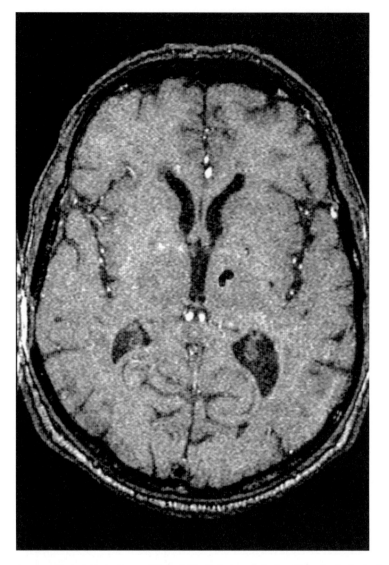

Figure 9.4.   A magnetic resonance image (T1-weighted) demonstrated a strategic stroke in the left thalamus in a patient with cognitive deficits, particularly in working memory and calculations. (Reprinted with permission from Mendez *et al.*, 2003.)

The major connections of the lateral dorsal nucleus are with the cingulate and parietal cortices. The larger and more posterior lateral posterior nucleus projects to the inferior parietal lobule. The pulvinar forms the most caudal portion of the thalamus and overhangs the dorsal surface of the midbrain. The pulvinar has connections with the visual cortex and is believed to be involved in the control of eye movements. The medial subdivision of the pulvinar includes cells that project to the posterior cingulate cortex (see Chapter 12). The pulvinar contains several nuclei that are retinotopically organized and is implicated in procesing behaviorally salient visual targets. It has direct projections to the lateral amygdala and is proposed to form part of a secondary extrageniculostriate visual system (Morris *et al.*, 2001; Vuilleumier *et al.*, 2003).

The pulvinar has been implicated in "blind sight" (see Chapter 4). An increase in bilateral pulvinar relative cerebral blood flow (rCBF) has been reported upon alleviation of chronic pain by anesthetic blocks and by direct thalamic stimulation (Kupers *et al.*, 2000). An increase in rCBF in the left pulvinar was reported in response to suboccipital stimulation for relief of the pain of migraine headache (Matharu *et al.*, 2003). Pulvinotomy and electrical stimulation of the pulvinar have been used successfully in the past for the control of chronic pain (Yoshii *et al.*, 1980). The pulvinar receives nociceptive input and projects to the superior parietal lobule but it is unknown whether the pulvinar mediates pain or is just associated with it (Matharu *et al.*, 2003).

It is hypothesized that abnormalities in the lateral thalamic nuclei, especially those regions that serve the temporoparietal association areas, may be responsible for sensory overload experienced by schizophrenic patients (Andreasen *et al.*, 1994).

Medial and lateral geniculate bodies

The medial geniculate body relays auditory signals from the inferior colliculus to the temporal cortex. The lateral geniculate body relays visual signals from the retina to the occipital cortex. Damage to the lateral geniculate body can result in visual field disturbances (Bogousslavsky *et al.*, 1988a).

Reticular nucleus

A sheet of myelinated fibers called the *external medullary lamina* covers the lateral, anterolateral, and ventrolateral surfaces of the thalamus and lies between the thalamus and the internal capsule. Embedded within the external medullary lamina is a group of small nuclei, collectively called the reticular nuclei, or more simply the *reticular nucleus*. Neurons of the reticular nucleus are GABA ergic and make extensive reciprocal connections with all the nuclei of the dorsal thalamus. They receive fibers from, but do not project fibers to, the cerebral cortex. The reticular nucleus receives collateral input from the thalamocortical, corticothalamic, thalamostriate, and pallidothalamic fibers.

The reticular nucleus is believed to serve as an attentional valve or gate for thalamocortical transmission. There appear to be as many gates as there are sensory modalities with individual cell groups within the reticular nucleus that are sensitive to specific sensory modalities or to portions of sensory modalities. The reticular nucleus is believed to mediate the inhibitory influences from the frontal lobes as well as the excitatory impact of the brainstem reticular formation. It provides a possible mechanism for autohypnosis and voluntary pain control (Mesulam, 1985; Scheibel, 1997).

Intralaminar nuclei

The intralaminar nuclei represent a rostral continuation of the brainstem reticular formation (see Chapter 10). In addition to reticular afferents, projections from spinal and brainstem pain systems are important inputs to the intralaminar nuclei. The pattern of projection from the intralaminar nuclei is diffuse and widespread, and reaches all areas of the cerebral cortex. The intralaminar nuclei provide significant input to the basal ganglia as well as to cells located in the thalamus itself. The centromedian is the largest of the intralaminar nuclei.

The diffusely projecting intralaminar nuclei are part of a system that governs the level of arousal of the brain. A vascular lesion that affects the intralaminar nuclei usually also involves the mediodorsal nucleus (Bogousslavsky, 1995).

Lesions placed in the medial portion of the centromedian nucleus produce a reduction in aggression. Lesions located laterally in this nucleus are less effective in reducing aggression (Andy *et al.*, 1975). Transient loss of consciousness usually seen after a paramedian infarction may be due to involvement of the intralaminar nuclei (Karabelas *et al.*, 1985).

Limbic thalamus

The limbic thalamus is defined as that portion of the thalamus that serves the limbic cortex (Bentivoglio *et al.*, 1993). Based on this definition, the limbic thalamus originally was made up of only the anterior thalamic nuclear group. Results of more recent studies have broadened the content of the limbic thalamus to include parts of a number of thalamic nuclei (see Table 9.1). The lateral dorsal nucleus projects to the cingulate cortex. In addition, the diffuse group of nuclei that project to many areas of the cortex include cell groups that project to the cingulate cortex. The midline and intralaminar nuclei, in particular, contain cells that project to the cingulate cortex. The ventral anterior nucleus is generally considered one of the motor nuclei and is associated with the basal ganglia and cerebellum. The ventral anterior nucleus also projects to the cingulate cortex, however, thus establishing a close link between motor systems and limbic cortex (Vogt *et al.*, 1987). Some cells in the medial pulvinar also project to the cingulate cortex (Musil and Olson, 1988). The mediodorsal nucleus projects heavily to the prefrontal cortex. It also sends fibers to the cingulate cortex and is included by some as part of the limbic thalamus (Bentivoglio *et al.*, 1993). The cingulate cortex projects back to all of the components of the limbic thalamus. Anterior, mediodorsal, and midline nuclei project to the ventral anterior portion of the cingulate cortex. These thalamic nuclei receive much of their information from brainstem and hypothalamic nuclei that are recognized as autonomic centers. The regulation of visceral and autonomic function is one of the prominent roles of the ventral anterior cingulate cortex (see Chapter 12).

Further behavioral considerations

One of the primary functions of the thalamus is to filter or gate sensory input. A defect in this function could explain difficulties in the interpretation of sensory input, which may include some of the symptoms of schizophrenia.

Distractibility, loss of associations, and shifting attentional focus commonly seen in schizophrenic patients may result from sensory overload. The inability to screen out irrelevant stimuli may be a

3-1_3-1 P   X = −13mm   Y = −66mm   Z =   1mm

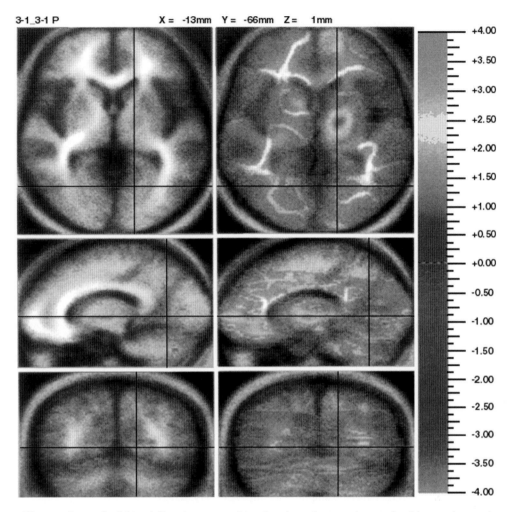

Figure 9.5. Difference in cerebral blood flow between schizophrenic patients and control subjects using positron emission tomography (PET) while they recalled Story A from the Weschler Memory Scale. Three orthogonal views are shown, with transaxial at the top, sagittal in the middle, and coronal at the bottom. The crosshairs show the location of the slice. Structures are as if standing at the foot of the bed (transaxial view) or facing the patient (coronal view). The left column shows differences using the "peak map." The right column demonstrates differences using the "t map." Significantly higher blood flow corresponds with lighter areas and is seen in the anterior frontal pole, thalamus, and cerebellum of control subjects. (Reproduced by permission from Andreasen, N.C. 1997. The role of the thalamus in schizophrenia. *Can. J. Psychiatry* **42**:27–33.)

failure of the gating function of the thalamus (Braff, 1993). Regional blood flow to the thalamus increases bilaterally during auditory hallucinations (but not during visual hallucinations) experienced by schizophrenic patients (Silversweig *et al.*, 1995).

One hypothesis advanced to explain the variety of symptoms of schizophrenia is that the midline neural circuits that mediate attention and information processing are dysfunctional.

When magnetic resonance images (MRIs) of normal individuals were averaged together and then compared with the averaged MRIs of schizophrenic patients, specific regional abnormalities were observed in the thalamus and adjacent white matter. The lateral and ventrolateral areas of the thalamus, which project to the cingulate gyrus, parietal cortex, and temporal cortex, were seen to be most involved (Andreasen *et al.*, 1994). The reduction in size of the thalamus may produce an abnormality in the normal gating and filtering function of the thalamus and allow a bombardment of the cortex by sensory stimuli, resulting in difficulty in distinguishing "self" from "not self." Figure 9.5 illustrates a decrease in blood flow in the thalamus seen in schizophrenic patients (Andreasen, 1997).

The thalamus is involved in many functions, including the storage and retrieval of memory. As stated by Silversweig and associates (1995), "The thalamus is believed to generate an internal representation of reality, in the presence or absence of sensory input." The anterior nuclei and the lateral dorsal nucleus in particular are involved in memory. **Memory disturbance in Korsakoff's disease corresponds with loss of cells in the medial portion of the dorsal medial nucleus as well as cells in the nearby midline nuclei.**

It has been hypothesized that a medial and a lateral pain system exist (Albe-Fessard et al., 1985). The medial pain system includes the periaqueductal gray of the midbrain and the intralaminar and midline thalamic nuclei, which project to the cingulate cortex and to the prefrontal cortex. The medial pain system is responsible for the affective component of pain. Ablation of the midline and intralaminar nuclei has been used to relieve chronic pain. The lateral pain system involves the ventral posteromedial and ventral posterolateral nuclei, which project onto the parietal cortex. The lateral system is responsible for the localization of pain.

SELECT BIBLIOGRAPHY

K. Kultas-Ilinsky and I. A. Ilinsky, eds. *Basal ganglia and thalamus in health and movement disorders.* (New York: Kluwer Academic/Plenum Publishers, 2000.)

REFERENCES

Albe-Fessard, D., Berkeley, K. J., Kruger, L., Ralston, H. J. III, and Willis, W. D. Jr. 1985. Diencephalic mechanisms of pain sensation. *Brain Res.* **356**:217–296.

Andreasen, N. C. 1997. The role of the thalamus in schizophrenia. *Can. J. Psychiatry* **42**:27–33.

Andreasen, N. C., Arndt, S., Swayze V., Cizadlo, T., Flaum, M., O'Leary, D., Ehrhardt, J. C., and Yuh, W. T. C. 1994. Thalamic abnormalities in schizophrenia visualized through magnetic resonance image averaging. *Science* **266**:294–297.

Andy, O. J., Jurko, M. F., and Giurintano, L. P. 1975. Behavioral changes correlated with thalamotomy site. *Confin. Neurol.* **36**:106–112.

Baleydier, C., and Mauguiere, F. 1987. Network organization of the connectivity between parietal area 7, posterior cingulate cortex and medial pulvinar nucleus: a double fluorescent tracer study in monkey. *Exp. Brain Res.* **66**:385–393.

Baxter, L. R. 1990. Brain imaging as a tool in establishing a theory of brain pathology in obsessive compulsive disorder. *J. Clin. Psychiatry* **51** (Suppl.):22–26.

Bentivoglio, M., Kultas-Llinsky, D., and Llinsky, I. 1993. Limbic thalamus: structure, intrinsic organization, and connections. In: B. A. Vogt and M. Gabriel (eds.) *Neurobiology of Cingulate Cortex and Limbic Thalamus*: A Comprehensive Handbook. Boston, Mass.: Birkhauser.

Bogousslavsky, J. 1991. Thalamic dementia and pseudo-dementia. In: A. Hartmann, W. Kuschinsky, and S. Hoyer (eds.) *Cerebral Ischemia and Dementia*. Berlin: Springer-Verlag.

— 1995. Thalamic infarcts. In: G. A. Donnay, B. Norrving, J. M. Bamford, and J. Bogousslavsky (eds.) *Lacunar and Other Subcortical Infarctions*. New York: Oxford University Press.

Bogousslavsky, J., Regli, F., and Assal, G. 1986. The syndrome of unilateral tuberothalamic artery territory infarction. *Stroke* **17**:434–441.

Bogousslavsky, J., Regli, F., and Uske, A. 1988a. Thalamic infarcts: clinical syndromes, etiology, and prognosis. *Neurology* **38**:837–848.

Bogousslavsky, J., Ferrazzini, M., Regli, F., Assal, G., Tanabe, H., and Delaloye-Bischof, A. 1988b. Manic delirium and frontal-like syndrome with paramedian infarction of the right thalamus. *J. Neurol. Neurosurg. Psychiatry* **51**:116–119.

Bogousslavsky, J., Regli, F., Delaloye, B., Delaloye-Bischof, A., Assal, G., and Uske, A. 1991. Loss of psychic self activation with bithalamic infarction: neurobehavioural, CT, MRI and SPECT correlates. *Acta Neurol. Scand.* **83**:309–316.

Bovie, J., Leijon, G., and Johansson, I. 1989. Central post-stroke pain – a study of the mechanisms through analyses of the sensory abnormalities. *Pain* **37**:173–185.

Braff, D. L. 1993. Information processing and attention dysfunctions in schizophrenia. *Schizophr. Bull.* **19**:233–259.

Clarke, W., Assal, G., Bogousslavsky, J., Regli, F., Townsend, D. W., Leenders, K. L., and Blecic, S. 1994. Pure amnesia after unilateral left polar thalamic infarct: topographic and sequential neuropsychological and metabolic (PET) correlations. *J. Neurol. Neurosurg. Psychiatry* **57**:27–34.

Corey-Bloom, J., Jernigan, T., Archibald, S., Harris, M. J., and Jeste, D. V. 1995. Quantitative magnetic resonance imaging in late-life schizophrenia. *Am. J. Psychiatry* **152**:447–449.

Cummings, J. L., and Mendez, M. F. 1984. Secondary mania with focal cerebrovascular lesions. *Am. J. Psychiatry* **141**:1084–1087.

Duncan, G. H., Kupers, R. C., Marhand, S., Villemure, J.-G., Gybels, J. M., and Bushnell, M. C. 1998. Stimulation of human thalamus for pain relief: possible modulatory circuits revealed by positron emission tomography. *J. Neurophysiol.* **80**(6):3326–3330.

Graff-Radford, N. R., Eslinger, P. J., Damasio, A. R., and Yamada, T. 1984. *Nonhemorrhagic infarction of the thalamus: behavioral, anatomic, and physiologic correlates. Neurology* **34**:14–23.

Graff-Radford, N. R., Damasio, H., Yamada, T., Eslinger, P. J., and Damasio, A. R. 1985. Nonhaemorrhagic thalamic infarction: clinical, neuropsychological and electrophysiological findings in four anatomical groups defined by computerized tomography. *Brain* **108**:485–516.

Graff-Radford, N. R., Tranel, D., Van Hoesen, G., and Brandt, J. P. 1990. Diencephalic amnesia. *Brain* **113**:1–25.

Head, H., and Holmes, G. 1911. Sensory disturbances from cerebral lesions. *Brain* **34**:102–254.

Jeste, D. V., Galasko, D., Corey-Bloom, J., Walens, S., and Granholm, E. 1996. Neuropsychiatric aspects of the schizophrenias. In: B. S. Fogel, R. B. Schiffer, and S. M. Rao (eds.) *Neuropsychiatry*. Baltimore, Md.: Williams and Wilkins.

Karabelas, T., Kalfakis, N., Kasvikis, I., and Vassilopoulos, D. 1985. Unusual features in a case of bilateral paramedian thalamic infarction. *J. Neurol. Neurosurg. Psychiatry* **48**:186.

Kupers, R. C., Gybels, J. M., and Gjedde, A. 2000. Positron emission tomography study of a chronic pain patient successfully treated with somatosensory thalamic stimulation. *Pain* **87**:295–302.

Martuza, R. L., Chiocca, E. A., Jenike, M. A., Girivnas, I. E., and Ballantine, H. T. 1990. Stereotactic radiofrequency thermal cingulotomy for obsessive compulsive disorder. *J. Neuropsychiatry Clin. Neurosci.* **2**:331–336.

Matharu, M. S., Bartsch, T., Ward, N., Frackowiak, R. S. J., Weiner, R., and Goadsby, P. J. 2003. Central neuromodulation in chronic migraine patients with suboccipital stimulators: a PET study. *Brain* **127**:220–230.

Melo, T. P., and Bogousslavsky, J. 1992. Hemiataxia–hypesthesia: a thalamic stroke syndrome. *J. Neurol. Neurosurg. Psychiatry* **55**:581–584.

Mendez, M. F., Papasian, N. C., Lim, G. T., and Swanberg, M. 2003. Thalamic acalculia. *J. Neuropsychiatry Clin. Neurosci.* **15**:115–116.

Mesulam, M. M. 1985. Attention, confusional states and neglect. In: M. M. Mesulem (ed.) Principles of Behavioral Neurology. Philadelphia, Pa.: Davis, pp. 125–168.

Morris, J. S., DeGelder, B., Weiskrantz, L., and Dolan, R. J. 2001. Differential extrageniculostriate and amygdala responses to presentation of emotional faces in a cortically blind field. *Brain* **124**:1241–1252.

Musil, S. Y., and Olson, C. R. 1988. Organization of cortical and subcortical projections to anterior cingulate cortex in the cat. *J. Comp. Neurol.* **227**:109–120.

Nadeau, S. E., Roeltgen, D. P., Sevush, S., Ballinger, W. E., and Watson, R. T. 1994. Apraxia due to a pathologically documented thalamic infarction. *Neurology* **44**:2133–2137.

Pakkenberg, B. 1992. The volume of the mediodorsal thalamic nucleus in treated and untreated schizophrenics. *Schizophr. Res.* **7**:95–100.

Partlow, G. D., del Carpio-O'Donovan, R., Melanson, D., and Peters, T. M. 1992. Bilateral thalamic glioma: review of eight cases with personality change and mental deterioration. *Am. J. Neuroradiol.* **13**:1225–1230.

Scheibel, A. B. 1997. The thalamus and neuropsychiatric illness. *J. Neuropsychiatry Clin. Neurosci.* **9**:342–353.

Silversweig, D. A., Stern, E., Frith, C., Cahill, C., Holmes, A., Groutoonik, S., Seaward, J., McKenna, P., Chua, S. E., Schnorr, L., Jones, T., and Frackowiak, R. S. J. 1995. A functional neuroanatomy of hallucinations in schizophrenia. *Nature* **378**:176–179.

Vuilleumier, P., Armony, J. L., Driver, J., and Dolan, R. J. 2003. Distinct spatial frequency sensitivities for processing faces and emotional expressions. *Nature Neurosci.* **6**(6):624–631.

Vogt, B. A., Pandya, D. N., and Rosene, D. L. 1987. Cingulate cortex of the rhesus monkey: I. Cytoarchitecture and thalamic afferents. *J. Comp. Neurol.* **262**:256–270.

Yoshii, N., Mizokami, T., Ushikubo, T., Kuramitsu, T., and Fukuda, S. 1980. Long-term follow-up study after pulvinotomy for intractable pain. *Appl. Neurophysiol.* **43**:128–132.

Zubieta, J.-K., Smith, Y. R., Bueller, J. A., Xu, Y., Kilbourn, M. R., Jewett, D. M., Meyer, C. R., Koeppe, R. A., and Stohler, C. S. 2002. μ-Opioid receptor-mediated antinociceptive responses differ in men and women. *J. Neurosci.* **22**(12):5100–5107.

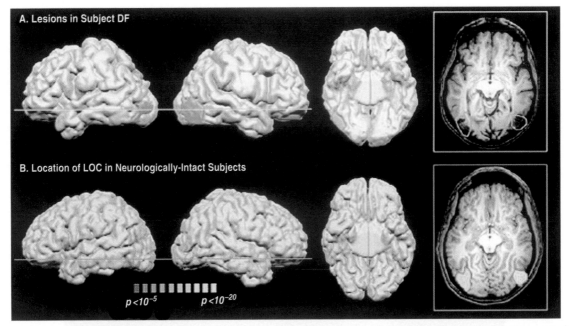

Figure 4.3.　A, B. The ventral visual stream lesions in a patient with visual agnosia (subject DF) are compared to the expected region (lateral occipital complex) for object recognition. A. Lesions in subject DF. Her lesions were traced on slices that indicated tissue damage and rendered on the pial surface in pale blue. Lateral views of the left and right hemispheres are shown, as is a ventral view of the underside of the brain. B. The expected location of the lateral occipital complex based on functional magnetic resonance imaging data from seven neurologically intact participants. The activation of the slice is shown in orange in A for comparison with the lesions in patient DF's brain. (Reproduced with permission from Oxford University Press from James *et al.*, 2003.)

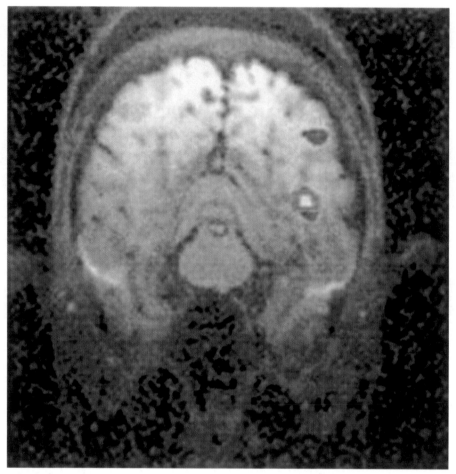

Figure 5.7.   This functional magnetic resonance image shows activation of the "fusiform face area" responsive to human faces. The right hemisphere appears on the left. The brain images at the left show in color the voxels that produced a significantly higher magnetic resonance signal intensity during the epochs containing faces than during those containing objects. These significance images are overlaid on a T1-weighted anatomical image of the same slice. In each image, the region of interest is shown outlined in green. (Reproduced with permission Kanwisher *et al.*, 1997.)

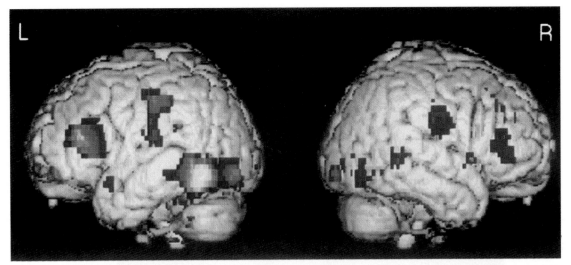

Figure 6.5. Functional magnetic resonance images demonstrating greater activation to words than to consonant letter strings during a nonlinguistic visual feature detection task. The images illustrate a left hemisphere language network for reading probably including temporal–occipital visual word form and lexical regions, an inferior parietal phonological encoding region, and Broca's area in the inferior frontal lobe. The right hemisphere also participates but to a much smaller degree than the left hemisphere. (Reproduced with permission from Price *et al.*, 1996.)

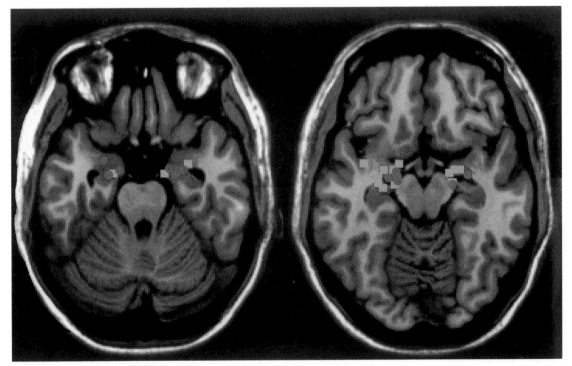

Figure 11.8. Functional magnetic resonance imaging demonstrates activation of both the left and right amygdalae when processing facial expressions of fright (green) as well as during conditioned fear (red). Expressions of fright produce activity more in the left side of the upper amygdala than in the right side, whereas the response to conditioned fear is more evenly distributed. (Reproduced with permission from Vass, 2004.)

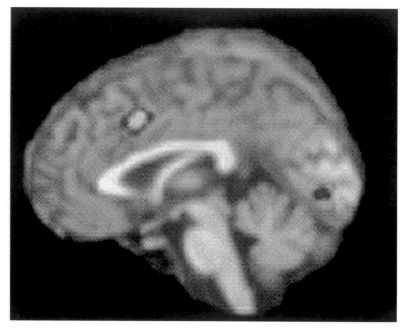

Figure 12.6. Functional magnetic resonance study demonstrates activation of the anterior cingulate gyrus region in the monitoring of conflict (incongruent trials). (Reproduced with permission from Kerns *et al.*, 2004.)

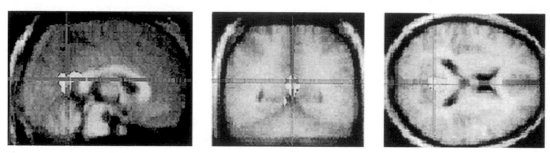

Figure 12.8. Functional magnetic resonance study demonstrates activation of the posterior cingulate gyrus region (including retrosplenial cortex) in assessing the familiarity of a person (faces or voices). (Reproduced with permission from Shah *et al.*, 2001.)

10 Brainstem

The brainstem is the connection between the spinal cord, the cerebellum, and the cerebrum. Only recently has it been implicated in behavior. The brainstem is anatomically comprised of three areas: (1) the medulla, (2) the pons, and (3) the midbrain (see Figure 2.1). The medulla, the inferior segment of the brainstem, represents a conical, expanded continuation of the upper cervical spinal cord. The pons lies between the medulla and the midbrain. The midbrain is the smallest and least differentiated division of the brainstem. The nuclei of cranial nerves III through XII are located in the brainstem along with long sensory and motor tracts that pass between the brain and spinal cord. Several regions of the brainstem, however, seem to be significantly involved in behavior. These behaviorally active regions include: (1) the reticular formation, (2) the parabrachial nucleus, (3) the raphe nuclei, (4) the periaqueductal gray, (5) the nucleus locus ceruleus, (6) the lateral tegmental nucleus, and (7) the ventral tegmental area (VTA). The VTA is considered to be one of the basal ganglia (see Chapter 7).

Anatomy and behavioral considerations

Reticular formation

The reticular formation is one of the oldest portions of the brain and represents the core of the brainstem. It is composed of complex collections of cells that form both diffuse cellular aggregations and more defined nuclei.

The ascending reticular activating system (ARAS) is a physiological concept. It is represented anatomically by the central core region of the brainstem (Figure 10.1), including the raphe nuclei (Figure 10.2). This region contains a number of nuclei. The ARAS receives collateral fibers from the surrounding specific sensory systems. The main long ascending pathway of the brainstem reticular formation is the central tegmental tract (Figure 10.3). This tract projects to the intralaminar nuclei of the thalamus (see Table 9.1, Chapter 9). The reticular formation extends rostrally from the brainstem into the hypothalamus. Ascending reticular fibers to the hypothalamus are distinct from those that go to the thalamus.

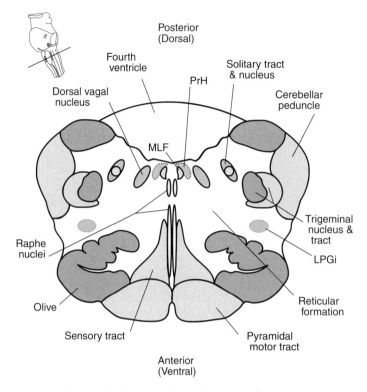

Figure 10.1.   A cross-section typical of the medulla. The brainstem diagram in the upper left indicates the level of the cross-section. Behaviorally significant nuclei are highlighted in red. LPGi, caudal extent of nucleus paragigantocellularis lateralis (positions approximate); MLF, medial longitudinal fasciculus; PrH, nucleus prepositus hypoglossi.

The continuous sensory input into the ARAS plays an important role in wakefulness, alertness, and arousal. Lesions in the rostromedial midbrain tegmentum abolish the electroencephalographic (EEG) arousal reaction elicited by sensory stimulation even though the long ascending sensory pathways remain intact. The cerebral cortex also plays a role in altering the state of consciousness by influencing the reticular neurons. Such a role has been suggested by the well-known arousing effect of psychic stimuli. Areas of the cerebral cortex from which the arousing effect can be obtained by electrical stimulation include the orbital prefrontal cortex, the lateral surface of the frontal lobe, the sensory motor cortex, the superior temporal gyrus, and the cingulate gyrus. The reticular formation has three more important functions: regulation of muscle reflexes, coordination of autonomic functions, and modulation of pain sensation. It is of interest to note that reticular formation neurons involved in the control of breathing and cardiac function are influenced by higher centers, including the hypothalamus and prefrontal association areas.

The pedunculopontine tegmental nucleus (PPTg) is a cholinergic nucleus of the ARAS that is involved in sleep mechanisms (Figure 10.3). It is recognized as important in the induction and maintenance of rapid eye movement (REM) sleep (Semba, 1993). It is considered to be a striatal output station and is a component of the "mesencephalic locomotor region" (Mogenson *et al.*, 1989; Winn *et al.*, 1997). A decrease in choline acetyltransferase has been reported in this nucleus in schizophrenic patients, which suggests a reduction in brainstem

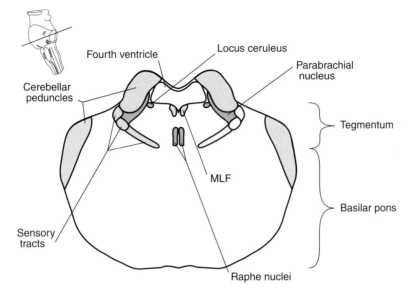

Figure 10.2.   A cross-section typical of the pons. Behaviorally significant nuclei are highlighted in red. The sensory tracts from medial to lateral are the medial lemniscus, the spinal lemniscus, and the lateral lemniscus. MLF, medial longitudinal fasciculus.

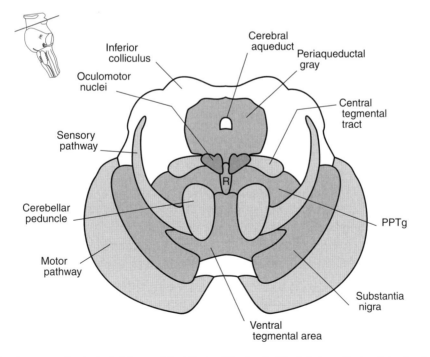

Figure 10.3.   A cross-section typical of the caudal midbrain at the level of the inferior colliculus. Behaviorally significant nuclei are highlighted in red. PPTg, pedunculopontine tegmental nucleus; R, raphe nucleus.

acetylcholine activity in this disorder (Karson *et al.*, 1993). See Chapter 7 for a more complete discussion of the importance of the pedunculopontine tegmental nucleus in the regulation of behavior.

Parabrachial nucleus

The parabrachial nucleus lies medial to the superior cerebellar peduncle and medial to the sensory (lemniscal) tracts in the pons and midbrain (Figure 10.3). It receives visceral sensory information from the spinal cord and brainstem. It gives rise to ascending fibers that project to the hypothalamus (see Chapter 8) and the amygdala (see Chapter 11) and to the raphe nuclei (Holstege, 1988).

The parabrachial nucleus is a general integrative site for visceral information, including taste, cardiorespiratory signals, and visceral pain (Craig, 1996). It links these sensations with the central nucleus of the amygdala and with the hypothalamus (see "autonomic sensory nuclei" in Figure 11.6). It is proposed that the parabrachial nucleus is important in the emotional and autonomic responses to incoming visceral signals, especially visceral pain (Bernard *et al.*, 1996).

Clinical vignette

A 15-year-old boy underwent resection of a cerebellar astrocytoma arising from the fourth ventricle and adherent to the brainstem. Postoperatively he developed a sleep disorder where he suddenly sat up in bed, screamed, and appeared to be staring in fright. During these episodes he was agitated and would try going over the rails or would thrash about in bed screaming. After 1 or 2 min, he promptly fell back to sleep. The patient had incomplete recollections of these episodes. Sometimes the only evidence of an episode was injury or blood on the floor. At other times, he recalled being frightened by images of parts of people sticking out of walls or by the belief that the bedposts were his room-mates restraining him.

The patient's evaluation was consistent with night terrors, or pavor nocturnus, associated with his brainstem lesion. Polysomnography documented his night terrors with spontaneous arousals punctuating all stages of sleep, particularly stage three and four sleep. His episodes of night terrors decreased with the addition of clonazepam at bedtime (Mendez, 1992).

Raphe nuclei

Several groups of cells situated along the midline of the medulla, pons, and midbrain are collectively called the *raphe nuclei* (Figures 10.1–10.4). They are part of the brainstem reticular formation but produce a particular neurotransmitter, serotonin (5-hydroxytryptamine (5-HT)). Neurons from different raphe nuclei contain specific cotransmitters (peptides). Areas that project fibers to the raphe nuclei include the amygdala, hypothalamus, and periaqueductal gray as well as other brainstem nuclei (Figure 10.5).

Rostral pontine and midbrain raphe nuclei project to the periaqueductal gray (PAG) and to structures in the cerebrum. Most pontine raphe nuclei have long ascending projections that are located in the medial forebrain bundle. Fibers project to the hypothalamus, nigral complex, intralaminar thalamic nuclei, stria terminalis, septum, hippocampus, amygdala, and cerebral cortex. Of particular interest are raphe projections to the ventral tegmental

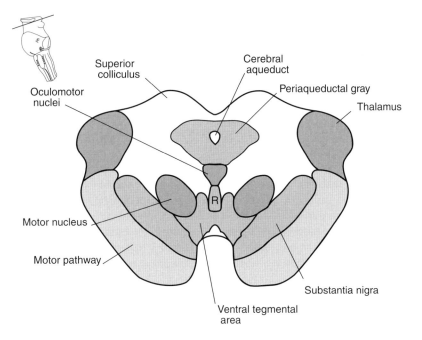

Figure 10.4.   A cross-section typical of the rostral midbrain at the level of the superior colliculus. Behaviorally significant nuclei are highlighted. R, raphe nucleus.

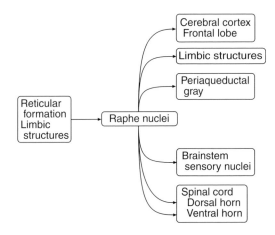

Figure 10.5.   The raphe nuclei are a major source of serotonin. Descending influences can block pain stimuli (dorsal horn) and facilitate motor activity (ventral horn). Ascending projections inhibit nonmeaningful stimuli and facilitate meaningful signals.

area and to the nucleus accumbens. Cortical projections are confined largely to the frontal lobe, although fibers to other neocortical areas have been demonstrated.

  Medullary and caudal pontine raphe nuclei project to other parts of the brainstem and to all levels of the cord. Targets include the trigeminal nuclei and the dorsal and ventral spinal cord gray. These descending projections of the raphe nuclei are ideally situated to regulate incoming sensory stimuli. The raphe spinal tract which terminates in the spinal trigeminal nucleus and in the spinal cord dorsal horn regulates (inhibits) incoming pain signals (Mason and Leung, 1996). The nucleus raphe magnus, which gives rise to the raphe spinal tract, is controlled by neurons in the PAG. Periaqueductal gray neurons, in turn, receive input from the limbic system thus providing a link between emotion, pain, and defense behaviors (see the following section, "Periaqueductal gray"). Other raphe spinal projections that terminate in the ventral horn are thought to function in a neuromodulatory role to facilitate locomotion.

Serotonin and the raphe nuclei have been implicated in the regulation of sleep, aggressive behavior, pain, and a variety of visceral and neuroendocrine functions. Raphe neurons decrease their firing rate from waking to sleep and cease firing during REM sleep. Destruction of serotonin neurons or blockade of serotonin receptors consistently produces an animal that is hypersensitive to virtually all environmental stimuli and is hyperactive in all situations. Serotonin inhibits sensory stimuli that have a waking effect (see next section, "Locus ceruleus and lateral tegmental nucleus"). It may help to facilitate meaningful sensory stimuli and to inhibit non-meaningful sensory stimuli. In this way serotonin aids in maintaining behavior within specific limits.

Clinical vignette

A 59-year-old man was found dead from a self-inflicted gunshot wound. Three years before his death he developed left-sided hemianesthesia. A computed tomographic (CT) scan taken at the time showed a lesion in the tegmentum of the upper pons on the right side. Over the following few months further neurological deficits developed but he was not incapacitated. Five months after the initial episode, severe depression with paranoid ideations developed. The patient had no past or family history of affective disorders. He failed to respond to a number of antidepressants that were tried over a period of 2 years. Postmortem examination revealed a cavernous hemangioma impinging on the upper pontine region of the raphe nuclei on the right side and extending to partially involve the raphe on the left side. It was believed that the lesion caused depletion of the ascending serotonergic system to the forebrain (Kline and Oertel, 1997).

Clinical vignette

A 55-year-old right-handed male presented with acute, uncontrolled crying spells and numbness over his left face and arm. Around 6:00 a.m. he awoke with a diffuse, pressure headache and suddenly started crying for no apparent reason. This crying abruptly ceased after 5 min. Over the next 2–3 h, he had five more crying spells, each lasting 5–10 min, occurring out-of-context, without precipitating factors or sadness, with an acute onset and offset, and without alteration of consciousness. The patient's left face and arm numbness persisted during and between these crying spells but abruptly resolved shortly after his last crying spell.

After an extensive neurological evaluation, his diagnosis was transient ischemic attacks with crying spells. The transient ischemic attacks could have involved the right brainstem and the raphe nuclei. This patient may have had a temporary activation or stimulation of ischemic areas or alterations in serotonergic neurons (Mendez and Bronstein, 1999).

Serotonergic neurons may have a priming effect on the cells of the nucleus locus ceruleus (LC), which are responsible for triggering the REM sleep stage(Jacobs, 1994). In contrast to the LC neurons, which increase their firing rate during periods of intense environmental stimuli, the serotonergic neurons fire more rapidly during periods of quiet, rhythmical behaviors such as grooming or chewing, behaviors associated with a relaxed state (Jacobs and Fornal, 1993).

Activity in the dorsal raphe nuclei raises the threshold that activates defensive behaviors controlled by the periaqueductal gray of the midbrain. Medullary raphe nuclei play a similar role in the modulation of cardiovascular responses to stress (Lovick, 1996). Projections from the raphe nuclei to the mesolimbic structures (ventral tegmental area and nucleus accumbens) provide a link between serotonin and dopamine. It is hypothesized that the raphe nuclei play an important regulatory role in the control of dopamine release. Because of this relationship the raphe nuclei may play a role in schizophrenia (Mylecharane, 1996).

A loss of the serotonergic neurons of the raphe nuclei has been documented in Alzheimer's disease (Aletrino *et al.*, 1992). However, the concentration of cortical serotonin was found to be in the normal range, suggesting that sprouting of raphe axon terminals in the cortex makes up for the deficiency of serotonin due to raphe neuron loss (Chen *et al.*, 1996).

Blood levels of serotonin are elevated in autistic and in retarded individuals. The significance of this finding is obscure since cerebrospinal fluid (CSF) levels do not correlate with blood levels. It has been suggested that the abnormal serotonin levels may reflect a role played by serotonin in brain development.

Uncontrolled crying is a behavior commonly seen after stroke (1-year incidence is 20%). Successful treatment by selective serotonin reuptake inhibitor drugs has led to the suggestion that this behavior results from stroke-induced partial destruction of raphe nuclei or of their ascending projections to the cerebral hemispheres (Andersen, 1995).

Periaqueductal gray

The periaqueductal gray (PAG) surrounds the cerebral aqueduct in the midbrain (see Figures 10.3 and 10.4). It is connected with many forebrain structures above as well as with brainstem structures below. It has reciprocal connections with the central nucleus of the amygdala. Descending fibers from the PAG include those to the raphe nuclei involved in the suppression of incoming pain signals. The PAG is centrally located between the limbic system and somatic and visceral motor control centers. The central nucleus of the amygdala of the limbic system is also an important source of fibers to the PAG (see Chapter 11; Figure 11.6).

The PAG is important in eliciting many somatic and visceral stereotypical behaviors. It is the major center through which the hypothalamus enacts behaviors critical to the survival of the self and of the species. These behaviors include regulation of heart rate and respiration, urination, grooming, and defensive and reproductive behaviors (Craig, 1996). Other behaviors elicited by stimulating the PAG include threat, freezing, escape, and vocalization (Bandler and Keay, 1996).

Stimulation of the PAG evoked "feelings of fear and death" (Nashold *et al.*, 1974). Facial blushing, sweating, and other autonomic responses were noted. It has been suggested that the PAG may play a key role in triggering panic (Gorman *et al.*, 1989: see Chapter 11).

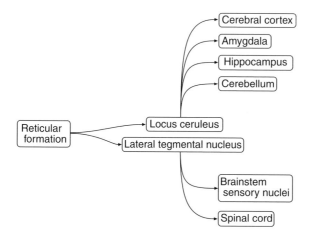

Figure 10.6.   The locus ceruleus and lateral tegmental nucleus provide norepinephric projections to the entire neuraxis. Novel environmental stimuli act through norepinephrine to direct the brain to alert, orient, and attend to selective stimuli. The two specific reticular nuclei that contact the locus ceruleus are nucleus hypoglossi prepositus and nucleus paragigantocellularis.

Locus ceruleus and lateral tegmental nucleus

The LC is represented by a group of distinct nerve cell bodies that make up a nucleus near the ventrolateral corner of the fourth ventricle in the pontine tegmentum (see Figure 10.2). It extends rostrally into the periaqueductal gray of the midbrain. Cells of the LC are rich in norepinephrine (NE), and the LC contains half the NE neurons found in the brain.

Input to the LC is provided largely by two reticular nuclei, the nucleus prepositus hypoglossi and the nucleus paragigantocellularis (see PrH and LPGi, Figures 10.1 and 10.6; Aston-Jones *et al.*, 1995). The nucleus prepositus hypoglossi provides inhibitory input whereas the nucleus paragigantocellularis provides strong excitatory input (Aston-Jones *et al.*, 1990, 1991a). The prepositus hypoglossi nucleus receives input from the nucleus of the solitary tract, which conveys information about the vegetative state of the body. The prepositus also receives input from other brainstem sensory nuclei and from the spinal cord (Aston-Jones *et al.*, 1991a). The nucleus paragigantocellularis receives signals from diverse sites throughout the brainstem and spinal cord that are associated with autonomic and integrative functions (Aston-Jones *et al.*, 1991b). Other fibers to the LC arrive from the parabrachial nucleus, the PAG, and the hypothalamus. It was suggested that one or more of these sources may be important in the inhibition of neuron discharge seen in the LC during paradoxical sleep (Luppi *et al.*, 1995).

The ascending projection from the LC represents the majority of the output of the LC. This group of fibers passes rostrally through the midbrain, lateral to the medial longitudinal fasciculus. The fibers accompany the medial forebrain bundle to and through the lateral hypothalamus. This ascending pathway continues rostrally to levels of the anterior commissure, where it divides into fibers that innervate midline portions of the thalamus, the amygdaloid nuclear complex, the hippocampus, and vast regions of the cortex (Foote *et al.*, 1983). Other fibers from the LC pass via the fornix to the hippocampal formation and as a component of the cingulum to the cingulate cortex. A contingent of fibers even terminates in the cerebellum (see Chapter 2). Descending fibers from the LC are relatively sparse. Efferent fibers from the LC to the caudal brainstem terminate on sensory nuclei, and fibers to the spinal cord end in both the dorsal and the ventral horn (Holets, 1988).

One of the most profuse projections of the LC is to the thalamus, where terminals are found in the intralaminar and anterior nuclei (see Table 9.1). These thalamic nuclei are included as part of the limbic thalamus. They project to all cortical areas and have been linked to arousal and selective attention. The NE system that arises in the LC "is unique in the brain in that it innervates more CNS areas than any other single nucleus" (Aston-Jones *et al.*, 1995). The remarkable feature of the LC projection is its wide distribution throughout the brain. Each LC neuron may contact thousands of cortical neurons. The most rostrally projecting fibers of the LC exit from the medial forebrain bundle and distribute to the rostral, dorsal, and lateral cortex of the frontal lobe, where they terminate in the most superficial cortical layer, which is considered an important site for cortical integration.

The lateral tegmental nucleus is represented by scattered NE neurons that extend ventrolaterally from the LC to the ventral aspect of the brainstem. Although these cells may appear to be only a ventrolateral extension of the LC, the connections of the lateral tegmental nucleus differ from those of the LC. Targets of the fibers from the lateral tegmental nucleus generally do not overlap those of the LC, thus justifying the recognition of the lateral tegmental nucleus as more than just an extension of the LC. Major projections descend and terminate in the spinal cord and brainstem. More diffuse projections terminate in the thalamus, hypothalamus, amygdala, and cerebellar cortex (Burstein, 1996). *Like the NE neurons of the LC, lateral tegmental nucleus neurons also cease firing during sleep.*

The locus ceruleus regulates arousal, attention and related autonomic tone. Locus ceruleus neurons respond with increased rates of firing to novel environmental stimuli but not to routine environmental stimuli (Jacobs, 1990). Stimuli that are effective in producing a response in the neurons of the LC are stimuli that disrupt ongoing behavior and elicit an orienting response. The largest response in LC activity occurs during an abrupt transition from sleep to waking (Aston-Jones *et al.*, 1996).

The ascending LC system is believed to function in arousal. It determines the salience of a target and is speculated to facilitate some types of learning. A relatively low tonic level of LC activity is associated with inattention. A high tonic level of LC activity is associated with labile attention and poor task performance – behavior often seen in attention deficit-hyperactivity disorder. Phasic discharge of LC neurons in response to a specific task against a background of low tonic activity results in improved performance. The locus ceruleus and sympathetic nervous system are activated at the same time to deal with perceived emergency situations (Aston-Jones et al., 1997). It is interesting to note that alcohol activates the norepinephrine system through a system that involves serotonin (Blum and Kozlowski, 1990).

Norepinephrine facilitates long-term potentiation of hippocampal neurons, indicating that it can influence memory. NE functions in the cortex to inhibit ongoing random neuron activity and to potentiate neuron response to selective stimuli, thus increasing the signal-to-noise ratio for incoming sensory signals. Actions of NE on the thalamus and cortex enhance the signal processing ability of the forebrain (Berridge, 1993). Norepinephrine produces a slow excitatory postsynaptic potential (EPSP) in neurons of the hippocampus and over a wide area of the cerebral cortex (Nicoll *et al.*, 1987).

The LC is believed to play an important role in the initiation of REM sleep. Locus ceruleus neurons are inactive during sleep, and electrical stimulation of the LC and subsequent release of NE produce an increase in the state of arousal (Aston-Jones and Bloom, 1981). The administration of NE is known to increase the state of arousal and also to increase the level of anxiety. Both arousal and anxiety, therefore, may be linked to the LC. Monoamine oxidase (MOA) inhibitors and tricyclic agents, which are effective in treating depression in patients, inhibit the firing of LC neurons in experimental animals. The high level of anxiety and loss of pleasure reported by depressed patients may be related to the loss of regulation of NE by LC neurons.

Acute exposure to opiates inhibits the action of LC neurons by binding μ receptors that are coupled to G protein (see Chapter 3) (Williams *et al.*, 2001). In contast, chronic exposure to opiates increases the excitability of the LC neurons by up regulation of the intracellular cAMP pathway (Nestler and Aghajanian, 1997). This is an expected response that brings the LC firing rate back toward a normal level. When opiates are withdrawn, the LC is activated. This activation is responsible for some of the behavioral signs of withdrawal.

A loss of cells is seen in the LC of patients with Parkinson' s disease or Alzheimer' s disease (Zweig *et al.*, 1993). These individuals are often diagnosed with depression, and cell loss in the LC correlates with depressive signs and symptoms (Forstl *et al.*, 1992). One model of depression recognizes the degeneration or retraction, or both, of LC neurons as part of the pathophysiology of this disorder (Kitayama *et al.*, 1994). Locus ceruleus neurons are sensitive to corticotropin-releasing factor (CRF), and the hypothalamic–pituitary–adrenal (HPA) axis is activated in depression and altered in panic disorder (see Chapter 8). The increase in CRF production during activation of the HPA axis may involve the LC in these disorders. Some antidepressant drugs may act by blocking CRF activation of the LC (Curtis and Valentino, 1994). In contrast, loss of cells in the LC was seen in patients with Alzheimer's disease, but there was no additional loss of LC neurons in patients with both Alzheimer's disease and depression (Hoogendijk *et al.*, 1999).

The effect of alcoholism on the loss of LC neurons remains in question (Halliday and Baker, 1996). Locus ceruleus neurons increase their firing rate during opiate withdrawal (Self and Nestler, 1995). No change was seen in the number of LC neurons in patients with schizophrenia, but a significant reduction in neuron size was reported (Karson *et al.*, 1991).

A model has been proposed which suggests that an increase in LC activity is involved in attention-deficit hyperactivity disorder. The model proposes that LC neurons fire at an abnormally high level as a result of a biochemical defect in the brainstem systems that regulate the LC (Mefford and Potter, 1989).

SELECT BIBLIOGRAPHY

V. Arango, M.D. Underwood, and J.J. Mann, Biological alterations in the brainstem of suicides. *Psychiatric Clinics of North America*, **20** (1997), 581–594.

M.B. Carpenter, and J. Sutin, *Human Neuroanatomy.* (Baltimore, Md.: Williams and Wilkins, 1983).

R.E. Hales, and S.C. Ydofsky. *Textbook of Neuropsychiatry.* (Washington D.C.: American Psychiatric Association Press, 1987.)

G. Holstege, R. Bandler, and C.B. Saper, The emotional motor system. *Progress in Brain Research*, **107**, (1996).

REFERENCES

Aletrino, M. A., Vogels, D. J. M., Van Doinburg, P. H. M. F., and Ten Donkelaar, H. J. 1992. Cell loss in the nucleus raphe dorsalis in Alzheimer's disease. *Neurobiol. Aging* **13**:461–468.

Andersen, G. 1995. Treatment of uncontrolled crying after stroke. *Drugs Aging* **6**:105–111.

Aston-Jones, G., and Bloom, F. E. 1981. Norepinephrine containing locus coeruleus neurons in behaving rats exhibit pronounced responses to non-noxious environmental stimuli. *J. Neurosci.* **1**:887–900.

Aston-Jones, G., Shipley, M. T., Ennis, M., Williams, J. T., and Pieribone, V. A. 1990. Restricted afferent control of locus coeruleus neurons revealed by anatomical, physiological, and pharmacological studies. In: D. J. Heal, and C. A. Marsden (eds.) *The Pharmacology of Noradrenaline in the Central Nervous System.* Oxford: Oxford University Press, pp. 187–247.

Aston-Jones, G., Chiang, C., and Alexinsky, T. 1991a. Discharge of noradrenergic locus coeruleus neurons in behaving rats and monkeys suggests a role in vigilance. *Prog. Brain Res.* **88**:501–520.

Aston-Jones, G., Shipley, M. T., Chouvet, G., Ennis, M., van Bockstaele, E., Pieribone, V., Shiekhattar, R., Akaoka, H., Drolet, G., Astier, B., Charlety, P., Valentino, R. J., and Williams, J. T. 1991b. Afferent regulation of locus coeruleus neurons: anatomy, physiology and pharmacology. *Prog. Brain Res.* **88**:47–75.

Aston-Jones, G., Shipley, M. T., and Grzanna, R. 1995. The locus coeruleus, A5 and A7 noradrenergic cell groups. In: G. Paxinos (ed.) *The Rat Nervous System*, 2nd edn. San Diego, Calif.: Academic Press, pp. 183–213.

Aston-Jones, G., Rajkowski, J., Kubiak, P., Valentino, R. J., and Shipley, M. T. 1996. Role of the locus coeruleus in emotional activation. In: G. Holstege, R. Bandler, and C. B. Saper (eds.) The emotional motor system. *Prog. Brain Res.* **107**:379–402.

Aston-Jones, G., Rajkowski, R., and Kubiak, P. 1997. Conditioned responses of monkey locus coeruleus neurons anticipate acquisition of discriminative behavior in a vigilance task. *Neuroscience* **80**:697–715.

Bandler, R., and Keay, K. A. 1996. Columnar organization in the midbrain periaqueductal gray and the integration of emotional expression. In: G. Holstege, R. Bandler, and C. B. Saper (eds.) The emotional motor system. *Prog. Brain Res.* **107**:285–300.

Bernard, J. F., Bester, H., and Besson, J. M. 1996. Involvement of the spino-parabrachio-amygdaloid and -hypothalamic pathways in the autonomic and affective emotional aspects of pain. In: G. Holstege, R. Bandler, and C. B. Saper (eds.) The emotional motor system. *Prog. Brain Res.* **107**:243–255.

Berridge, D. W. 1993. Noradrenergic modulation of cognitive function: clinical implications of anatomical, electrophysiological and behavioural studies in animal models. *Psychol. Med.* **23**:557–564.

Blum, K., and Kozlowski, G. P. 1990. Ethanol and neuromodulator interactions: a cascade model of reward. *Prog. Alcohol Res.* **2**:131–149.

Burstein, R. 1996. Somatosensory and visceral input to the hypothalamus and limbic system. In: G. Holstege, R. Bandler, and C. B. Saper (eds.) The emotional motor system. *Prog. Brain Res.* **107**:257–267.

Chen, C. P., Adler, J. T., Bowen, D. M., Esiri, M. M., McDonald, B., Hope, T., Jobst, K. A., and Francis, P. T. 1996. Presynaptic serotonergic dysfunction in patients with Alzheimer's disease: correlations with depression and neuroleptic medication. *J. Neurochem.* **66**:1592–1598.

Craig, A. D. 1996. An ascending general homeostatic afferent pathway originating in lamina I. In: G. Holstege, R. Bandler, and C. B. Saper (eds.) The emotional motor system. *Prog. Brain Res.* **107**:226–242.

Curtis, A. L., and Valentino, R. J. 1994. Corticotropin-releasing factor neurotransmission in locus coeruleus: a possible site of antidepressant action. *Brain Res. Bull.* **35**:581–587.

Foote, S. L., Bloom, F. E., and Aston-Jones, G. 1983. Nucleus locus ceruleus: new evidence of anatomical and physiological specificity. *Physiol. Rev.* **63**:844–901.

Forstl, H., Burns, A., Luthert, P., Cairns, N., Lantos, P., and Levy, R. 1992. Clinical and neuropathological correlates of depression in Alzheimer's disease. *Psychol. Med.* **22**:877–884.

Gorman, J. M., Liebowitz, M. R., Fyer, A. J., and Stein, J. 1989. A neuroanatomical hypothesis for panic disorder. *Am. J. Psychiatry* **146**:148–161.

Halliday, G., and Baker, K. 1996. Noradrenergic locus coeruleus neurons. *Alcohol Clin. Exp. Res.* **20**:191–192.

Holets, V. R. 1988. Locus coeruleus neurons in the rat containing neuropeptide Y, tyrosine hydroxylase or galanin and their efferent projections to the spinal cord, cerebral cortex and hypothalamus. *Neuroscience* **24**:893–906.

Holstege, G. 1988. Anatomical evidence for a strong ventral parabrachial projection to nucleus raphe magnus and adjacent tegmental field. *Brain Res.* **447**:154–158.

Hoogendijk, W. J. G., Sommer, I. E. C., Pool, C. W., Kamphorst, W., Hofman, M. A., Eikelnboom, P., and Swaab, D. F. 1999. Lack of association between depression and loss of neurons in the locus coeruleus in Alzheimer disease. *Arch. Gen. Psychiatry* **56**:45–51.

Jacobs, B. L. 1990. Locus coeruleus neuronal activity in behaving animals. In: D. J. Heal, and C. A Marsden (eds.) *The Pharmacology of Noradrenaline in the Central Nervous System*. Oxford: Oxford University Press, pp. 248–265.

— 1994. Serotonin, motor activity and depression-related disorders. *Am. Sci.* **82**:456–463.

Jacobs, B. L., and Fornal, C. A. 1993. 5-HT and motor control: a hypothesis. *Trends Neurosci.* **16**:346–352.

Karson, C. N., Garcia-Rill, E., Biedermann, J., Mrak, R. E., Husain, M. M., and Skinner, R. D. 1991. The brain stem reticular formation in schizophrenia. *Psychiatry Res.* **40**:31–48.

Karson, C. N., Casanova, M. F., Kleinman, J. E., and Griffin, W. S. T. 1993. Choline acetyltransferase in schizophrenia. *Am. J. Psychiatry* **50**:454–459.

Kitayama, I., Nakamura, S., Yaga, T., Murase, S., Nomura, J., Kayahara, T., and Nakano, K. 1994. Degeneration of locus coeruleus axons in stress-induced depression model. *Brain Res. Bull.* **35**:573–580.

Kline, P., and Oertel, J. 1997. Depression associated with pontine vascular malformation. *Biol. Psychiatry* **42**:519–521.

Lovick, T. A. 1996. Midbrain and medullary regulation of defensive cardiovascular functions. In: G. Holstege, R. Bandler, and C. B. Saper (eds.) The emotional motor system. *Prog. Brain Res.* **107**:301–313.

Luppi, P.-H., Aston-Jones, G., Akaoka, H., Chouvet, G., and Jouvet, M. 1995. Afferent projections to the rat locus coeruleus demonstrated by retrograde and anterograde tracing with cholera-toxin B subunit and *Phaseolus vulgaris* leucoagglutinin. *Neuroscience* **65**:119–160.

Mason, P., and Leung, C. G. 1996. Physiological functions of pontomedullary raphe and medial reticular neurons. In: G. Holstege, R. Bandler, and C. B. Saper (eds.) The emotional motor system. *Prog. Brain Res.* **107**:269–282.

Mefford, I. N., and Potter, W. Z. 1989. a neuroanatomical and biochemical basis of attention deficit disorder with hyperactivity in children: a defect in tonic adrenaline mediated inhibition of locus coeruleus stimulation. *Med. Hypotheses* **29**:33–42.

Mendez, M. F. 1992. Pavor nocturnus from a brainstem glioma. *J. Neurol. Neurosurg. Psychiatry* **55**:860.

Mendez, M. F., and Bronstein, Y. L. 1999. Crying spells presenting as a transient ischemic attack. *J. Neurol. Neurosurg. Psychiatry* **67**:255.

Mogenson, G. J., Wu, M., and Tsai, C. T. 1989. Subpallidal-pedunculopontine projections but not subpallidal-mediodorsal thalamus projections contribute to spontaneous exploratory locomotor activity. *Brain. Res.* **485**:396–398.

Mylecharane, E. J. 1996. Ventral tegmental area 5-HT receptors: mesolimbic dopamine release and behavioural studies. *Behav. Brain Res.* **73**:1–5.

Nashold, B. S. Jr., Wilson, W. P., and Slaugher, G. 1974. The midbrain and pain. In: J. J. Bonica (ed.) International Symposium on Pain. *Adv. Neurol.* **4**:191–196.

Nestler, E. J., and Aghajanian, G. K. 1997. Molecular and cellular basis of addiction. *Science* **278**:58–63.

Nicoll, R. A., Madison, D. V., and Lancaster, B. 1987. Noradrenergic modulation of neuronal excitability in mammalian hippocampus. In: H. Y. Meltzer (ed.) *Psychopharmacology: The Third Generation of Progress.* New York: Raven Press, pp. 105–112.

Self, D. W., and Nestler, E. J. 1995. Molecular mechanisms of drug reinforcement and addiction. *Annu. Rev. Neurosci.* **18**:463–495.

Semba, K. 1993. Aminergic and cholinergic afferents to REM sleep induction regions of the pontine reticular formation in the rat. *J. Comp. Neurol.* **330**:543–556.

Williams, J. T., Christie, M. J., and Manszoni, O. 2001. Cellular and synaptic adaptations mediating opioid dependence. *Physiol. Rev.* **81**:299–343.

Winn, P., Brown, V. J., and Inglis, W. L. 1997. On the relationships between the striatum and the pedunculopontine tegmental nucleus. *Crit. Rev. Neurobiol.* **11**:241–261.

Zweig, R. M., Cardillo, J. E., Cohen, M., Giere, S., and Hedreen, J. C. 1993. The locus coeruleus and dementia in Parkinson's disease. *Neurology* **43**:986–991.

11 Limbic system: temporal lobe

The temporal lobe can be divided into two subdivisions. The newer lateral portion (neo-cortical) is responsible for audition, for speech, and for the integration of sensory information from a variety of sensory modalities and is the topic of Chapter 5. The other division of the temporal lobe is the ventromedial portion, which is older cortex (archicortex and paleocortex) and consists of regions that have become recognized as components of the limbic system. The limbic system structures that are part of the temporal lobe include the parahippocampal gyrus (see Figures 5.2 and 13.1), the entorhinal cortex, the hippocampal formation (Figure 11.1), the uncus (see Figure 13.2), the amygdala, and the cortex of the temporal pole (Martin, 1996). All sensory information from the external world passes through unimodal and multimodal association areas before finally converging on the hippocampus and amygdala. These structures can be considered to be supramodal centers. Chapter 13 provides an overall picture of the limbic system.

The hippocampus is important in memory and for learning the importance of specific external stimuli. The amygdala appears to be important in emotional conditioning and in learning the relationship between internal and external cues related to emotion and affect (Bechara *et al.*, 1995).

Hippocampal formation

The hippocampal formation occupies a central position in the limbic system (Figures 11.1–11.3). Superficially, cortex near the rostral end of the parahippocampal gyrus is the entorhinal cortex and corresponds with BA 28 (Figures 13.1 and 13.2). The parahippocampal gyrus rolls medially deep to the surface to produce the parahippocampal sulcus. The hippocampal formation lies deep within the parahippocampal sulcus and forms a portion of the medial wall of the temporal horn of the lateral ventricle (Figure 11.2). The hippocampal formation consists of the subiculum, the hippocampus proper, and the dentate gyrus.

The entorhinal cortex is the gateway to the hippocampal formation (Figure 11.3). It receives input from the olfactory bulb, prepyriform area, amygdala, and multimodal association areas of the temporal and frontal lobes. The entorhinal cortex is made up of six layers. However, its cellular structure differs significantly from that of other

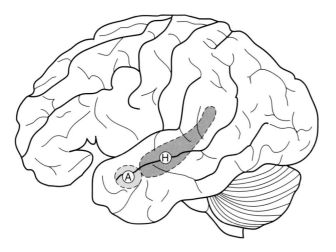

Figure 11.1.   The approximate location of the amygdala (A) and hippocampus (H) in the temporal lobe is indicated. Compare
with Figure 2.2.

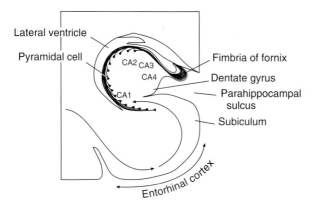

Figure 11.2.   A diagrammatic cross-section through the ventromedial temporal lobe and the entorhinal cortex of the
parahippocampal gyrus. The hippocampal formation consists of the subiculum, the dentate gyrus, and the
hippocampus proper. The hippocampus proper is made up of four longitudinal zones, CA1–CA4. Information
enters the hippocampal formation via the entorhinal cortex and exits via the fornix.

six-layered neocortical regions, and it is probably a form of transitional cortex. Two
pathways conduct signals from the entorhinal cortex to the hippocampal formation.
Axons pass from the medial entorhinal cortex to the hippocampal formation as the
alvear pathway and terminate in the subiculum and CA1. Axons from the lateral entorhinal cortex make up the perforant pathway that terminates in the dentate gyrus
and all sectors of the hippocampus except CA4. The perforant pathway has been
described as the "single most vulnerable circuit in the cerebral cortex" (Morrison
and Hof, 1997).

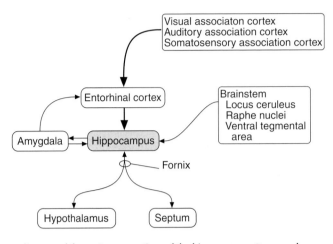

Figure 11.3. A diagram of the major connections of the hippocampus. Processed sensory information arrives at the hippocampus via the entorhinal cortex. Major hippocampal efferents project to the amygdala, hypothalamus, and septum.

The hippocampus is more primitive than the entorhinal cortex and consists of only three cell layers. Four subdivisions within the hippocampus are recognized (Figure 11.2). These longitudinally oriented zones are referred to as CA1, CA2, CA3, and CA4. CA refers to cornu ammonis, or Ammon's horn, an early name for the hippocampus. CA1 lies ventrolaterally, and CA4 lies medially near the origin of the fornix. The pyramidal cell is the most distinctive cell of the hippocampal formation. Moderate amounts of dopamine, norepinephrine, and acetylcholine are present in the hippocampal formation. In addition to the entorhinal cortex, other sources of input to the hippocampal formation include the septal nuclei, hypothalamus, and thalamus as well as the brainstem (Figure 11.3).

Two functional separate circuits involve these sectors. A direct entorhinal-CA1 circuit is important for recollection-based recognition memory. The CA3 sector coupled with CA1 is necessary for recall (Brun *et al.*, 2002).

The glutamatergic hypothesis of schizophrenia suggests that there is a disruption of glutamate-mediated transmission within the hippocampus. Antagonism of the glutamatergic *N*-methyl-ᴅ-aspartic acid (NMDA) receptor has produced behavioral and cognitive effects in normal subects similar to schizophrenia (Krystal *et al.*, 1999). A reduction in excitatory transmission, especially in CA1, is proposed to result in decreased glutamatergic stimulation of the anterior cingulate cortex, the nucleus accumbens, and the temporal cortex (Tamminga,1998, 1999). Hippocampal neurons appear to be particularly vulnerable following traumatic brain injury (McCarthy, 2003).

Signals leave the hippocampus by way of the axons of the pyramidal cells (Figure 11.2). These axons accumulate medially to form the fimbria of the fornix (Figures 11.2 and 11.3). Efferent fibers from the hippocampus project to the septal area and to the hypothalamus. Reciprocal (back-and-forth) connections exist between the hippocampus and the amygdala (Amaral *et al.*, 1992).

The hippocampal formation is well known for its role in memory. It is responsible for the formation of declarative memory, which is the memory of facts, experiences, and information about events. The hippocampus will retain the memory for weeks to months before it is consolidated elsewhere in the cortex.

One hypothesis of memory involving the hippocampal formation is based on the concept of a "cognitive map" (Jacobs and Schenk, 2003). This hypothesis proposes that the original need for memory was for a mechanism that would provide for the ability to return to home. It seems to contain a world-centered map as opposed to the egocentric map found in the posterior parietal lobe. Declarative memory grew from the map mechanism and much of declarative memory is based on a stepwise sequence of events similar to those experienced as one journeys away from home. It may be speculated that one role of the hippocampus is to establish meaningful relationships between various stimuli such as objects, faces, names, etc. Large ensembles of neurons from the CA1 region of the rat were recorded during spatial exploration (Wilson and McNaughton, 1993). The investigators could determine the location of the rat by analyzing the pattern of ensemble firing. Expression of a gene (Zif268) in the hippocampus promotes the consolidation of memory in rats (Izquierdo and Cammarota, 2004).

Clinical vignette

A 40-year-old right-handed man was hospitalized for delirium and generalized seizures. On examination, he was confused, disoriented, and febrile. He was treated for presumed herpes simplex encephalitis with aciclovir and phenytoin. Magnetic resonance imaging subsequently showed hyperintense lesions in the left mesial temporal lobe with significant swelling consistent with herpes encephalitis (Figure 11.4).

After recovery, the patient was left with a severe amnestic disorder from damage to the left hippocampal formation and parahippocampal gyrus. He had difficulty learning any new information and an inability to recall any items on delayed recall tests. His remote memory, however, remained intact.

The posterior hippocampal gray matter volume is greater in experienced London taxi drivers compared with control subjects and the gray matter volume of the right posterior hippocampus volume varies positively with the time driving (Maguire *et al.*, 2000). This difference appears to be the result of experience and not innate navigational expertise (Maguire *et al.*, 2003).

Sleep may be important in consolidating memories. Changes seen between training sessions are believed to be due to increased synaptic connections formed when sessions were replayed in the hippocampus when the animals slept (Skaggs and McNaughton, 1996).

Hippocampal structures have been implicated in both cognitive and emotional processes. It is speculated that the hippocampal formation deals with two forms of information. One form arrives from other areas of the cortex, is cognitive in nature, and enters by way of the entorhinal cortex. The other form arrives from the septum, hypothalamus, and brainstem and is related to the behavioral/emotional state (Swanson *et al.*, 1987). The hippocampal-septal "corridor" is believed to have an important modulatory effect on hypothalamic–brainstem structures involved in various endocrine, autonomic and somatomotor aspects of emotional behavior (Alheid and Heimer, 1996).

The hippocampus is activated during rapid eye movement (REM) sleep, and it is likely that it contributes significantly to the REM sleep phenomenon. It appears that limbic activation may be necessary in order to bring to a conscious level percepts that are being processed in the temporal lobe.

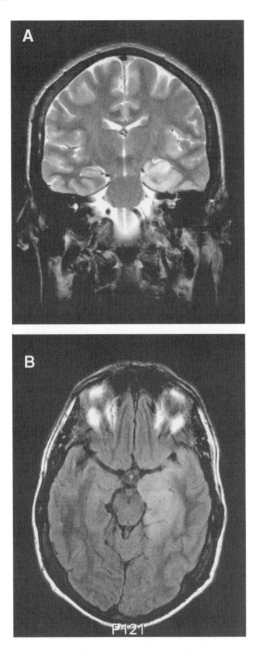

Figure 11.4. A. A coronal cut showed an area of hyperintensity in the left medial temporal lobe on T2-weighted magnetic resonance imaging. B. A horizontal view revealed mass effect from the left medial temporal inflammation. (Reprinted with permission from Mendez and Cummings, 2003.)

The dentate gyrus is a source of new neurons throughout life but production decreases dramatically in old age (Cameron and McKay, 1999). The stem cells migrate rostrally into the olfactory bulb, some migrate into the granular cell layer and others enter into CA1 of the hippocampus (Jin *et al.*, 2004). Jacobs (2002) suggests the new cells may be maintained following a process termed "use it or lose it." It has been estimated that upwards of 10 000 new cells are added each day to the dentate gyrus in the adult rat (Cameron and McKay, 2001). (Neurogenesis declines when corticosterone levels increase (Gould *et al.*, 1997) but increases with higher levels of estrogen (Tanapat *et al.*, 1999).) Other factors including haloperidol (Eisch *et al.*, 2000), glutamate antagonists (Gould *et al.*, 1994), serotonin (Brezun and Daszuta, 1999), and even electroconvulsive shock (Madsen *et al.*, 2000) promote neurogenesis.

Jacobs (2002) hypothesized that a decrease in neurogenesis may provoke clinical depression. The importance of serotonin in the support of neurogenesis as well as the role of the immune system were included in the hypothesis.

Lesions restricted to the hippocampus proper, the fornix, the subiculum or the dentate gyrus each produce deficits in declarative memory (Squire *et al.*, 1990). None of these restricted lesions is as disruptive to memory as is a lesion that involves all of these plus the surrounding temporal cortex (Delis and Lucas, 1996). In addition to temporal lobe structures, lesions involving the fornix, the mamillary body, and the medial thalamus can produce amnesia. Patients who present with severe amnesia without dementia typically have lesions in the medial temporal lobe. The amnesia is anterograde; that is, the ability to store and recall information is lost subsequent to the date of the damage to the medial temporal lobe. Events that took place up to several years before the date of the lesion may be hazy. Childhood memories remain intact.

Imaging studies have revealed differences between control subjects and schizophrenic patients in a number of cortical regions. The most consistent findings are in the region of the medial temporal lobe (Kotrla and Weinberger, 1995). Abnormalities in the histology of the entorhinal cortex have played an important role in discussions of the neuroanatomical substrates of schizophrenia. A bilateral reduction in overall volume of the hippocampus is reported in patients with schizophrenia (Nelson *et al.*, 1998). Decreases in mean neuronal density have been reported (Krimer *et al.*, 1995, 1997) along with disruption of cortical layers and a decrease in mean neuronal size (Heckers and Heinsen, 1991; Jakob and Beckmann, 1994). If it is true that the numbers of neurons remain constant while the volume of tissue is reduced, then this suggests that there is abnormal connectivity ("wiring"). The areas most affected include the entorhinal area, the subiculum, and the left anterior and mid-regions of CA1 and CA2 in the hippocampus (Arnold *et al.*, 1995; Narr *et al.*, 2004). These abnormalities are compatible with neurodevelopmental models of schizophrenia that describe abnormal synaptic pruning (Figure 6.7) and abnormal embryological migration of neurons (Arnold *et al.*, 1997). However, there is also reported to be a selective decrease in the actual number of nonpyramidal cells of CA2 in schizophrenics and manic depressives which indicates that cell loss in the hippocampus may be a contributing factor in the pathophysiology of major psychoses (Benes *et al.*, 1998).

Heckers (2001) summarizes hippocampal findings in schizophrenic in three points. First, most studies found a decrease in volume in schizophrenia patients. This reduction is subtle and is in the order of 4% as compared to healthy controls. This is significantly different from the pronounced volume reduction seen in neurodegenerative disorders such as Alzheimer's disease. Second, this reduction is seen early in the disease process with evidence of subsequent slow progression of volume loss. Third, volume loss may be affecting certain parts of the hippocampus more than others (some studies report the volume loss to affect mainly the anterior half of the hippocampus). This finding suggests that not all hippocampal functions are impaired in schizophrenia.

Recent studies extended the findings to at-risk children (children of schizophrenic parents). Pantelis *et al.* (2003) followed 75 high-risk subjects for one year. Subjects with smaller right hippocampal formation, prefrontal, and cingulate cortical regions (23 subjects) developed psychotic symptoms. These subjects had no psychotic symptoms upon entry to the study. Fifty-two other subjects with more normal cortical volumes (also high-risk subjects) did not develop psychotic symptoms within the follow-up period.

Decreased hippocampal volume has also been reported in other psychiatric disorders such as unipolar depression (Sheline *et al.*, 1996), posttraumatic stress disorder (Gurvits *et al.*, 1996), bipolar disorder (Hirayasu *et al.*, 1998) and alcohol dependence (De Bellis *et al.*, 2000).

Acetylcholine is important in the operation of the hippocampus. During high cholinergic activity, old memory is recalled. During low cholinergic activity, new memory is formed (Hasselmo *et al.*, 1995). It is proposed that a defect in a cholinergic receptor could result in perceptual difficulties such as those seen in schizophrenia (Adler *et al.*, 1998).

Clinical vignette

A 30-year-old woman with normal IQ suffered a bilateral loss of the amygdala. Testing revealed that she was able to recognize the personal identity of faces and could learn the identity of new faces (Adolphs *et al.*, 1994). She was able to recognize prototypical fear from facial expression but was unable to assess the intensity of the fear expressed. She had experienced failure in social and marital relations and was unable to hold a job but was not a social outcast, as is the case with monkeys with loss of the amygdala (Adolphs *et al.*, 1995).

The hippocampus and portions of the amygdala were found to show increased neuronal density and reduced neuron size in children with autism (Bauman and Kemper, 1985). Pyramidal cells in CA1 (Sommer's sector) are highly sensitive to anoxia and ischemia, including epileptic seizure-induced damage.

Amygdala

The amygdala is a nuclear complex located inside the temporal lobe, deep to the uncus (see Figures 5.2 and 11.1). It is one of the most studied limbic structures, and such a mountain of evidence has accumulated implicating its role in our emotional life that it has been dubbed "the heart and soul of the brain's emotional network" (LeDoux, 1992).

The degree of craving experienced by cocaine addicts paralleled an increase in cerebral glucose metabolism in the frontal cortex and the amygdala (London *et al.*, 1996). It is proposed that increased levels of glutamate in the amygdala may mediate the craving experienced by cocaine addicts (Kalivas *et al.*, 1998).

Blood flow to the right limbic and paralimbic structures including the amygdala was increased in patients with posttraumatic stress disorder under provoked conditions (Figure 11.5). The activation of these brain areas is hypothesized to reflect intense emotions or emotional memory and may not be specific to posttraumatic stress disorder (Rauch *et al.*, 1996). The amygdala was seen to be enlarged in patients with bipolar disorder (Altshuler *et al.*, 1998).

Blood flow to the left amygdala was increased significantly in patients with unipolar major depression. A circuit involving the prefrontal cortex, the amygdala, and related parts of the basal ganglia and medial thalamus has been proposed to describe the functional neuroanatomy of depression (Drevets *et al.*, 1992). The amygdala was found to be significantly larger in patients with bipolar disorder than in control subjects. Other structures (thalamus, pallidum, and striatum) showed modest enlargement (Strakowski *et al.*, 1999).

Atrophy of regions of the amygdala containing large neurons which have reciprocal connections with the basal nucleus of Meynert was reported in Alzheimer's disease (Scott *et al.*, 1991). This is consistent with reduced acetylcholinesterase activity in the amygdala in Alzheimer's disease (Shinotoh *et al.*, 2000). It is hypothesized that functional changes in the neocortex and amygdala are early and leading events in Alzheimer's disease rather than a consequence of degeneration elsewhere (Herholz *et al.*, 2004).

It is convenient to recognize three nuclear areas within the amygdala, although each of these three may be subdivided (Price *et al.*, 1987). These areas are the lateral (basolateral) nuclei, the central nucleus, and the medial (corticomedial) nuclei (Figure 11.6).

Lateral nuclei

Sensory input to the lateral nuclei of the amygdala arises from third-order unimodal sensory cortex, especially the visual association cortex of the temporal lobe. Other sensory areas that project to the amygdala include the multimodal sensory areas of the frontal lobe, with those from the temporal lobe being particularly dense (Amaral *et al.*, 1992; Figures 5.3, 11.6 and 11.7). It is via this route that sensory information from the external environment reaches the amygdala. Other fibers arrive from the insular cortex, which provides sensory information from the internal environment (see Chapter 5). There are also reciprocal connections with the orbital cortex of the prefrontal lobe.

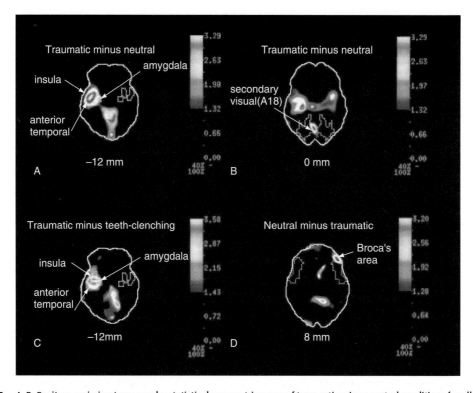

Figure 11.5.   A–D. Positron emission tomography statistical parametric maps of traumatic minus control conditions for all subjects ($n = 8$; 16 scans per condition) are displayed with a Sokoloff color scale reproduced in black and white in units of z score. Patients were presented with 30- to 40-s audio tapes of two separated traumatic experiences based on past personal events (traumatic condition) or two neutral scripts (e.g., brushing one's teeth, emptying the dishwasher; neutral condition). Dashed outlines reflecting boundaries of specified brain regions, as defined via a digitized version of the Talairach atlas, are superimposed for anatomical reference. Whole-brain slice outlines are demarcated with solid lines. All images are transverse sections parallel to the intercommissural plane, shown in conventional neuroimaging orientation (top = anterior, bottom = posterior, right = left, left = right). Each transverse section is labeled with its z coordinate, denoting its position with respect to the intercommissural plane (superior > 0). For the traumatic minus neutral condition, activation is located within right anterior temporal and insular cortex, the amygdala (A), and secondary visual cortex (B). C. For the traumatic minus teeth-clenching condition, the pattern of activation shown parallels that seen in panel B. D. For the neutral minus traumatic condition, activation is located within the left Broca's area (representing a decrease in relative blood flow associated with the traumatic condition). (Modified with permission from Rauch, S. L., van der Kolk, B. A., Fisler, R. E., Alpert, N. M., Orr, S. P., Savage, C. R., Fischman, A. J., Jenike, M. A., and Pitman, R. K. 1996. A symptom provocation study of posttraumatic stress disorder using positron emission tomography and script-driven imagery. *Arch. Gen. Psychiatry* **53**:380–386.)

    Projections from the lateral division of the amygdala go to both cortical and subcortical areas. Cortical areas include the orbital cortex, temporal pole, and hippocampus as well as the cingulate gyrus. Many of these projections are direct. All of these areas could be involved in the perception of anxiety and fear (Davis, 1997). Subcortical targets include the central and medial amygdala nuclei, and the mediodorsal nucleus of the thalamus. The mediodorsal nucleus projects fibers to all areas of the prefrontal cortex. Therefore, there are both direct and indirect routes from the lateral amygdala to the prefrontal

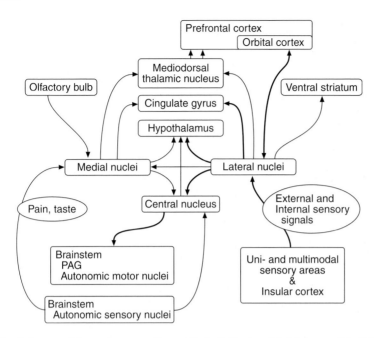

Figure 11.6.   A diagram of the major connections of the individual nuclei of the amygdala (lateral nuclei, central nucleus and medial nuclei). Behaviorally preeminent pathways are highlighted in red. The lateral nuclei evaluate integrated sensory information with regard to emotional content and interconnect with the prefrontal cortex, cingulate gyrus, and ventral striatum for somatic response and emotional appreciation. The medial nuclei associate taste and pain signals with emotions. The central nucleus connects with brainstem autonomic centers for motor and autonomic response to emotional stimuli. All three nuclei of the amygdala have connections with the hypothalamus for expression of emotion by way of the autonomic and endocrine systems. PAG, periaqueductal gray.

cortex. Connections with the lateral hypothalamus provide a route by which the lateral amygdala can regulate autonomic tone. A behaviorally sensitive region in which a large number of amygdala efferents terminate, including those from the lateral amygdala, is the ventral striatum (see Chapter 7; Figure 7.2), which includes the nucleus accumbens (Russchen *et al.*, 1985).

The lateral nuclei of the amygdala are believed to attach emotional significance to specific incoming somatic and visceral sensory stimuli. Connections with the hippocampus may provide the substrate for learning the emotional significance of specific spatial and sensory cue stimuli (McGaugh *et al.*, 1996). The amygdala can search for past stimuli of a similar nature in order to tag the current stimulus with the same emotion. Connections with the prefrontal cortex and cingulate gyrus allow for appreciation of the emotion, for memory of the emotional situation and for the formulation of appropriate somatic and autonomic responses. Connections with the central nucleus provide the basis of direct control of brainstem motor and autonomic nuclei.

Portions of the lateral nuclei closely allied with the hippocampus demonstrate abundant pathology in Alzheimer's disease (Van Hoesen, 1997). The nucleus basalis (of Meynert), which projects to widespread areas of the cortex and which has been implicated in Alzheimer's disease, receives fibers from the amygdala (see Chapter 7; Price *et al.*, 1987).

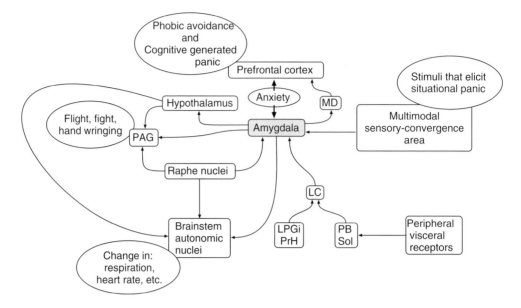

Figure 11.7.   Neuroanatomical structures related to panic disorder. The amygdala is believed to play a central role in panic disorder. Sensory cues that trigger panic may originate internally or externally (right side of figure). Anxiety is the result of excitation of the amygdala. Phobic avoidance may originate in the prefrontal lobes. Somatic and motor behaviors typical of panic are effected by the periaqueductal gray (PAG) and brainstem autonomic nuclei. LC, locus ceruleus; LPGi, nucleus paragigantocellularis lateralis; MD, mediodorsal thalamic nucleus; PB, parabrachial nucleus; PrH, nucleus prepositus hypoglossi; Sol, solitary nucleus.

Medial nuclei

The most prominent source of fibers that enter the medial division of the amygdala is the olfactory bulb (see Figure 11.6). Other afferents arise from brainstem areas that are related to visceral sensations, taste, and pain.

These connections may contribute to the emotional aspects of smell, taste, and pain.

Efferents from the medial nuclei terminate in the hypothalamus, especially in the ventromedial nucleus, which is related to feeding behavior. Hypothalamic efferents influenced by the medial amygdala include those that regulate the anterior pituitary (see Chapter 8).

Central nucleus

The central nucleus of the amygdala receives input from the lateral and medial amygdala nuclei as well as from brainstem autonomic sensory nuclei (solitary and parabrachial nuclei; see Chapter 10). The central nucleus is the predominant output channel for the amygdala (Bohus *et al.*, 1996). Efferents from the central nucleus terminate in the dorsal nucleus of the vagus as well as other brainstem parasympathetic motor nuclei and in the brainstem reticular formation, including the periaqueductal gray (see Chapter 10; Figure 10.3). Other efferents also control autonomic activity by way of efferent fibers to the hypothalamus (Figure 11.6).

Signals are processed over parallel pathways through the amygdala. These pathways converge in the central nucleus (Pitkanen *et al.*, 1997). The central nucleus is closely tied with the emotional responsiveness of parasympathetic tone. It copes with environmental challenges by promoting responses that have been successful in the past and by assigning emotional significance to current events (Hatfield *et al.*, 1996). Fight or flight responses or defensive freezing behaviors can be elicited by the central nucleus and its connections with the periaqueductal gray (see Chapter 10; Figure 10.3).The central nucleus plays a key role in monitoring the level of autonomic tone by way of feedback from the viscera. Connections with the brainstem autonomic motor nuclei provide a route by which the amygdala directly modifies the autonomic nervous system. Stimulation of the central nucleus in the cat produced electroencephalographic (EEG) changes indicative of arousal (Kreindler and Steriade, 1964). Rats with a lesion in the central nucleus fail to benefit from procedures that normally improve response to conditioned stimuli. (Holland and Gallagher, 1993)

Functional and behavioral considerations

The overall function of the amygdala is to assign emotional significance to a current experience, especially as that experience relates to anxiety or fear (Deakin and Graeff, 1991). It helps focus attention on the critical stimulus at the expense of irrelevant stimuli. The loss of fear seen in the Kluver–Bucy syndrome is attributed to bilateral destruction of the amygdala (see below). The sensation of anxiety is appreciated in the orbital prefrontal cortex and possibly the cingulate gyrus by way of projections from the amygdala. Projections from the amygdala to the hypothalamus as well as reciprocal hypothalamic-prefrontal connections are the basis of the endocrine, autonomic, and behavioral reactions to anxiety-producing situations. The location of the amygdala with respect to the prefrontal cortex and autonomic centers is consistent with the role it plays in learning relationships between stimuli and socially important behavior (Aggleton, 1993). Evidence indicates the fifth to the seventh year of age is a critical period for the development of emotion-related facial recognition (Tremblay *et al.*, 2001). As adults age, they pay less attention to negative emotional stimuli than to positive emotional stimuli. Collaborating evidence showed the amygdala of both younger and older adults was activated when viewing emotional images. But compared with younger adults, activation in older adults was greater for positive than for negative emotional pictures (Mather *et al.*, 2004). In contrast, Schwartz *et al.* (2003) have shown that infants with an inhibited social temperament tend to mature into adults with a similar personality. As adults, these inhibited individuals showed significantly greater activation of the amygdala bilaterally to novel faces than do uninhibited individuals. Although the amygdala appears to respond preferentially to fearful expressions, left amygdala activation correlated positively with the degree of extraversion of the subject (Canli *et al.*, 2002). The results suggest that the personality of extraversion may influence the brain response to emotionally important stimuli.

The amygdala responds to fearful faces and other emotionally important images independent of the current focus of attention (figure 11.8.) (Vuilleumier *et al.*, 2001, 2002; Morris *et al.*, 2002). Evidence indicates that it not only detects facially communicated threat, but determines if the threat is directed at the subject or elsewhere (Adams *et al.*, 2003). There appear to be at least two routes by which sensory signals reach the amygdala. A cortical route involves the striate cortex. A more direct route involves a subcortical extrastriate pathway that includes the superior colliculus and pulvinar (see Chapter 9)(Morris *et al.*, 1999). The amygdala discriminates between emotional and nonemotional visual targets, even if the image is viewed so quickly that the subject is not consciously aware of having viewed it (Morris *et al.*, 1998; Whalen *et al.*, 1998; Killgore and Yurgelun-Todd, 2004). Activation of the amygdala provides evidence for context enhancement of

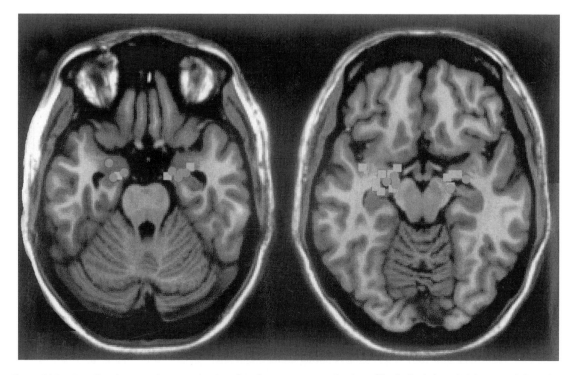

Figure 11.8.   Functional magnetic resonance imaging demonstrates activation of both the left and right amygdalae when processing facial expressions of fright (green) as well as during conditioned fear (red). Expressions of fright produce activity more in the left side of the upper amygdala than in the right side, whereas the response to conditioned fear is more evenly distributed. (Reproduced with permission from Vass, 2004.) See also color plate.

emotionally important visual targets. It sends feedback projections to the visual pathway that can draw attention to emotionally important targets (see Figure 4.3). The left amygdala more than the right responds when sexually explicit visual images are seen and more activation is seen in men than in women (Hamann *et al.*, 2004). The amygdala in cooperation with the hippocampus is responsible for fear conditioning, that is the coupling of a neutral stimulus with one that evokes fear (Dolan, 2002). The amygdala does not appear to be critical for species-typical social behavior, but is important in inhibiting social behavior when evaluating new individuals for signs of threat (Amaral, 2003).

Morris *et al.* (1998) speculated that the right amygdala is more involved in the nonconscious detection of meaningful emotional stimuli, whereas the left amygdala is related to the conscious processing of emotional stimuli. There is evidence that the right amygdala is critical in processing inherent emotional content of stimuli (Phelphs *et al.*, 2001; Nomura *et al*, 2004). The right showed more rapid habituation to fearful stimuli than did the left amygdala, especially during processing facial expressions (Hariri *et al.*, 2002).

The amygdala is lateralized based on sex. Enhanced memory for emotional films viewed in an experimental setting correlated with increased activity in the right amygdala for men. The same situation correlated with increased activity in the left amygdala for women (Cahill *et al.*, 2001).

Clinical vignette

A 40-year-old man with a history of posttraumatic epilepsy developed hyperoral and other behavioral changes after a period of status epilepticus. On resolution of the abnormal epileptiform activity, he demonstrated a voracious appetite and indiscriminate eating habits which included paper towels, plants, styrofoam cups, and feces. At one point, he drank urine from a catheter bag. The patient would also wander about the ward and touch many objects. He frequently wandered into the rooms of other patients and touched them inappropriately. Although initially aggressive, he became quite agreeable and docile.

The patient had the Kluver–Bucy syndrome from damage to amygdala. His hyperoral behavior resulted in death from asphyxiation. The patient had a respiratory arrest after stuffing his mouth with surgical gauze. Neuropathology revealed the virtual absence of the left amygdaloid complex and atrophy of the right amygdala (Mendez and Foti, 1997).

Electrical stimulation of the amygdala in humans elicits feelings of fear and anxiety as well as autonomic reactions consistent with fear (Gloor *et al.*, 1981). Electrical stimulation of the medial division of the amygdala in female mammals results in ovulation and uterine contraction. It induces penile erection in the male. Exaggerated and indiscriminate sexual activity may result from bilateral damage to the amygdala (Sachs and Meisel, 1994). The descending raphe spinal pathway that regulates incoming pain signals is also a target of fibers from the amygdala. Projections from the amygdala to brainstem motor and autonomic nuclei mediate the autonomic and facial reactions to fearful stimuli. Electrical stimulation of the central nucleus of the amygdala in cats results in behavioral and autonomic changes that resemble a state of fear, including an increase in heart and respiration rate and an increase in blood pressure. Chronic stimulation produces stomach ulcers in rats. Electrical stimulation of the medial division also produces an increase in plasma levels of corticosterone, possibly by way of projections to the hypothalamus. Dopaminergic fibers that project from the amygdala to the hippocampus are part of a behaviorally significant reward system (Blum *et al.*, 1996).

In 13 of 15 patients with ictal (epileptic) fear, the abnormal EEG activity originated from the right temporal lobe limbic structures, especially the amygdala (Hermann *et al.*, 1992). It is easy to speculate how ictal activity in this region can lead to an increase in anxiety and psychiatric manifestations such as are seen in panic attacks or pathological aggression.

Hallucinations have been experienced during temporal lobe stimulation. The most complex forms of hallucinations are associated with lesions in the anterior portion of the temporal lobe, which contains the amygdala, the uncus, and the anterior hippocampus. Epileptic activity in the different temporal–limbic regions can result in the generation of syndromes that are very similar to many "functional" psychiatric disorders. A "must read" paper by Mesulam (1981) describes 12 such cases in detail. In this series patients exhibited multiple personalities, panic-like attacks, and delusions of possession. In most of the cases, structural imaging (computed tomography (CT) or magnetic resonance imaging (MRI)) were normal and EEG revealed the abnormal electrical activity.

Because the highest incidence of psychiatric complications among patients with temporal lobe epilepsy is in those with spike foci in the anterior temporal area, it is assumed that these spikes cause abnormal activation in the amygdaloid complex. It should be noted, however, that the evidence does not support the notion that directed or organized aggression can be a direct consequence or a manifestation of ongoing seizure activity. Surgical amygdalectomy has been performed to alleviate severe and intractable aggression.

Bilateral destruction of the amygdala and surrounding structures in the monkey produces the Kluver–Bucy syndrome (see Chapter 13). This disorder is characterized by excessive docility, lack of fear response, and hypersexuality (Delis and Lucas, 1996). Bilateral temporolimbic damage in humans produces a similar behavioral pattern, frequently accompanied by amnesia, aphasia, and visual agnosia (Aggleton, 1992). Patients show few strong responses to provocative stimuli, and aggression is rare (Saver et al., 1996).

Uncus

The uncus is found superficial to the amygdala on the ventromedial aspect of the temporal lobe (see Figure 5.2). It is continuous caudally with the entorhinal area and is continuous rostrally with the periamygdaloid area and the prepyriform area. Its dorsal surface is the amygdaloid (semilunar) gyrus. The amygdala lies deep to the surface of the uncus (see Figures 11.3 and 13.2). The uncus represents the bulk of the body of the "pear" after which the pyriform (pear-shaped) lobe is named.

Schizophrenia

Ventricular enlargement of up to 33% has been reported in schizophrenia (Pakkenberg, 1987). The greatest enlargement is seen in the temporal horn of the lateral ventricle (Brown et al., 1986). Ventricular enlargement is a reflection of brain tissue loss. The greatest loss of tissue in schizophrenics is seen in the hippocampal formation, the amygdala, and the parahippocampal gyrus (Bogerts et al., 1985; Nelson et al., 1998; Velakoulis et al., 1999). Lower volumes have been reported in the temporal lobes of schizophrenics when compared with normal control subjects. Compared longitudinally over an average of 15 months (schizophrenics) and 68 months (controls), the temporal lobe volumes of both groups declined. This decline in volume was viewed as age related and correlated with a decline in neurocognitive performance in the control subjects. Interestingly, the decline in temporal lobe volume in the schizophrenic group correlated with an improvement in delusions and thought disorder (Gur et al., 1998).

The organization of pyramidal cells in the hippocampus is thought to be disturbed in the schizophrenic brain. The degree of reduction of the tissue volume of both the hippocampus and the amygdala in patients with schizophrenia as compared to normal control subjects correlates with the severity of positive psychotic symptoms (Guze and Gitlin, 1994). Delusions, hallucinations, and paranoid ideas (positive symptoms of schizophrenia) are associated with temporolimbic dysfunctions (Bogerts, 1998). Reality distortion (delusions and hallucinations) correlated with increased blood flow in the left mesiotemporal lobe structures (Liddle et al., 1992).

Panic disorder

Panic disorder has been viewed alternately as either a biological or a psychological disorder. Recent advances in the understanding of the neurobiological basis of panic attacks has allowed researchers to speculate on the neuroanatomical origins of panic/agoraphobic symptoms (see Figure 11.7). There are three main components of panic disorder: the acute panic attack, anticipatory anxiety, and phobic avoidance (Gorman et al., 1989). When cerebral blood flow (CBF) was examined in patients with panic disorder in the absence of a panic attack, a significant decrease in CBF was noted in the left parahippocampal gyrus as compared to the right parahippocampal gyrus (Reiman *et al.*, 1984). It is hypothesized that the parahippocampal and hippocampal regions serve as an external alarm center in contrast to the anterior insular area, which serves as an internal alarm center (Reiman, 1997). Depression develops in up to 70% of patients with panic disorder, and metabolic study results may be unable to separate the neuroanatomical basis of these two disorders (Gorman *et al.*, 1989). Neuroanatomical substrates of components of panic disorder are identified, but an accurate overall model is not yet complete.

The vagus nerve monitors the internal environment ("peripheral visceral receptors" in Figure 11.7) and contributes to visceral tone. Visceral sensory information is passed to the solitary and parabrachial nuclei of the brainstem (Sol and PB in Figure 11.7). Other interoceptive information is channeled through the nucleus prepositus hypoglossi and nucleus paragigantocellularis (see Chapter 10, Figure 10.1, and PrH and LPGi in Figure 11.7). The subsequent activation of the locus ceruleus (see Chapter >10) increases the level of anxiety as controlled by the amygdala. Assessment of the parasympathetic nervous system including measures reflecting the vagus nerve suggests that there may (Friedman *et al.*, 1993) or may not be aberrant parasympathetic function in panic disorder (Asmundson and Stein, 1994).

The parabrachial nucleus (see Figure 10.2; PB in Figure 11.7) receives and integrates incoming visceral signals. It also functions in the control of respiratory rate. Overactivity of the parabrachial/locus ceruleus axis may be responsible for spontaneous and nocturnal panic attacks (Goddard and Charney, 1997).

Electrical stimulation of the locus ceruleus in monkeys produces signs of severe anxiety but not of panic (Redmond, 1987).

It was concluded that the locus ceruleus does not play a central role in panic, but it may play an important role in mediating anticipatory anxiety by way of its connections with the amygdala (Grove *et al.*, 1997).

Electrical stimulation of the amygdala in humans evokes strong fear responses (Graeff, 1990). It is hypothesized that the amygdala attaches emotional significance to sensory stimuli (Deakin and Graeff, 1991). Overactivity of the central nucleus of the amygdala is believed to function in anticipatory anxiety and in fear, but not in frank panic (Graeff, 1990). The amygdala–hippocampus system may assess the magnitude of a particular threat based on past experience (Deakin and Graeff, 1991). These structures may underlie anticipatory anxiety. Phobic avoidance is believed to be a learned behavior mediated by the prefrontal cortex (Gorman *et al.*, 1989).

Excitation of neurons in the dorsal periaqueductal gray of the midbrain may be a key event in triggering panic (see Chapter 10; Grove *et al.*, 1997). Patients who received electrical stimulation of the dorsal periaqueductal gray reported feelings of fear and death (Nashold *et al.*, 1974). Input from the locus ceruleus may prime panic through connections with the periaqueductal gray. In contrast, serotonin from the raphe nuclei has an inhibitory effect on the periaqueductal gray, the locus ceruleus, and the amygdala (Sheehan *et al.*, 1993; Jenke *et al.*, 1995).

The ventromedial temporal lobe includes limbic structures that are important in emotional processing. The hippocampal formation is critical in the storage and recall of memory events. The amygdala is the "emotional heart and soul" of the brain and is instrumental in generating anxiety. Close ties between the hippocampus, amygdala, and prefrontal cortex link specific situations with emotions. The amygdala appears to hold center stage in panic disorder. It controls anxiety, and connections between it and the periaqueductal gray and brainstem autonomic nuclei are believed to be responsible for the motor component of panic disorder.

SELECT BIBLIOGRAPHY

J. P. Aggleton ed. *The Amygdala: A Functional Analysis.* (Oxford, U.K.: Oxford University Press, 2000.)

P. F. Buckley ed. Schizophrenia. *Psychiatric Clinics of North America,* **21** (1998).

S. A. Christianson ed. *The Handbook of Emotion and Memory: Research and Theory.* (Hillsdale, N. J.: Lawrence Erlbaum Associates, 1992.)

P. Ekman, J. J. Campos, R. J. Davidson, and F. B. M. deWaal, Emotions inside out. *Annals of the New York Academy of Sciences,* **1000** (2003).

P. Gloor, *The Temporal Lobe and Limbic System.* (New York: Oxford University Press, 1997.)

G. Holstege, R. Bandler, and C. B. Saper, eds. The emotional motor system. *Progress in Brain Research,* **107** (1996).

M. R. Johnson, and R. B. Lydiard, The neurobiology of anxiety disorders. In Anxiety disorders; longitudinal course and treatment. *Psychiatric Clinics of North America,* **18** (1995), 681–725.

W. A. Lishman, *Organic Psychiatry.* (Oxford, England: Blackwell Scientific Publications, 1987.)

J. F. McGinty, ed. *Advancing From the Ventral Striatum to the Extended Amygdala,* vol. **877**. (New York: New York Academy of Sciences, 1999.)

J. Rhawn, *Neuropsychology, Neuropsychiatry, and Behavioral Neurology.* (New York: Plenum Press, 1989.)

D. L. Schacter, *Searching for Memory: The Brain, the Mind, and the Past.* (New York: Basic Books, 1996.)

M. R. Trimble, and T. G. Bolwiged. *The Temporal Lobes and the Limbic System.* (Petersfield, UK: Wrightson Biomedical Publishing, 1992.)

REFERENCES

Adams, R. B. Jr., Gordon, H. L., Baird, A. A., Ambady, N., and Kleck, R. E. 2003. *Science* **300**:1536.

Adler, L. E., Olincy, A., Waldo, M., Harris, J. G., Griffith, J., Stevens, K., Flach, K., Nagamoto, H., Bickford, P., Leonard, S., and Freedman, R. 1998. Schizophrenia, sensory gating, and nicotinic receptors. *Schizophr. Bull.* **24**:189–202.

Adolphs, R., Tranel, D., Damasio, H., and Damasio, A. 1994. Impaired recognition of emotion in facial expressions following bilateral damage to human amygdala. *Nature* **372**:669–672.

— 1995. Fear and the human amygdala. *J. Neurosci.* **15**:5879–5891.

Aggleton, J. P. 1992. The functional effects of amygdala lesions in humans: a comparison with findings from monkeys. In: J. P. Aggleton (ed.), *The Amygdala: Neurobiological Aspects of Emotion, Memory, and Mental Dysfunction.* New York: Wiley-Liss, pp. 485–503.

— 1993. The contribution of the amygdala to normal and abnormal emotional states. *Trends Neurosci.* **16**:328–333.

Alheid, G. F., and Heimer, L. 1996. Theories of basal forebrain organization and the "emotional motor system". *Prog. Brain Res.* **107**:461–484.

Altshuler, L. L., Bartzokis, G., Grieder, T., Curran, J., and Mintz, J. 1998. Amygdala enlargement in bipolar disorder and hippocampal reduction in schizophrenia: an MRI study demonstrating neuro-anatomic specificity. *Arch. Gen. Psychiatry* **55**:663–664.

Amaral, D. G. 2003. The amygdala, social behavior, and danger detection. *Ann. N.Y. Acad. Sci.* **1000**:337–347.

Amaral, D. G., Price, J. L., Pitkanen, A., and Carmichael, S. T. 1992. Anatomical organization of the primate amygdaloid complex. In: J. P. Aggleton (ed.) *The Amygdala.* New York: Wiley, pp. 1–66.

Arnold, S. E., Franz, B. A., Gur, R. C., Gur, R. E., Shapiro, R. M., Moberg, P. J., and Trojanowski, J. Q. 1995. Smaller neuron size in schizophrenia in hippocampal subfields that mediate cortico-hippocampal interactions. *Am. J. Psychiatry* **152**:738–748.

Arnold, S. E., Ruscheinsky, D. D., and Han, L.-Y. 1997. Further evidence of abnormal cytoarchitecture of the entorhinal cortex in schizophrenia using spatial point pattern analyses. *Biol. Psychiatry* **42**:639–647.

Asmundson, G. J., and Stein, M. B. 1994. Vagal attenuation in panic disorder: an assessment of parasympathetic nervous system function and subjective reactivity to respiratory manipulation. *Psychosom. Med.* **56**(3):187–193.

Bauman, N. M., and Kemper, T. L. 1985. Histoanatomic observations of the brain in early infantile autism. *Neurology* **35**:866–874.

Bechara, A., Tranel, D., Damasio, H., Adolphs, R., Rockland, C., and Damasio, A. R. 1995. Double dissociation of conditioning and declarative knowledge relative to the amygdala and hippocampus in humans. *Science* **269**:1115–1118.

Benes, F. M., Kwok, E. W., Vincent, S. L., and Todtenkopf, M. S. 1998. A reduction of nonpyramidal cells in sector CA2 of schizophrenics and manic depressives. *Biol. Psychiatry* **44**:88–97.

Blum, K., Cull, J. G., Braverman, E. R., and Comings, D. E. 1996. Reward deficiency syndrome. *Am. Sci.* **84**:132–145.

Bogerts, B. 1998. The temporolimbic system theory of positive schizophrenic symptoms. *Schizophr. Bull.* **23**(3):423–443.

Bogerts, B., Meertz, E., and Schonfeldt-Bausch, R. 1985. Basal ganglia and limbic system pathology in schizophrenia: a morphometric study of brain volume and shrinkage. *Arch. Gen. Psychiatry* **42**:784–791.

Bohus, B., Koolhaas, J. M., Luiten, P. G. M., Korte, S. M., Roozendaal, B., and Wiersma, A. 1996. The neurobiology of the central nucleus of the amygdala in relation to neuroendocrine and autonomic outflow. In: G. Holstege, R. Bandler, and C. B. Saper (eds.) The emotional motor system. *Prog. Brain Res.* **107**:447–460.

Brezun, J. M., and Daszuta, A. 1999. Depletion in serotonin decreases neurogenesis in the dentate gyrus and the subventricular zone of adult rats. *Neuroscience.* **89**:999–1002.

Brown, R., Colter, N., Corsellis, J. A. N., Crow, T. J., Frith, C. D., Jagoe, R., Johnstone, E. C., and Marsh, L. 1986. Post-mortem evidence of structural brain changes in schizophrenia: differences in brain weight, temporal horn area and parahippocampal gyrus compared with affective disorder. *Arch. Gen. Psychiatry* **43**:36–42.

Brun, V. H., Otnaess, M. K., Molden, S., Steffenach, H.-A., Witter, M. P., Moser, M.-B., and Moser, E. I. 2002. Place cells and place recognition maintained by direct entorhinal-hippocampal circuitry. *Science* **296**:2243–2246.

Cahill, L., Haier, R. J., White, N. S., Fallon, J., Kilpatrick, L., Lawrence, C., Potkin, S. G., and Alkire, M. T. 2001. Sex-related difference in amygdala activity during emotionally influenced memory storage. *Neurobiol. Learn. Mem.* **75**:1–9.

Cameron, H. A., and McKay, R. D. G. 1999. Restoring production of hippocampal neurons in old age. *Nat. Neurosci.* **2**(10):894–897.

— 2001. Adult neurogenesis produces a large pool of new granule cells in the dentate gyrus. *J. Comp. Neurol.* **435**(4):406–417.

Canli, T., Sivers, H., Whitfield, S. L., Gotlib, I. H., and Gabrieli, J. D. E. 2002. Amygdala response to happy faces as a function of extraversion. *Science* **296**:2191.

Davis, M. 1997. Neurobiology of fear responses: the role of the amygdala. *J. Neuropsychiatry Clin. Neurosci.* **9**:82–402.

Deakin, J. F. W. and Graeff, F. G. 1991. 5-HT and mechanisms of defense. *J. Psychopharmacol.* **5**:305–315.

De Bellis, M. D., Clark, D. B., Beers, S. R., Soloff, P. H., Boring, A. M., Hall, J., Kersn, A., and Keshavan, M. S. 2000. Hippocampal volume in adolescent-onset alcohol use disorders. *Am. J. Psychiatry* **157**(5):737–744.

Delis, D. C., and Lucas, J. A. 1996. Memory. In: B. S. Fogel, R. B. Schiffer, and S. M. Rao (eds.) *Neuropsychiatry*. Baltimore, Md.: Williams and Wilkins, pp. 365–399.

Dolan, R. J. 2002. Emotion, cognition and behavior. *Science* **298**:1191–1194.

Drevets, W. C., Videen, T. O., Price, J. L., Preskorn, S. H., Carmichael, S. T., and Raichle, M. E. 1992. A functional anatomical study of unipolar depression. *J. Neurosci.* **12**:3628–3641.

Eisch, A. J., Barrot, M., Schad, C. A., Self, D. W., and Nestler, E. J. 2000. Opiates inhibit neurogenesis in the adult rat hippocampus. *Proc. Natl. Acad. Sci. U.S.A.* **97**:7579–7584.

Friedman, B. H., Thayer, J. F., Borkovec, T. D., Tyrrell, R. A., Johnson, B. H., and Colombo, R. 1993. Autonomic characteristics of nonclinical panic and blood phobia. *Biol. Psychiatry* **34**:298–310.

Gloor, P., Olivier, A., and Quesney, L. F. 1981. The role of the amygdala in the expression of psychic phenomena in temporal lobe seizures. In: Y. Ben-Ari (ed.) *The Amygdaloid Complex*. New York: Elsevier, pp. 489–507.

Goddard, A. W., and Charney, D. S. 1997. Toward an integrated neurobiology of panic disorder. *J. Clin. Psychiatry* **58** (Suppl. 2):4–11.

Gorman, J. M., Liebowitz, M. R., Fyer, A. J., and Stein, J. 1989. A neuroanatomical hypothesis for panic disorder. *Am. J. Psychiatry* **146**:148–161.

Gould, E., Cameron, H. A., and McEwen, B. S. 1994. Blockade of NMDA receptors increases cell death and birth in the developing dentate gyrus. *J. Comp. Neurol.* **340**:551–565.

Gould, E., McEwen, B. S., Tanapat, P., Galena, L. A. M., and Fuchs, E. 1997. Neurogenesis in the dentate gyrus of the adult tree shrew is regulated by psychosocial stress and NMDA receptor activation. *J. Neurosci.* **17**:2492–2498.

Graeff, F. B. 1990. Brain defence systems and anxiety. In: M. Roth, G. D. Burrows, and R. Noyes (eds.) *Handbook of Anxiety*, vol. 3. Amsterdam: Elsevier Science, pp. 307–357.

Grove, G., Coplan, J. D., and Hollander, E. 1997. The neuroanatomy of 5-HT dysregulation and panic disorder. *J. Neuropsychiatry Clin. Neurosci.* **9**:198–207.

Gur, R. E., Cowell, P., Turetsky, B. I., Gallacher, F., Cannon, T., Bilker, W., and Gur, R. C. 1998. A follow-up magnetic resonance imaging study of schizophrenia. *Arch. Gen. Psychiatry* **55**:145–152.

Gurvits, T. V., Shenton, M. E., Hokama, H., Ohta, H., Lasko, N. B., Gilbertson, M. W., Orr, S. P., Kikinis, R., Jolesz, F. A., McCartey, R. W., and Pitman, R. K. 1996. Magnetic resonance imaging study of hippocampal volume in chronic, combat-related posttraumatic stress disorder. *Biol. Psychiatry* **40 (11)**:1091–1099.

Guze, B. H., and Gitlin, M. 1994. The neuropathologic basis of major affective disorders: neuroanatomic insights. *J. Neuropsychiatry* **6**:114–119.

Hamann, S., Herman, R. A., Nolan, C. L., and Wallen, K. 2004. Men and women differ in amygdala response to visual sexual stimuli. *Nature Neurosci.* **7**:411–416.

Hariri, A. R., Tessitore, A., Matty, V. S., Fera, F., and Weinberger, D. R. 2002. The amygdala response to emotional stimuli: a comparison of faces and scenes. *Neuroimage* **17**:317–323.

Hasselmo, M. E., Schnett, E., and Barkai, E. 1995. Dynamics of learning and recall at excitatory recurrent synapses and cholinergic modulation in rat hippocampal region CA3. *J. Neurosci.* **15**:5249–5262.

Hatfield, T., Han, J.-S., Conley, M., Gallagher, M., and Holland, P. 1996. Neurotoxic lesions of basolateral, but not central, amygdala interfere with Pavlovian second-order conditioning and reinforcer devaluation effects. *J. Neurosci.* **16**:5256–5265.

Heckers, S. 2001. Neuroimaging studies of the hippocampus in schizophrenia. *Hippocampus* **11**:520–528.

Heckers, S., and Heinsen, H. 1991. Hippocampal neuron number in schizophrenia. A stereological study. *Arch. Gen. Psychiatry* **48**:1002–1008.

Herholz, K., Weisenbach, S., Zündorf, G., Lenz, O., Schröder, H., Bauer, B., Kalbe, E., and Heiss, W. D. 2004. In vivo study of acetylcholine esterase in basal forebrain, amygdala, and cortex in mild to moderate Alzheimer disease. *Neuroimage* **21**:136–143.

Hermann, B. P., Wyler, A. R., Blumer, D., and Richey, E. T. 1992. Ictal fear: lateralizing significance and implications for understanding the neurobiology of pathological fear states. *Neuropsychiatry Neuropsychol. Brain Neurol.* **5**:203–210.

Hirayasn, Y., Shenton, M. E., Salisbury, D. F., Dickey, C. C., Fischer, I. A., Mazzoni, P., Kisler, T., Arakaki, H., Kwon, J. S., Anderson, J. E., Yurgelun-Todd, D., Tohen, M., and McCartey, R. W. 1998. Lower left temporal lobe MRI volumes in patients with first-episode schizophrenia compared with psychotic patients with first-episode affective disorder and normal subjects. *Am. J. Psychiatry.* **155(10)**:1384–1391.

Holland, P. C., and Gallagher, M. 1993. Amygdala central nucleus lesions disrupt increments, but not decrements, in conditioned stimulus processing. *Behav. Neurosci.* **107**:246–253.

Izquierdo, I., and Cammarota, M. 2004. Zif and the survival of memory. *Science* **304**:829–830.

Jacobs, B. L. 2002. Adult brain neurogenesis and depression. *Brain Behav. Immun.* **16**:602–609.

Jacobs, L. F., and Schenk, F. 2003. Unpacking the cognitive map: the parallel map theory of hippocampal function. *Psychol. Rev.* **110(2)**:285–315.

Jakob, H., and Beckmann, H. 1994. Circumscribed malformation and nerve cell alterations in the entorhinal cortex of schizophrenics. Pathogenetic and clinical aspects. *J. Neural Transm.* **98**:83–106.

Jenke, F., Moreau, J. L., and Martin, J. R. 1995. Dorsal periaqueductal gray-induced aversion as a simulation of panic anxiety: elements of face and predictive validity. *Psychiatry Res.* **57**:181–191.

Jin, K., Peel, A. L., Mao, X. O., Xie, L., Cottrell, B. A., Henshall, D. C., and Greenberg, D. A. 2004. Increased hippocampal neurogenesis in Alzheimer's disease. *Proc. Natl. Acad. Sci. U.S.A.* **101(1)**:343–347.

Kalivas, P. W., Pierce, R. C., Cornish, J., and Sorg, B. A. 1998. A role for sensitization in craving and relapse in cocaine addiction. *J. Psychopharmacol.* **12**:49–53.

Killgore, W. D., and Yurgelun-Todd, D. A. 2004. Activation of the amygdala and anterior cingulate during nonconscious processing of sad versus happy faces. *Neuroimage* **21**:1215–1223.

Kotrla, K. J., and Weinberger, D. R. 1995. Brain imaging in schizophrenia. *Annu. Rev. Med.* **46**:113–122.

Kreindler, A., and Steriade, M. 1964. EEG patterns of arousal and sleep induced by stimulating various amygdaloid levels in the cat. *Arch. Ital. Biol.* **102**:576–586.

Krimer, L. S., Herman, M. M., and Saunders, R. C. 1995. Qualitative and quantitative analysis of the entorhinal cortex cytoarchitectural organization in schizophrenia. *Soc. Neurosci. Abstr.* **21**:239.

Krimer, L. S., Herman, M. M., Saunders, R. C., Boyd, J. C., Hyde, T. M., Carter, J. M., Kleinman, J. E., and Weinberger, D. R. 1997. A qualitative and quantitative analysis of the entorhinal cortex in schizophrenia. *Cerebr. Cortex* **7**:732–739.

Krystal, J. H., D'Souza, D. C., Petrakis, I. L., Belger, A., Berman, R., Charney, D. S., Abi-Saab, W., and Madonick, S. 1999. NMDA agonists and antagonists as probes of glutamatergic dysfunction and pharmacotherapies for neuropsychiatric disorders. *Harv. Rev. Psychiatry* **7**:125–133.

LeDoux, J. E. 1992. Brain mechanisms and emotional learning. *Curr. Opin. Neurobiol.* **2**:191–197.

Liddle, P. F., Friston, K. J., Frith, C. D., Hirsch, S. R., Jones, T., and Frackowiak, R. S. J. 1992. Patterns of cerebral blood flow in schizophrenia. *Br. J. Psychiatry* **160**:179–186.

London, E. D., Stapleton, J. M., Phillips, R. L., Grant, S. J., Villemagne, V. L., Liu, X., and Soria, R. 1996. PET studies of cerebral glucose metabolism: acute effects of cocaine and long-term deficits in brains of drug abusers. *NIDA Res. Monogr.* **163**:146–158.

Madsen, T. M., Treschow, A., Bengzon, J., Bolwig, T. G., Lindvall, O., and Tingström, A. 2000. Increased neurogenesis in a model of electroconvulsive therapy. *Biol. Psychiatry.* **47**:1043–1049.

Maguire, E. A., Gadian, D. G., Johnsrude, I. S., Good, C. D., Ashburner, J., Frackowiak, R. S. J., and Frith, C. D. 2000. Navigation-related structural change in the hippocampi of taxi drivers. *Proc. Natl. Acad. Sci. U.S.A.* **97**:4398–4403.

Maguire, E. A., Spiers, H. J., Good, C. D., Hartley, T., Frackowiak, R. S. J., and Burgess, N. 2003. Navigational expertise and the human hippocampus: a structural brain imaging analysis. *Hippocampus* **13**:250–259.

Martin, J. H. 1996. *Neuroanatomy: Text and Atlas*, 2nd edn. Stamford, Conn.: Appleton and Lange, p. 449.

Mather, M., Canli, T., English, T., Witfiled, S., Wais, P., Ochsner, K., Gabrieli, J. D. E., and Carstensen, L. L. 2004. Amygdala responses to emotionally valenced stimuli in older and younger adults. *Psychol. Sci.* **15(4)**:259–263.

McCarthy, M. M. 2003. Stretching the truth: why hippocampal neurons are so vulnerable following traumatic brain injury. *Exp. Neurol.* **184**:40–43.

McGaugh, J. L., Cahill, L., and Roozendaal, B. 1996. Involvement of the amygdala in memory storage: interaction with other brain systems. *Exp. Neurol.* **93**:13508–13524.

Mendez, M. F., and Cummings, J. L. 2003. *Dementia: A Clinical Approach*, 3rd edn. Philadelphia, Pa.: Butterworth-Heinemann.

Mendez, M. F., and Foti, D. J. 1997. Lethal hyperoral behaviour from Kluver–Bucy syndrome. *J. Neurol. Neurosurg. Psychiatry* **62(3)**:293–294.

Mesulam, M. M. 1981. Dissociative states with abnormal temporal lobe EEG: multiple personality and the illusion of possession. *Arch. Neurol.* **38**:176–181.

Morris, J. S., Öhman, A., and Dolan, R. J. 1998. Conscious and unconscious emotional learning in the human amygdala. *Nature* **393**:467–470.

— 1999. A subcortical pathway to the right amygdala mediating "unseen" fear. *Proc. Natl. Acad. Sci. U.S.A.* **96**:1680–1685.

Morris, J. S., deBonis, M. and Dolan, R. J. 2002. Human amygdala responses to fearful eyes. *Neuroimage* **17(1)**:214–222.

Morrison, J. H., and Hof, P. R. 1997. Life and death of neurons in the aging brain. *Science* **278**:412–419.

Narr, K. L., Thompson, P. M., Szeszko, P., Robinson, D., Jang, S., Woods, R. P., Kim, S., Hayashi, K. M., Asunction, D., Toga, A. W., and Bilder, R. M. 2004. Regional specificity of hippocampal volume reductions in first-episode schizophrenia. *Neuroimage* **21**:1563–1575.

Nashold, B. S. Jr., Wilson, W. P., and Slaughter, G. 1974. The midbrain and pain. In: J. J. Bonica (ed.) *International symposium on pain. Adv. Neurol.* **4**:191–196.

Nelson, M. D., Saykin, A. J., Flashman, L. A., and Riordan, H. J. 1998. Hippocampal volume reduction in schizophrenia as assessed by magnetic resonance imaging. *Arch. Gen. Psychiatry* **55**:433–440.

Nomura, M., Ohira, H., Haneda, K., Iidaka, T., Sadato, N., Okada, T., and Yonekura, Y. 2004. Functional association of the amygdala and ventral prefrontal cortex during cognitive evaluation of facial expressions primed by masked angry faces: an event-related fMRI study. *Neuroimage* **21**:352–363.

Pakkenberg, B. 1987. Post-mortem study of chronic schizophrenic brains. *Br. J. Psychiatry* **151**:744–752.

Pantelis, C., Velakoulis, D., McGorry, P. D., Wood, S. J., Suckling, J., Phillips, L. J., Yung, A. R., Bullmore, E., Brewer, W., Soulsby, B., Desmond, P., and McGuire, P. K. 2003. Neuroanatomical abnormalities before and after onset of psychosis: a cross sectional and longitudinal MRI comparison. *Lancet* **361**:281–288.

Phelphs, E. A., O'Connor, K. J., Gatenby, J. C., Gore, J. C., Grillon, C., and Davis, M. 2001. Activation of the left amygdala to a cognitive representation of fear. *Nat. Neurosci.* **4**:437–441.

Pitkanen, A., Savander, V., and LeDoux, J. E. 1997. Organization of intra-amygdaloid circuitries in the rat: an emerging framework for understanding functions of the amygdala. *Trends Neurosci.* **20**:517–523.

Price, J. L., Russchen, F. T., and Amaral, D. G. 1987. The limbic region. II: the amygdaloid complex. In: A. Bjorklund and T. Hokfelt (eds.) *Handbook of chemical neuroanatomy*, vol. 5. *Integrated Systems of the CNS, Part I. Hypothalamus, Hippocampus, Amygdala, Retina*. New York: Elsevier.

Pritchard, P. B. III, Holmstrom, V. L., and Roitzsch, J. C. 1985. Epileptic amnestic attacks: benefits from antiepileptic drugs. *Neurology* **35**:1188–1189.

Rauch, S. L., van der Kolk, B. A., Fisler, R. E., Alpert, N. M., Orr, S. P., Savage, C. R., Fischman, A. J., Jenike, M. A., and Pitman, R. K. 1996. A symptom provocation study of posttraumatic stress disorder using positron emission tomography and script-driven imagery. *Arch. Gen. Psychiatry* **53**:380–387.

Redmond, D. E. Jr. 1987. Studies of the nucleus locus coeruleus in monkeys and hypotheses for neuropsychopharmacology. In: H. Y. Meltzer (ed.) *Psychopharmacology: The Third Generation of Progress*. New York: Raven Press, pp. 967–975.

Reiman, E. M. 1997. The application of positron emission tomography to the study of normal and pathological emotions. *J. Clin. Psychiatry* **58** (Suppl. 16):4–12.

Reiman, E. M., Raichel, M. E., Butler, F. K., Herscovitch, P., and Robins, E. 1984. A focal brain abnormality in panic disorder, a severe form of anxiety. *Nature* **310**:683–685.

Russchen, F. T., Amaral, D. G., and Price, J. L. 1985. The afferent connections of the substantia innominata in the monkey, *Macaca fascicularis. J. Comp. Neurol.* **242**:1–27.

Sachs, B. D., and Meisel, R. L. 1994. The physiology of male sexual behavior. In: E. Knobil and J. D. Neill (eds.) *The Physiology of Reproduction*. New York: Raven Press, pp. 3–105.

Saver, J. L., Salloway, S. P., Devinsky, O., and Bear, D. M. 1996. Neuropsychiatry of aggression. In: B. S. Fogel, R. B. Schiffer, and S. M. Rao (eds.) *Neuropsychiatry*. Baltimore, Md.: Williams and Wilkins, pp. 523–548.

Schwartz, C. E., Wright, C. I., Shin, L. M., Kagan, J., and Rauch, S. L. 2003. Inhibited and uninhibited infants "grown up": adult amygdalar response to novelty. *Science* **300**:1952–1954.

Scott, S. A., Dekosky, S. T., and Scheff, S. W. 1991. Volumetric atrophy of the amygdala in Alzheimer's disease: quantitative serial reconstruction. *Neurology* **41**:351–356.

Sheehan, D. V., Raj, B. A., Trehan, R. R., and Knapp, E. L. 1993. Serotonin in panic disorder and social phobia. *Int. Clin. Psychopharmacol.* **8**(Suppl. 2):163–77.

Sheline, Y. I., Wang, P. W., Gado, M. H., Csernansky, J. G., and Vannier, M. W. 1996 Hippocampal atrophy in recurrent major depression. *Proc. Natl. Acad. Sci. U.S.A.* **93(9)**:3908–3913.

Shinotoh, H., Namba, H., Fukushi, K., Nagatsuka, S., Tanaka, N., Aotsuka, A., Ota, T., Tanada, S., and Irie, T. 2000. Progressive loss of cortical acetylcholinesterase activity in association with cognitive decline in Alzheimer's disease: a positron emission tomography study. *Ann. Neurol.* **48**:194–200.

Skaggs, W. E., and McNaughton, B. L. 1996. Replay of neuronal firing sequences in rat hippocampus during sleep flowing spatial exposure. *Science* **271**:1870–1873.

Squire, L. R., Amaral, D. G., and Press, G. A. 1990. Magnetic resonance measurements of hippocampal formation and mammillary nuclei distinguish medial temporal lobe and diencephalic amnesia. *J. Neurosci.* **19**:3106–3117.

Strakowski, S. M., DelBello, M. P., Sax, K. W., Zimmerman, M. E., Shear, P. K., Hawkins, J. M., and Larson, E. R. 1999. Brain magnetic resonance imaging of structural abnormalities in bipolar disorder. *Arch. Gen. Psychiatry* **56**:254–260.

Swanson, L. W., Kohler, D., and Bjorklund, A. 1987. The limbic region. I: the septohippocampal system. In: A. Bjorklund and T. Hokfelt (eds.) *Handbook of chemical neuroanatomy*, vol. 5. *Integrated Systems of the CNS, Part I. Hypothalamus, Hippocampus, Amygdala, Retina.* New York: Elsevier.

Tamminga, C. A. 1998. Schizophrenia and glutamatergic transmission. *Crit. Rev. Neurobiol.* **12**:21–36.

— 1999. Glutamatergic aspects of schizophrenia. *Br. J. Psychiatry* **174** (Suppl. 37):12–15.

Tanapat, P., Hastings, N. B., Reeves, A. J., and Gould, E., 1999. Estrogen stimulates a transient increase in the number of new neurons in the dentate gyrus of the adult female rat. *J. Neurosci.* **19**:5792–5801.

Tremblay, C., Kirouac, G., and Dore, F. Y. 2001. The recognition of adults' and children's facial expressions of emotions. *J. Psychol.* **121(4)**:341–350.

Van Hoesen, G. W. 1997. Ventromedial temporal lobe: anatomy, with comments on Alzheimer's disease and temporal injury. *J. Neuropsychiatry* **9**:331–341.

Vass, R. 2004. Fear not. *Sci. Am.* **14**:62–69.

Velakoulis, D., Pantelis, C., McGorry, P. E., Dudgeon, P., Brewer, W., Cook, M., Desmond, P., Bridle, N., Tierney, P., Murrie, V., Singh, B., and Copolov, D. 1999. Hippocampal volume in first-episode psychoses and chronic schizophrenia. *Arch. Gen. Psychiatry* **56**:133–140.

Vuilleumier, P., Armony, J. L., Driver, J., and Dolan, R. J. 2001. Effects of attention and emotion on face processing in the human brain: an event related fMRI study. *Neuron* **30(3)**:829–841.

Vuilleumier, P., Armony, J. L., Clarke, R., Husain, M., Driver, J., and Dolan, R. J. 2002. Neural response to emotional faces with and without awareness: event-related fMRI in a parietal patient with visual extinction and spatial neglect. *Neuropsychologia* **40(12)**:2156–2166.

Whalen, P. J., Rauch, S. L., Etcoff, N. L., McInerney, S. C., Lee, M. B., and Jenike, M. A. 1998. Masked presentations of emotional facial expressions modulate amygdala activity without explicit knowledge. *J. Neurosci.* **18(1)**:411–418.

Wilson, M. A., and McNaughton, B. L. 1993. Dynamics of the hippocampal ensemble code for space. *Science* **261**:1055–1058.

12 Limbic system: cingulate cortex

Several brain regions have emerged relatively recently as major contributors to the human psychological system. A good example is the cingulate cortex. As early as the 1930s, it was observed that cats become mute and akinetic after the occurrence of lesions of the cingulate cortex. However, it was not until the 1950s that the cingulate gyrus was examined more carefully. Together with the parahippocampal gyrus, which lies below it, the cingulate gyrus (Figure 12.1) forms a large arcuate convolution that surrounds the rostral brainstem and constitutes what Broca referred to as the *grande lobe limbique* (see Figure 13.1).

Anatomy and behavioral considerations

The cingulate cortex lies deep within the longitudinal cerebral fissure and spans the corpus callosum like a great arc (see Figure 12.1). It is separated from the frontal and parietal cortex above by the cingulate sulcus, within which much of the cingulate cortex lies. Two major subdivisions of the cingulate cortex and a connecting bundle can be identified:

- The anterior cingulate cortex (ACC) forms a large region around the genu of the corpus callosum. The majority of the ACC consists of BA 24 and lies just beneath the supplementary motor area. The smaller paragenu area of the ACC wraps around the front and underside of the genu of the corpus callosum and corresponds largely with BA 25 (see Figures 2.3 and 12.1). The terms *infralimbic, subcallosal* and *anterior limbic* have been applied to all or parts of the paragenu area located below the genu (IL and PG, Figure 12.1). The gyrus that lies in front of BA 24 is the prelimbic area (PL, Figure 12.1). Much of the prelimbic area corresponds with BA 32. All these areas are currently considered anterior cingulate cortex (Devinsky *et al.*, 1995). Up until recently some authors have considered the prelimbic, infralimbic, and anterior limbic cortex as part of the prefrontal lobe (Musil and Olson, 1991). The ACC has been subdivided into the rostral cingulate zone (RCZ) and the caudal cingulate zone (CCZ) (Picard and Strick, 1996). The ACC has large layer V pyramidal neurons that project into motor systems, giving it control over body movement. The ACC also controls aspects of autonomic behavior.
- The posterior cingulate cortex (PCC) is continuous with the anterior cingulate cortex and includes the retrosplenial area and parasplenial area, which wrap around behind and below the splenium of the corpus callosum (RS and PS, Figure 12.1). The PCC

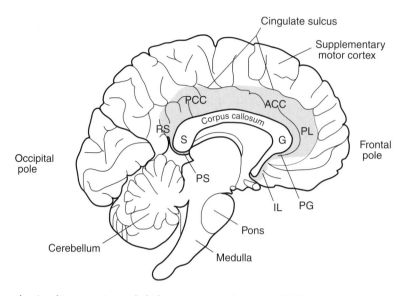

Figure 12.1.   The cingulate cortex is stippled. The anterior cingulate cortex (ACC) consists of Brodmann's area 24, the prelimbic area (PL), the paragenu area (PG), and the infralimbic area (IL). The posterior cingulate cortex (PCC) consists of Brodmann's area 23, the retrosplenial area (RS), and the parasplenial area (PS). The paragenu area is continuous laterally with the parahippocampal gyrus located on the ventromedial aspect of the temporal lobe (see Figure 5.2). G, genu of corpus callosum; S, splenium of corpus callosum. See Figure 1.1 for general orientation.

includes BA 23, 29, and 30. The cellular structure and connections of the PCC differ from those of the ACC. The PCC is involved with spatial aspects of eye movement control and associated memory.

• The cingulum is a large bundle of fibers that parallels the arc of the cingulate gyrus (Figures 12.2 and 12.3). The cingulum appears in some publications as the "sagittal bundle of the gyrus fornicatus". It is an association bundle and contains short fibers that interconnect different areas of the cingulate cortex. Long fibers located within the cingulum project to the occipital cortex and to the hippocampus (Figures 12.3 and 12.4). The cingulum also contains fibers that connect the cingulate cortex reciprocally with the prefrontal, temporal, and parietal areas.

Anterior cingulate cortex

The ACC lies in a position to filter and control the relationship between the emotional limbic system and the skeletomotor and autonomic portions of the nervous system. It is considered to be a key element in the "rostral limbic system" (see Chapter 13). In contrast with the PCC, cortical layer IV (internal granular layer) of the ACC is poorly developed. For this reason the cortex of the ACC is called *agranular cortex*. Layer IV is the target of axons that arise from relay nuclei of the thalamus. A number of subdivisions of the ACC deal with different aspects of emotionally related behavior, including the motor aspects of those behaviors. The posterior prelimbic area (BA 32) and the more posterior portion of BA 24 are called the *cognitive division* (Figure 12.5). More anterior portions, including BA 25 and 33

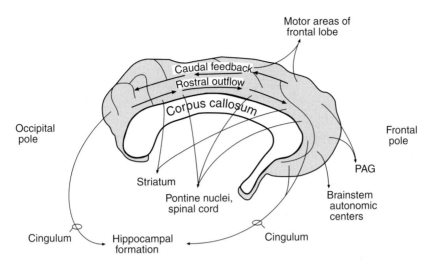

Figure 12.2.   Some of the major efferent projections of the cingulate cortex. Fibers to the motor areas of the frontal lobe arise from the skeletomotor control region of the anterior cingulate cortex. The general flow of information within the cingulate cortex is from caudal to rostral effector regions (rostral outflow) with other fibers providing "caudal feedback" from the effector regions. These fibers are found within the cingulum. The periaqueductal gray of the midbrain (PAG) is important in the regulation of pain.

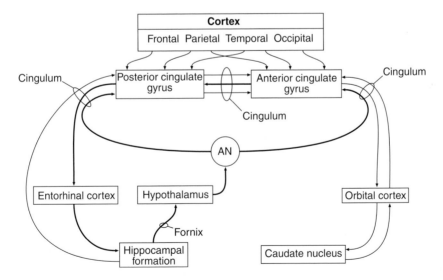

Figure 12.3.   An overview of the connections associated with the cingulate gyrus. The circuit of Papez is highlighted in red (compare with Figure 13.8). The cingulum is an association bundle that interconnects one part of the cingulate gyrus with the other as well as with other cortical areas. Many fibers course ventrocaudally in the cingulum to terminate in the entorhinal cortex (right). Others course rostroventrally to terminate in the orbital cortex, caudate nucleus, and other structures (left). The majority of the fibers from the hippocampus to the hypothalamus terminate in the mammillary nucleus. Many cortical connections are reciprocal (see text). AN, anterior nucleus of the thalamus, a major component of the "limbic thalamus."

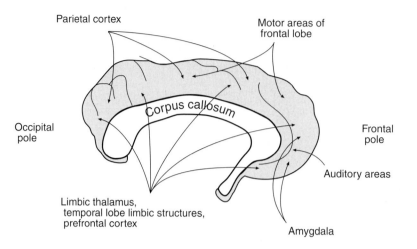

Figure 12.4. Some of the major projections to the cingulate cortex. The area served by the amygdala is restricted to the "affect" portion of the cingulate cortex and does not overlap the area served by the parietal cortex (see Figure 12.2).

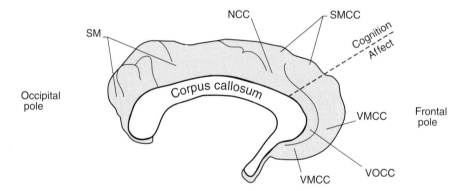

Figure 12.5. The cingulate cortex can be divided functionally into regions that subserve vocalization (VOCC), visceromotor functions (VMCC), skeletomotor functions (SMCC), and nociception (NCC) as well as a posterior region that appears to function in spatial orientation and spatial memory (SM). The anterior cingulate cortex can be divided into regions that serve affect and cognition. The border between these two regions is indicated by the dashed line (after Devinsky *et al.*, 1995).

(paragenu area) and anterior area 24, have been termed the *affect division* (Devinsky *et al.*, 1995). The affect division regulates autonomic and endocrine functions, assesses the motivational and emotional content of internal and external stimuli, and plays a role in maternal–infant interactions. The cognitive division of the ACC includes the skeletomotor and nociceptive regions (Figure 12.5) and is involved in response selection and in cognitive aspects of problem solving. The ACC is important in providing motivation and in selecting appropriate skeletomotor responses to internal and external stimuli, including socially relevant stimuli (Carter *et al.*, 1997).

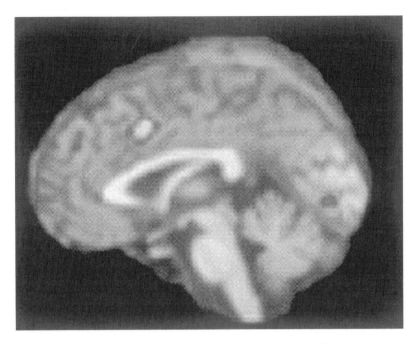

Figure 12.6. Functional magnetic resonance study demonstrates activation of the anterior cingulate gyrus region in the monitoring of conflict (incongruent trials). (Reproduced with permission from Kerns *et al.*, 2004.) See also color plate.

The ACC is involved with planning motor activity (premotor function) and with memory and the selection of motor and autonomic responses associated with affect, including responses to painful stimuli. It is important in the retrieval of remote fear memory (Frankland *et al.*, 2004). The ACC and parietal cortex may interact closely during directed attention (Mesulam, 1983). Activity in the ACC occurs well in advance of the execution of the behavior, suggesting that it functions in an executive and planning capacity.

The strategic anatomical location of the cingulate gyrus suggests that it plays an important gating (executive) function in goal-directed behavior, motivation, and neurovegetative functions. The ACC is associated with motivation and the initiation of behavior, whereas the PCC is involved with memory and spatial orientation (Musil and Olson, 1993). The ACC is activated during conflict monitoring (Figure 12.6). Once activated it recruits conflict control mechanisms that appear to take place in the dorsolateral prefrontal cortex (Kerns *et al.*, 2004).

The ACC along with the basal ganglia represent the anterior attention system. This system plays an executive role in selecting and controlling various brain areas in order to perform complex cognitive tasks. This system can, for example, scan available visual objects and select those with particular properties defined by a set of instructions. It works by recruiting and controlling the posterior attention system (see Chapter 4) as well as other brain systems. One region under its executive control is the dorsolateral prefrontal cortex in which past events are represented and transformed as a part of working memory (Posner and Dehaene, 1994). The ACC plays a central role in shifting attention during working memory. Connections between the ACC and left prefrontal (BA 46, 44 and 9) are particularly important (Kondo *et al.*, 2004).

Stimulation of the ACC elicits autonomic-related responses, including pupillary, cardiovascular, respiratory, gastrointestinal, and urinary changes, but without integrated forms of behavior. Studies with rats showed that ablation of the supracallosal cingulate cortex resulted in such severe deficits in maternal behavior that only 12% of the pups survived. These effects may be related to projections to the hypothalamus and the release of oxytocin by the hypothalamus which normally coincides with maternal behavior (Pedersen *et al.*, 1994). Similar studies with male rats showed the same negative effects of lesions on paternal behavior. Studies with hamsters demonstrated marked deficits in play behavior following the occurrence of cingulate cortex lesions (Murphy *et al.*, 1981). Play behavior has a unique role in the evolution of mammals, particularly as it has contributed to human acculturation, not only with respect to games and sports but also in regard to creative associations inspired by wit and humor in the various arts and sciences. In the course of evolution, nature assured the safety of offspring by developing a separation cry for audiovocal communication between mother and child (MacLean and Newman, 1988). In the meantime, the cingulate gyrus developed to contain high concentrations of opiate receptors (Panksepp *et al.*, 1978), suggesting that the cingulate gyrus may play a role in mother–child separation anguish.

Electrical stimulation in different parts of the ACC evokes different emotions, including euphoria, fear, pleasure, and agitation (Bancaud and Talairach, 1992). Lesions of the ACC may produce contralateral neglect, and blood flow to the ACC is significantly increased during performance of tasks that require considerable attention (Pardo *et al.*, 1990). Transient sadness is associated with an increase in blood flow in some limbic structures including the ACC (George *et al.*, 1995). The ACC has been reported to be significantly more active in patients with obsessive-compulsive disorder (Swedo *et al.*, 1989). The ACC, along with the orbital prefrontal cortex and the caudate nucleus, demonstrates increased blood flow in patients with obsessive-compulsive disorder when in a provoked state (Figure 12.7; Rauch *et al.*, 1994).

Visceromotor control

The cortex just below the genu of the corpus callosum (infralimbic cortex) regulates autonomic behavior. This region is included in the affect region of the ACC and has been called part of the "ventral anterior cingulate system" as well as visceral motor cortex (Neafsey *et al.*, 1993). It is reciprocally connected with the visceral sensory cortex of the insular area (Hurley *et al.*, 1991). It receives a large input from the amygdala (see Figure 12.4) and has efferent fibers that project to visceromotor centers, including the periaqueductal gray, the solitary nucleus, the motor nucleus of the vagus, the reticular formation motor nuclei, and the thoracic sympathetic lateral horn (see Figure 12.2; Hurley *et al.*, 1991). It also receives dopaminergic fibers from the ventral tegmental area of the midbrain (see Chapter 7). The ACC is not the anatomical site where emotion is experienced, but it does contribute to the overall emotional response by activation of visceral and somatic states that are important in the experience of emotion (Neafsey *et al.*, 1993). Vocalizations emitted by animals in response to threat, attack, or fear arise from this region. Since stimulation of the periaqueductal gray of the midbrain can produce these same vocalizations, the projections from the infralimbic area to the periaqueductal gray may be critical in

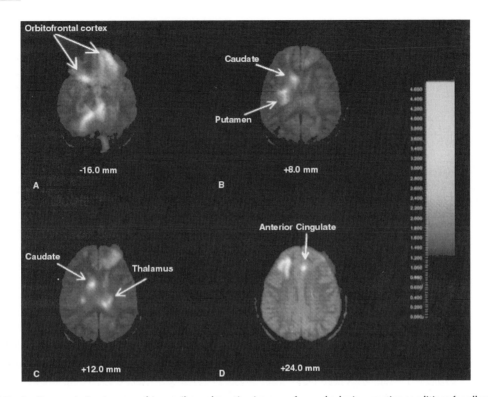

Figure 12.7.   Positron emission tomographic omnibus subtraction images of provoked minus resting conditions for all subjects ($n = 8$; 13 scans per condition) displayed with a "hot iron" scale in units of z score, superimposed over a normal magnetic resonance image transformed to Talairach space, for the purpose of anatomical reference. Patients with obsessive-compulsive disorder were provoked with stimuli tailored to each patient's symptoms. All images are transverse sections parallel to the anterior commissure-posterior commissure plane, shown in conventional neuroimaging orientation (top = anterior, bottom = posterior, right = left, and left = right). Areas of significant activation include the orbitofrontal cortex, caudate nucleus, and cingulate cortex. (Reproduced by permission from Rauch, S. L., Jenike, M. A., Alpert, N. M., Baer, L., Breiter, H. C. R., Savage, C. R., and Fischman, A. J. 1994. Regional cerebral blood flow measured during symptom provocation in obsessive-compulsive disorder using oxygen 15-labeled carbon dioxide and positron emission tomography. *Arch. Gen. Psychiatry* **51**:62–70.)

transmitting the signals from the affect division of the ACC to the brainstem (see Chapter 10; Figures 10.3 and 10.4).

Stimulation of the infralimbic region of the ACC in animals results in marked changes in blood pressure, and heart and respiratory rates as well as gonadal and adrenocortical hormone secretion, thirst, penile erection, and aggression (Buchanan and Powell, 1993). These areas appear to be involved in the autonomic responses seen during classical conditioning, suggesting that memory for these associations may be integrated here (Gibbs and Powell, 1991). Lesions in this area eliminate the conditioned emotional, respiratory and vocalization responses that normally accompany noxious footshock (Frysztak and Neafsey, 1991).

Stimulation of the infralimbic region in humans results in changes in autonomic tone. Respiratory arrest may occur. However, patients can voluntarily override the arrest. Increased activity in the ACC was seen during sympathetic-mediated heart rate increase during cognitive and motor tasks. Patients with ACC damage showed a blunted heart rate increase under the same conditions (Critchley *et al.*, 2003). In contrast to animals, involuntary vocalization rarely occurs in humans during stimulation of the ACC but rather is more common during cingulate seizures. Reduced blood flow is seen in the left paragenu area of the ACC in stutterers, demonstrating the importance of this region in verbal expression (Pool *et al.*, 1991). Conclusive evidence is not yet available to confirm that the ACC is involved in the production of emotionally evoked vocalizations in humans.

Skeletomotor control

The portion of the ACC that lies above the genu (BA 24) extends deep into the cingulate sulcus (see Figure 12.2). This region includes the cingulate motor area (effector area) and coincides with part of the cognition region of the ACC and with the "dorsal anterior cingulate system" (Neafsey *et al.*, 1993). This extensive cortical area contains projection neurons, the axons of which extend to the supplementary motor area, the primary motor area, and to the red nucleus, striatum, and spinal cord (Bates and Goldman-Rakic, 1993). These direct connections to important motor areas underscore the importance of the dorsal ACC in motor behavior. Motor behavior associated with the ACC includes attention to significant external stimuli; including orienting movements of the eyes and head toward a significant stimulus as well as inhibition of attention to less relevant internal and external stimuli. The cingulate motor area receives visuospatial information from the PCC ("rostral outflow" in Figure 12.2) as well as a small number of fibers directly from the visual cortex (Miller and Vogt, 1984). Efferents from the ACC include projections to the frontal eye fields, underscoring the importance of the cingulate cortex in attention and orientation to external stimuli.

Stimulation of the dorsal ACC produces simple and complex movements similar to those seen after stimulation of the premotor areas found on the lateral aspect of the frontal lobe (see Chapter 6; Luppino *et al.*, 1991). Behavioral changes are also seen and include primitive gestures such as kneading or pressing the hands together, lip-smacking, and picking at bedclothes. These movements can be modified with sensory stimulation and can be resisted by voluntary efforts of the patients (Devinsky *et al.*, 1995). Connections between the dorsal ACC and supplementary cortex may underlie these behaviors. Lesions that interrupt these connections may account for the motor neglect that is sometimes seen after damage to this region. Blood flow in the ACC is decreased in patients with primary depression (Bench *et al.*, 1992). Reduced metabolic activity in this region may account for the impaired initiation and organization of behavior seen in depression. A lesion of the ACC can produce hypokinesia and hypometria as well as contralateral neglect and akinetic mutism (see p. 214).

Nociception (pain)

The ACC is a major component of the medial pain system. The area of the ACC involved in pain lies behind and below the skeletomotor control region (see Figure 12.4; NCC, Figure 12.5). Neurons in this region respond to noxious stimuli. The region seems to have no localizing value since noxious stimuli applied anywhere on the body result in activation of these neurons. This generalized activation coupled with the fact that the ACC receives projections from medially located diffuse thalamic nuclei as opposed to laterally located relay nuclei (see Chapter 9; Table 9.1), makes the ACC part of the medial pain system (Vogt, 1993). The ACC appears to be involved in specifying the affective content of the noxious stimulus, in selecting a motor response to the stimulus, and with learning associated with the prediction and avoidance of noxious stimuli. It is speculated that the ACC organizes appropriate responses to pain. One response to pain is the inhibition of activity in the prefrontal cortex during noxious stimulation (Devinsky *et al.*, 1995). The ACC projects to the midbrain periaqueductal gray (PAG in Figure 12.2), an area known to regulate pain perception (see Chapter 10). These findings are consistent with the data showing that cingulotomy may be particularly effective in otherwise refractory pain.

The ACC is activated by application of noxious stimuli (Casey *et al.*, 1994). Response to noxious heat stimulus was seen to increase activity in the contralateral ACC in human subjects (Talbot *et al.*, 1991). Blood flow increases were observed in the ACC during application of noxious stimuli, while at the same time prefrontal cortex blood flow was seen to decrease (Derbyshire *et al.*, 1994). A lesion surgically introduced in the anterior cingulum bilaterally is referred to as cingulotomy. Patients suffering from chronic pain who were treated with cingulotomy reported that they continued to feel the pain but that the pain did not bother them and did not trigger an adverse emotional reaction (Foltz and White, 1962). Psychiatric patients who received surgical lesions of the cingulate cortex or cingulum, or both, reported relief from chronic, intractable pain (Ballantine *et al.*, 1967).

Social interactions

Social interactions require complex processing of information from a number of sources, including the memory of past events. The ACC appears to play a pivotal role in the generation of socially appropriate behavior. It lies in a position to evaluate the consequences of future behavior by the prefrontal cortex with motor and autonomic responses to ongoing social behavior.

Lesions of the ACC in animals commonly result in reduced aggressivity, diminished shyness, emotional blunting, impaired maternal–infant interactions, and inappropriate intraspecies social behavior. The fact that aggressive behavior is reduced following bilateral cingulotomy in animals led to the use of this procedure in humans in an attempt to reduce aggression, agitation, psychosis, and compulsive behavior (Devinsky *et al.*, 1995).

Patients with cingulate lesions or with cingulate epilepsy may express impulsivity, apathy, aggressive behavior, psychosis, and sexually deviant behavior as well as obsessions and compulsions. Hypometabolism seen in the ACC of patients with borderline personality disorder is speculated to be related to impulsiveness, a main characteristic of this disorder (De La Fuente *et al.*, 1997). Surgical cingulotomy, which removes cortex in the region of BA 24 and 32 and the cingulum, may produce impaired social behavior. In some cases the behavior of patients with cingulate lesions has resulted in institutionalization (Bancaud and Talairach, 1992). The skin conductance of one patient following bilateral cingulate and orbitofrontal cortex surgery showed no response to emotional stimuli (Damasio *et al.*, 1990). The concentration of serotonin (5-hydroxytryptamine (HT)$_{1A}$) receptors is increased in BA 24 in schizophrenics, whereas the concentration of serotonin 5-HT$_{2A,C}$ receptors is decreased in the same area. These findings correlate with hypofrontality (Gurevich and Joyce, 1997).

Memory

Thalamic projections carrying signals from the hippocampus and mamillary body of the hypothalamus (see Figure 12.3) project to portions of both the anterior and posterior cingulate cortex. The ACC is believed to be involved in early acquisition of memory in novel situations (Raichle *et al.*, 1994). The paragenu area appears to be more important in memory than are more caudal parts of the ACC. Grasby *et al.* (1993) hypothesized that the ACC responds to the attentional demands of response selection to memory tasks and may serve both short-term and long-term memory function. The ACC plays an active role during tasks that require the memorization of words, of faces, or of a series of connected events found in a story.

An increase in regional cerebral blood flow was seen in the ACC of subjects who performed an attention-demanding auditory addition test. It appeared that the increase occurred when internal information stores were being addressed. ACC blood flow decreased when the task required that internally stored information be suppressed (Deary *et al.*, 1994).

Clinical vignette
The following three clinical vignettes demonstrate the intertwined relationship between neurological and psychiatric aspects of abnormal brain processing, which involves brain regions that are responsible for emotional or cognitive regulation.

Case 1
An 11-year-old girl had started having seizures by age 2.5 years. At age 3 she developed obsessive features and by age 8 she was preoccupied with Satan, feared punishment for real and imagined behaviors, and spent long periods of time washing her hands, brushing her teeth, and showering. Depth electroencephalographic (EEG) recording documented seizure onset from the right anterior cingulate region. Surgical destruction of 4 cm of the affected cortex eliminated her seizures and markedly reduced her obsessive-compulsive behaviors during the first 15 postoperative months (Levin and Duchowny, 1991).

Case 2
A 43-year-old man had a long history of medically intractable complex partial seizures. The seizures were stereotyped and characterized by laughter, repetition of the phrase "oh my God," and bilateral arm extensions followed by repeated touching of the forehead and mouth. The seizures were short (< 10 s) and were without auras or postictal confusion. The patient was amnestic for the seizure. Eventually he became reclusive and lost his job. Depth EEG recording showed that the seizures originated from the right anterior cingulate region. After resection of this region, the seizures improved and the patient was able to live independently and entered into a romantic relationship (Devinsky *et al.*, 1995).

Case 3
A 42-year-old man similarly had a long history of intractable complex partial seizures. In addition he had a history of sociopathic behavior (15 years) that began about 1 year after a mild head injury. During a seizure

the patient would exhibit grotesque facial contortions, tongue thrusting, a strangulated yell, and bilateral arm and leg extensions with side-to-side thrashing. This patient similarly had no pre- or postictal problems. Consciousness was preserved unless the seizure generalized. Interictally, the patient was irritable and demonstrated poor impulse control with sexual preoccupation and deviance. Depth EEG recording showed that the seizures stemmed from the right cingulate cortical region. After surgery his family reported that his irritability was diminished and that he exhibited better social conduct. At last follow-up he was employed and married (Devinsky *et al.*, 1995).

Posterior cingulate cortex

In contrast to the anterior cingulate cortex, layer IV of the posterior cingulate cortex (PCC) is well developed, as is the same layer found in the primary somatosensory, primary visual, and primary auditory cortex. Because of the granular appearance of this layer, these areas of cortex are described as granular cortex. The PCC is a key element in the "caudal limbic system" (see Chapter 13). Inputs to the PCC include projections from the hippocampal formation and the anterior nuclear complex of the thalamus as well as from the medial pulvinar nuclei of the thalamus. The hippocampal formation is recognized to be important for memory (see Chapter 11). The anterior nuclear complex of the thalamus is part of the circuit of Papez (see Figures 12.3 and 13.8; see Chapter 13). The pulvinar is involved in the control of eye movements (see Chapter 9). The connections from the PCC to motor areas are much more limited than those of the ACC. Some projections from the PCC go directly to the striatum (see Chapter 7) and to the pontine nuclei. However, much of the outflow of the PCC is by way of the "rostral outflow" system, which consists of association fibers within the cingulum that connect the PCC with the effector regions of the ACC (see Figure 12.2). The "caudal feedback" system consists of reciprocal fibers that project back to the PCC (Van Hoesen *et al.*, 1993).

The PCC is involved in the performance of learned tasks. The ACC appears to be associated with short-term storage and recall of information, whereas the PCC becomes involved via reciprocal connections when needed in the storage and recall of some aspects of long-term information. The PCC plays a role in the memory of the past location of significant targets. Grasby *et al.* (1993) hypothesized that the activation seen in the parasplenial (retrosplenial) area in memory tasks reflects the activation of a prefrontal–hippocampal or a thalamic–hippocampal polysynaptic pathway that includes the posterior cingulate cortex. The PCC is involved in the control of phasic eye movements and associated head movements produced as part of an orienting response to a novel target. This orienting response occurs simultaneously with autonomic responses and cortical arousal (Steinfels *et al.*, 1983), indicating that the orienting responses generated by the PCC are closely coupled with emotional responses.

Cognitive impairment correlates with alterations in activity in the posterior cingulate cortex (Martinez-Bisbal *et al.*, 2004). Subjects with isolated memory impairment coupled with slight verbal and/or visuospatial impairments showed reduced cerebral blood flow in the posterior cingulate cortex. This group was at high risk for Alzheimer's disease (Elfgren *et al.*, 2003). Individuals with mild

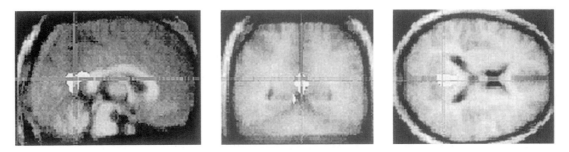

Figure 12.8.   Functional magnetic resonance study demonstrates activation of the posterior cingulate gyrus region (including retrosplenial cortex) in assessing the familiarity of a person (faces or voices). (Reproduced with permission from Shah *et al.*, 2001.) See also color plate.

cognitive impairment have a high risk to develop Alzheimer's disease. Subjects within a study group who developed Alzheimer's disease demonstrated significantly decreased rCBF in the left posterior cingulate cortex two years previously (Huang *et al.*, 2002).

Decreased activity was seen in the right posterior cingulate cortex when men reported sexual desire in response to viewing sexually stimulating photographs. Parietal areas (attention) and frontal areas (motor preparation and imagery) were also activated (Mouras *et al.*, 2003). The PCC also showed deactivation in subjects in response to photographs of individuals with whom they were in love (Bartels and Zeki, 2000).

Subjects viewed familiar faces and heard familiar voices. The fusiform gyrus responded to faces and the superior temporal gyrus responded to voices, but the PCC was activated only when a familiar stimulus was encountered (Figure 12.8) (Shah *et al.*, 2001).

A lesion of the anterior cingulum will interrupt most fibers going to and from the ACC, including reciprocal connections with the thalamus, amygdala, parahippocampus, and posterior cingulate gyrus. In contrast, a lesion of the posterior cingulum, which preferentially serves the PCC, will interrupt fewer projection pathways (Vogt, 1993).

Connections of the cingulate cortex

The limbic thalamus provides input to all regions of the cingulate cortex (see Figure 12.3; Bentivoglio *et al.*, 1993). The major component of the limbic thalamus is the anterior thalamic nucleus (see Chapter 9). The anterior nucleus is actually a nuclear complex that consists of the anterior ventral, anterior medial, and anterior dorsal nuclei. Projections from anterior ventral and anterior dorsal nuclei favor the PCC, whereas the anterior medial nucleus projects to the ACC. The anterior nuclear complex is part of the circuit of Papez and lies between the mamillary body and the cingulate cortex (see Figures 12.3 and 13.8; see Chapter 13). Although the entire cingulate cortex also receives afferents from the lateral dorsal thalamic nucleus, the lateral dorsal nucleus preferentially targets the PCC. The lateral dorsal nucleus is also part of the limbic thalamus and is a relay nucleus that transfers sensory information and especially visual information from the lateral geniculate body of the thalamus and from the pretectum of the midbrain. The pretectum of the midbrain is an area where vision, touch, and hearing converge. The pretectum–lateral dorsal nucleus connection is therefore a route by which visual, touch (somesthesis), and auditory signals can reach the cingulate cortex.

The ventral anterior nucleus and ventromedial nucleus are part of the motor thalamic region. Projections from both of these thalamic motor nuclei favor the ACC, which contains the effector region of the cingulate cortex. Midline and intralaminar thalamic nuclei, which are considered "diffuse" nuclei, project to all regions of the cingulate cortex with a preference for the ACC. The midline and intralaminar nuclei are significant structures in the medial pain system and play a role in the affective responses to painful stimuli (Vogt *et al.*, 1993).

Other input fibers to the cingulate gyrus arise from neuron cell bodies located in many areas of the cerebral cortex, including the temporal cortex and the orbital cortex of the frontal lobe. Reciprocal connections link the ACC with the motor cortex. Projections from the ACC also include fibers to the red nucleus, putamen, pontine gray, and spinal cord: all motor control centers. The amygdala is a major limbic emotional center, and the ventral amygdalofugal pathway also projects to the ACC (see Figure 12.4). These connections have led to the suggestion that the ACC coordinates activities between the limbic system and motor areas (Van Hoesen *et al.*, 1993).

The PCC receives a large number of fibers from the parietal lobe, including the primary somesthetic area. It has been suggested that the PCC coordinates activities between the limbic system and the somesthetic cortex (Van Hoesen *et al.*, 1993). Targets of fibers from the PCC are similar to those of the ACC with several exceptions. The PCC has reciprocal connections with the motor cortex, but they are much less extensive than those of the ACC. Both regions of the cingulate project to the neostriatum (caudate nucleus and putamen), but PCC projections favor the caudate nucleus. The caudate is recognized to function in emotionally related behaviors (see Chapter 7). Considering the connections with the hippocampus and mamillary bodies, it is not surprising that animal studies have shown that both the PCC and ACC are involved in memory. The inferior portion of the PCC (BA 29) in particular has been implicated in spatial memory (Sutherland and Hoesing, 1993).

Efferent fibers from the cingulate gyrus contribute heavily to the cingulum (see Figures 12.2 and 12.3). Many cingulum fibers curve ventrally in a caudal direction to terminate in the entorhinal cortex (see Figure 11.2). The cingulum is often depicted in diagrams of the circuit of Papez which emphasize the link between the cingulate gyrus and the hippocampus (see Figures 12.3 and 13.8). However, an equally large number of fibers course rostrally in the cingulum to make connections with other brain structures. These fibers also curve ventrally. Many fan out to terminate in the orbital cortex of the frontal lobe. Others continue to arch ventrocaudally to terminate in the striatum, the anterior and mediodorsal nuclei of the thalamus, and the hypothalamus (see Chapter 8). This account of the elaborate connections between the cingulate cortex and all areas of the limbic system highlights the important and central role that the cingulate cortex plays in mediating our emotion and cognitive function on the one hand and motor response on the other.

Behavioral disorders and neurosurgery

There is no clear-cut syndrome associated with cingulate lesions. Electrical stimulation of human cingulate cortex has been reported to produce a spectrum of behaviors, including speech arrest and involuntary vocalization, as well as autonomic, affective, and psycho-sensory phenomena (Devinsky and Luciano, 1993).

During the last two decades, highly refined neurosurgical procedures have emerged that can alleviate some of the most recalcitrant psychiatric symptoms (see Rapoport and Inoff-Germain (1997) for recent overview). Current procedures are usually labeled "functional neurosurgery" and depend on the ability to perform microsurgical proced-ures guided by stereotactic knowledge. The procedures are dramatically different from the old "lobotomy" in that the surgical lesions made are extremely small and are placed in very specific structures bilaterally. Surgery can be performed under local anesthesia, although general anesthesia is used most often. Such procedures have been developed for the treatment of depression, anxiety, and chronic pain. Four procedures are in current use.

Cingulotomy is the most commonly reported psychosurgical procedure used in the United States and Canada. It has proved effective in the relief of pain, anxiety, obsessive-compulsive disorder, and depression with minimal psychiatric, neurological, or general medical morbidity (Ballantine et al., 1987; Cosgrove and Rauch, 1995; Jenike et al., 1991; Marino and Cosgrove, 1997). A second operation is often necessary 6 months to a year after the initial procedure. Bilateral lesions are created that measure approximately 8–10 mm in lateral diameter and extend about 2cm dorsally from the corpus callosum. The lesion destroys the anterior cingulate gyrus and interrupts the cingulum (Ovsiew and Frim, 1997).

Subcaudate tractotomy, developed in the United Kingdom, is used to treat unresponsive affective disorder (Poynton et al., 1995). Bilateral lesions are placed in the white matter beneath and in front of the head of the caudate nucleus using either small radioactive rods or thermocoagulation. During the weeks after the surgery, patients show a significant but transient performance deficit on recognition memory tests (Kartsounis et al., 1991).

Capsulotomy was developed in Sweden and is sometimes performed in the United States. It is used to treat refractory anxiety disorders including obsessive-compulsive disorder. The lesion produced in the anterior one-third of the internal capsule is approxi-mately 4 mm wide and 16 mm long (Ovsiew and Frim, 1997).

Limbic leukotomy was developed in the UK (Figure 12.9). It consists of a subcaudate tractotomy bilaterally accompanied by cingulotomy (Mindus and Jenike, 1992).

Akinetic mutism

Akinetic mutism may be seen after bilateral damage to the ACC or to the adjacent supplementary motor cortex, or to both. One patient who showed recovery after one month reported that during the period of mutism "she did not talk because she had nothing to say," her mind was "empty," and she "felt no will to reply" (Damasio and Van Hoesen, 1983).

Gilles de la Tourette syndrome (GTS)

The pathogenesis and the exact anatomical basis of GTS remain unknown (see Chapter 7). It has been suggested that the ACC may play a central role in GTS since stimulation of the ACC in animals

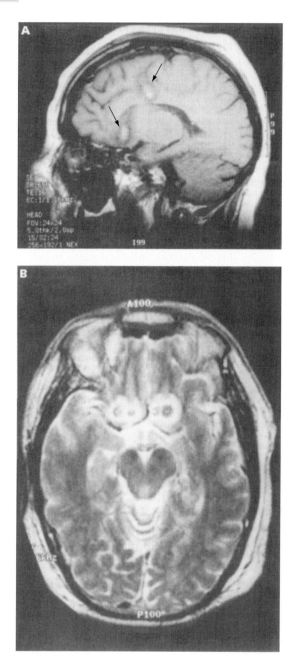

Figure 12.9.   Sagittal (A) and low axial (B) magnetic resonance imaging (MRI) of acute limbic leukotomy lesions. The dorsal
lesion (A, top arrow) involves the anterior cingulate gyrus in the same location as a cingulotomy. The ventral
lesion (A, bottom arrow) is located similarly to those produced in subcaudate tractotomy. (Modified from Ovsiew,
F., and Frim, D. M. 1997. Neurosurgery for psychiatric disorders. *J. Neurol. Neurosurg. Psychiatry* **63**:701–705.
Editorial.)

produces vocalizations. The targets of projections from the ACC include areas involved in vocalization, and dopaminergic hyperactivity is postulated as a primary cause of GTS. In addition, glucose utilization in the ACC of patients with GTS is decreased, and cingulotomy has successfully reduced obsessive-compulsive behaviors in these patients (Devinsky *et al.*, 1995).

Obsessive-compulsive disorder

For more on obsessive-compulsive disorder, please refer to chapters 4, 6, and 7. Increased metabolic activity in the ACC, along with the entire cerebral cortex, the orbital gyri, and heads of the caudate nuclei, was reported in patients suffering from obsessive-compulsive disorder (OCD) (Baxter *et al.*, 1988; Baxter, 1992; Swedo *et al.*, 1992). The ACC interacts with the orbital cortex of the frontal lobe and the striatum in OCD (see Chapters 4 and 7). The two main symptoms of OCD are obsessive-compulsive behaviors and anxiety. Anxiety is believed to be mediated through the hippocampus, amygdala, septal nuclei, mamillary bodies (hypothalamus), anterior thalamic nuclei, and cingulum. Cingulotomy has been used with some success in treatment of resistant OCD. The cingulum contains fibers that project from the ACC to the orbital cortex and to the caudate nucleus. Psychosurgical lesions limited to the ACC have resulted in reduced anxiety (Chiocca and Martuza, 1990). Obsessive-compulsive thoughts and sensations are more likely to be mediated through the interaction between the orbital cortex and the caudate nucleus (Baxter, 1992). It is theorized that a loop connecting the frontal region with the caudate nucleus and passing through the thalamus and back to the frontal area subserves obsessive-compulsive symptoms (see Figure 7.5). A lesion that interrupts the caudate-frontal axons (subcaudate tractotomy) would be expected to directly decrease obsessive-compulsive symptoms (Martuza *et al.*, 1990).

Schizophrenia

A number of studies have revealed abnormalities in the ACC as well as other areas, including the hippocampus and dorsolateral prefrontal cortex in schizophrenia. The volume of the ACC remains the same as well, as does the number of pyramidal neurons in schizophrenic patients, but the number of interneurons is significantly reduced (Benes *et al.*, 1991). These interneurons are believed to be GABAergic and function as inhibitory interneurons. They may play a role in organizing information that is received from regions such as the prefrontal cortex and the hippocampus. The loss of these inhibitory interneurons is believed to result in an overall increase in activity of the pyramidal neurons of the ACC that project to the hippocampus (Benes, 1996). In addition to a decrease in interneurons in schizophrenia, the number of axon terminals in the ACC is increased. It has been speculated that these are axons of glutamatergic nerve cell bodies located in the prefrontal cortex (Benes, 1996, 1998). Impairments in cognition may be due to dysfunction in the ACC that reflects the loss of the integrative and organizing function of the GABAergic interneurons (Dolan *et al.*, 1995). Patients with schizophrenia also demonstrate reduced glucose metabolism in the ACC that correlates with the attentional dysfunction seen in these patients (Tamminga *et al.*, 1992; Carter *et al.*, 1997). Both the prefrontal cortex and the ACC are implicated in the psychomotor poverty syndrome of schizophrenia (Liddle *et al.*, 1992). Poverty of movement and catatonia are consistent with a decrease in the motivational aspect of ACC function. The gray matter volume of the ACC was reduced bilaterally in subjects with schizophrenia (Job *et al.*, 2003a). Differences were seen between control and subjects at high risk for schizophrenia as well as first-episode patients (Job *et al.*, 2003b). The modulation of prefronto-temporal integration was abnormal as viewed by fMRI in schizophrenia (Fletcher *et al.*, 1999).

The left ACC along with other structures was activated when schizophrenic patients experienced auditory hallucinations. The PCC was prominently activated when a schizophrenic patient experienced visual hallucinations (Silbersweig *et al.*, 1995).

Schizophrenic patients demonstrate oculomotor abnormalities and use catch-up saccades during pursuit eye movements. The motor region of the ACC projects to the frontal eye fields. The frontal eye field of the prefrontal cortex is well known for its involvement in saccadic (fast) eye movements, but it is also involved in smooth pursuit tracking (MacAvoy *et al.*, 1991).

Depression

Depressed patients are reported to show both increased and decreased blood flow to the ACC as well as to the prefrontal cortex. It is suggested that patients with an increased metabolism before treatment go on to show a good response to therapy, whereas those with decreased metabolism remain significantly depressed after 6 weeks of treatment. It is proposed that the ACC, specifically BA 24, functions as a bridge, linking mood, motor, autonomic, and cognitive behaviors (Mayberg, 1997).

Cingulate cortex seizures

The description of seizures originating from the cingulate cortex provides strong evidence for the involvement of this region in affective regulation. A number of common features seem to characterize ictal events of cingulate cortex origin. While consciousness may be preserved in spite of bilateral motor involvement, in the majority of patients the level of attention or of consciousness is affected. Automatisms (complex oral, facial, or appendicular movements) occur early in the seizure. Patients may even assume a fetal position, utter brief phrases such as "oh my God," or exhibit hitting movements (Devinsky *et al.*, 1995).

Interictally, patients with cingulate seizures have been reported to show marked behavioral aberrations such as episodic outbursts or fixed and intermittent psychotic behavior. Patients with cingulate seizures have more paroxysmal aggressive outbursts, greater sociability, and less logor-rhea (increased speech) than patients with temporal lobe epilepsy. These behavioral aberrations frequently improve after removal of the abnormal cingulate cortical tissue by cingulotomy (Ledesma and Paniaqua, 1969).

SELECT BIBLIOGRAPHY

A. J. Bouckoms, Limbic surgery for pain. In *Textbook of Pain*, ed. P. D. Wall and R. Melzack. (Edinburgh: Churchill Livingstone, 1994.)

M. A. Jenike, Obsessional disorders. *Psychiatric Clinics of North America*, **15** (1992).

J. E. Rodgers, *Psychosurgery: Damaging the Brain to Save the Mind.* (New York: Harper Collins, 1992.)

B. A. Vogt, and M. Gabriel, eds. *Neurobiology of Cingulate Cortex and Limbic Thalamus: A Comprehensive Handbook.* (Boston, Mass.: Birkhauser, 1993.)

REFERENCES

Ballantine, H. T., Cassidy, W. L., Flanagan, N. B., and Marino, R. Jr. 1967. Stereotaxic anterior cingulotomy for neuropsychiatric illness and intractable pain. *J. Neurosurg.* **26**:488–495.

Ballantine, H. T., Bouckoms, A. J., Thomas, A. K., and Giriunas, I. E. 1987. Treatment of psychiatric illness by stereotactic cingulotomy. *Biol. Psychiatry* **22**:807–819.

Bancaud, J., and Talairach, J. 1992. Clinical semiology of frontal lobe seizures. *Adv. Neurol.* **57**:3–58.

Bartels, A., and Zeki, S. 2000. The neural basis of romantic love. *Neuroreport* **11**(17):3829–3834.

Bates, J. F., and Goldman-Rakic, P. S. 1993. Prefrontal connections of medial motor areas in the rhesus monkey. *J. Comp. Neurol.* **355**:211–228.

Baxter, L. R. Jr. 1992. Neuroimaging studies of obsessive compulsive disorder. *Psychiatr. Clin. North Am.* **15**:871–884.

Baxter, L. R., Schwartz, J. M., Mazziotta, J. C., Phelps, M. E., Pahl, J. J., Guze, B. H., and Fairbanks, L. 1988. Cerebral glucose metabolic rates in non-depressed obsessive-compulsives. *Am. J. Psychiatry* **45**:1560–1563.

Bench, C. J., Firston, K. J., Brown, R. G., Scott, L. C., Frackowiak, R. S. J., and Dolan, R. J. 1992. The anatomy of melancholia – focal abnormalities of cerebral blood flow in major depression. *Psychol. Med.* **22**:607–615.

Benes, F. M. 1996. Excitotoxicity in the development of corticolimbic alterations in schizophrenic brain. In: S. J. Watson (ed.) *Biology of Schizophrenia and Affective Disease*. Washington, D.C.: American Psychiatric Press.

— 1998. Model generation and testing to probe neural circuitry in the cingulate cortex of postmortem schizophrenic brain. *Schizophr. Bull.* **24**:219–230.

Benes, F. M., McSparren, J., Bird, E. D., SanGiovanni, J. P., and Vincent, S. L. 1991. Deficits in small interneurons in prefrontal and cingulate cortices of schizophrenic and schizoaffective patients. *Arch. Gen. Psychiatry* **48**:996–1001.

Bentivoglio, M., Kultas-Ilinsky, K., and Ilinsky, I. 1993. Limbic thalamus: structure, intrinsic organization, and connections. In: B. A. Vogt and M. Gabriel (eds.) *Neurobiology of Cingulate Cortex and Limbic Thalamus: A Comprehensive Handbook*. Boston, Mass.: Birkhauser, pp. 71–122.

Buchanan, S. L., and Powell, D. A. 1993. Cingulothalamic and prefrontal control of autonomic function. In: B. A. Vogt and M. Gabriel (eds.) *Neurobiology of Cingulate Cortex and Limbic Thalamus: A Comprehensive Handbook*. Boston, Mass.: Birkhauser, pp. 381–414.

Carter, C. S., Mintun, M., Nichols, T., and Cohen, J. D. 1997. Anterior cingulate gyrus dysfunction and selective attention deficits in schizophrenia: [^{15}O]H$_2$O PET study during single-trial stroop task performance. *Am. J. Psychiatry* **154**:1670–1675.

Casey, K. L., Minoshima, S., Berger, K. L., Koeppe, R. A., Morrow, T. J., and Frey, K. A. 1994. Positron emission tomographic analysis of cerebral structures activated specifically by repetitive noxious heat stimuli. *J. Neurophysiol.* **71**:802–807.

Chiocca, E. A., and Martuza, R. L. 1990. Neurosurgical therapy of obsessive-compulsive disorder. In: M. A. Jenike, L. Baer, and W. E. Minichiello (eds.) *Obsessive-Compulsive Disorders: Theory and Management*. Littleton, Mass: Year Book Medical Publishers.

Cosgrove, G. R., and Rauch, S. L. 1995. Psychosurgery. *Neurosurg. Clin. N. Am.* **6**:167–176.

Critchley, H. D., Mathias, C. J., Josephs, O., O'Doherty, J., Zanini, S., Dewar, B. K., Cipolotti, L., Shallice, T., and Dolan, R. J. 2003. Human cingulate cortex and autonomic control: converging neuroimaging and clinical evidence. *Brain* **125**(10):2139–2152.

Damasio, A. R., and Van Hoesen, G. W. 1983. Focal lesions of the limbic frontal lobe. In: K. M. Heilman, and P. Satz (eds.) *Neuropsychology of Human Emotion*. New York: Guilford Press.

Damasio, A. R., Tranel, D., and Damasio, H., 1990. Individuals with sociopathic behaviour caused by frontal damage fail to respond autonomically to social stimuli. *Behav. Brain. Res.* **41**(2):81–94.

De La Fuente, J. M., Goldman, S., Stanus, E., Vizuete, C., Morlan, I., Bobes, J., and Mendlewicz, J. 1997. Brain glucose metabolism in borderline personality disorder. *J. Psychiatr. Res.* **31**:531–541.

Deary, I. J., Ebmeier, K. P., MacLeod, K. M., Dougall, N., Hepburn, D. A., Grier, B. M., and Goodwin, G. M. 1994. PASAT performance and the pattern of uptake of $_{99m}$Tc-exametazime in brain estimated with single photon emission tomography. *Biol. Psychol.* **38**:1–18.

Derbyshire, S. W. G., Jones, A. K. P., Devani, P., Friston, K. J., Feinmann, C., Harris, M., Pearce, S., Watson, J. D., and Frackowiak, R. S. 1994. Cerebral responses to pain in patients with atypical facial pain measured by positron emission tomography. *J. Neurol. Neurosurg. Psychiatry* **57**:1166–1172.

Devinsky, O., and Luciano, D. 1993. The contributions of cingulate cortex to human behavior. In: B. A. Vogt, and M. Gabriel (eds.) *Neurobiology of Cingulate Cortex and Limbic Thalamus: A Comprehensive Handbook.* Boston, Mass.: Birkhauser, pp. 527–556.

Devinsky, O., Morrell, M. J., and Vogt, B. A. 1995. Contribution of anterior cingulate cortex to behaviour. *Brain* **118**:279–306.

Dolan, R. J., Fletcher, P., Frith, C. D., Friston, K. J., Frackowiak, R. S. J., and Grasby, P. M. 1995. Dopaminergic modulation of impaired cognitive activation in the anterior cingulate cortex in schizophrenia. *Nature* **378**:180–182.

Elfgren, C., Gustafson, L., Vestberg, S., Risberg, J., Rosen, I., Ryding, E., and Passant, U. 2003. Subjective experience of memory deficits related to clinical and neuroimaging findings. *Dement. Geriatr. Cogn. Disord.* **16**(2):84–92.

Fletcher, P., McKenna, P. J., Friston, K. J., Frith, C. D., and Dolan, R. J. 1999. Abnormal cingulate modulation of fronto-temporal connectivity in schizophrenia. *Neuroimage* **9**:337–342.

Foltz, E. L., and White, L. E. 1962. Pain "relief" by frontal cingulumotomy. *J. Neurosurg.* **19**:89–100.

Frankland, P. W., Bontempi, B., Talton, L. E., Kaczmarek, L., and Silva, A. J. 2004. The involvement of the anterior cingulate cortex in remote contextual fear memory. *Science* **304**:881–883.

Frysztak, R. J., and Neafsey, E. J. 1991. The effect of medial frontal cortex lesions on respiration, "freezing", and ultrasonic vocalizations during conditioned emotional responses in rats. *Cereb. Cortex* **1**:418–425.

George, M. S., Ketter, T. A., Parekh, P. L., Horwitz, B., Herscovitch, P., and Post, R. M. 1995. Brain activity during transient sadness and happiness in healthy women. *Am. J. Psychiatry* **152**:341–351.

Gibbs, C. M., and Powell, D. A. 1991. Single-unit activity in the dorsomedial prefrontal cortex during the expression of discriminative bradycardia in rabbits. *Behav. Brain Res.* **453**:79–92.

Grasby, P. M., Firth, C. D., Friston, K. J., Bench, C., Frackowiak, R. S. J., and Dolan, R. J. 1993. Functional mapping of brain areas implicated in auditory-verbal memory function. *Brain* **116**:1–20.

Gurevich, E. V., and Joyce, J. N. 1997. Alterations in the cortical serotonergic system in schizophrenia: a postmortem study. *Biol. Psychiatry* **42**:529–545.

Huang, C., Wahlund, L.-O., Svensson, L., Winblad, B., and Julin, P. 2002. Cingulate cortex hypoperfusion predicts Alzheimer's disease in mild cognitive impairment. *BMC Neurol.* **2**(1):9.

Hurley, K. M., Herbert, H., Moga, M. M., and Saper, C. B. 1991. Efferent projections of the infralimbic cortex of the rat. *J. Comp. Neurol.* **308**:249–276.

Jenike, M. A., Bear, L., Ballantine, H. T., Martuza, R. L., Tyners, S., Giriunas, I., Buttolph, M. L., and Cassem, N. H. 1991. Cingulotomy for refractory obsessive-compulsive disorder. A long-term follow-up of 33 patients. *Arch. Gen. Psychiatry* **48**:548–554.

Job, D. E., Whalley, H. C., McConnell, S., Glabus, M., Johnstone, E. C., and Lawrie, S. M. 2003a. Voxel-based morphometry of grey matter densities in subjects at high risk of schizophrenia. *Schizophr. Res.* **64**:1–13.

Job, D. E., Whalley, H. C., Yates, S. L., Glabus, M., Johnstone, E. C., and Lawrie, S. M. 2003b. Voxel based morphometry of grey matter reductions over time in subjects with schizophrenia. *Schizophr. Res. Suppl.* **60**:198.

Kartsounis, L. D., Poynton, A., Bridges, P. K., and Bartlett, J. R. 1991. Neuropsychological correlates of stereotactic subcaudate tractotomy. A prospective study. *Brain* **114**:2657–2673.

Kerns, J. G., Cohen, J. D., Macdonald III, A. W., Cho, R. Y., Stenger, V. Q., and Carter, C. S. 2004. Anterior cingulate conflict monitoring and adjustments in control. *Science* **303**:1023–1026.

Kondo, H., Morishita, M., Osaka, N., Osaka, M., Fukuyama, H., and Shibasaki, H. 2004. Functional roles of the cingulo-frontal network in performance on working memory. *Neuroimage* **21**:2–14.

Ledesma, J. A., and Paniaqua, J. L. 1969. Circunvolucion del cingulo y agrisividad. *Actas Luso Esp. Neurol. Psiquiatr. Cienc. Afines.* **28**:289–298.

Levin, B., and Duchowny, M. 1991. Childhood obsessive compulsive disorder and cingulate epilepsy. *Biol. Psychiatry* **30**:1049–1055.

Liddle, P. F., Friston, K. J., Frith, C. D., Hirsch, S. R., Jones, T., and Frackowiak, R. S. J. 1992. Patterns of cerebral blood flow in schizophrenia. *Br. J. Psychiatry* **160**:179–186.

Luppino, G., Matelli, M., Camarada, R. M., Gallese, V., and Rizzolatti, G. 1991. Multiple representations of body movements in mesial area 6 and the adjacent cingulate cortex: an intracortical microstimulation study in the macaque monkey. *J. Comp. Neurol.* **311**:463–482.

MacAvoy, M. G., Bruce, C. J., and Gottlieb, J. P. 1991. Smooth pursuit eye movement representation in the primate frontal eyefield. *Cereb. Cortex* **1**:95–102.

MacLean, P. D., and Newman, J. D. 1988. Role of midline frontolimbic cortex in production of the isolation call of squirrel monkeys. *Brain Res.* **45**:111–123.

Marino, R. Jr., and Cosgrove, G. R. 1997. Neurosurgical treatment of neuropsychiatric illness. *Psychiatr. Clin. North Am.* **20**:933–943.

Martinez-Bisbal, M. C., Arana, E., Marti-Bonmati, L., Molla, E., and Celda, B. 2004. Cognitive impairment: classification by 1H magnetic resonance spectroscopy. *Eur. J. Neurol.* **11**(3):187–193.

Martuza, R. L., Chiocca, E. A., Jenike, M. A., Giriunas, I. E., and Ballantine, H. T. 1990. Stereotactic radiofrequency thermal cingulotomy for obsessive compulsive disorder. *J. Neuropsychiatry Clin. Neurosci.* **2**:331–335.

Mayberg, H. S. 1997. Limbic-cortical dysregulation: a proposed model of depression. *J. Neuropsychiatry Clin. Neurosci.* **9**:471–481.

Mesulam, M.-M. 1983. The functional anatomy and hemispheric specialization of directed attention. The role of the parietal lobe and its commentary. *Trends Neurosci.* **6**:384–387.

Miller, M. W., and Vogt, B. A. 1984. Direct connections of rat visual cortex with sensory, motor and association cortices. *J. Comp. Neurol.* **226**:184–202.

Mindus, P., and Jenike, M. A. 1992. Neurosurgical treatment of malignant obsessive compulsive disorder. *Psychiatr. Clin. North Am.* **15**:921–938.

Mouras, H., Stoleru, S., Bittoun, J., Glutron, D., Pelegrini-Issac, M., Paradis, A.-L., and Burnon, Y. 2003. Brain processing of visual sexual stimuli in healthy men: a functional magnetic resonance imaging study. *Neuroimage* **20**(2):855–869.

Murphy, M. R., MacLean, P. D., and Hamilton, S. C. 1981. Species-typical behavior of hamsters deprived from birth of the neocortex. *Science* **213**:459–461.

Musil, S. Y., and Olson, C. R. 1991. Cortical areas in the medial frontal lobe of the cat delineated by quantitative analysis of thalamic afferents. *J. Comp. Neurol.* **308**:457–466.

— 1993. The role of cat cingulate cortex in sensorimotor integration. In: B. A. Vogt and M. Gabriel (eds.) *Neurobiology of Cingulate Cortex and Limbic Thalamus: A Comprehensive Handbook.* Boston, Mass.: Birkhauser, pp. 345–365.

Neafsey, E. J., Terreberry, R. R., Hurley, K. M., Ruit, K. G., and Frysztak, R. J. 1993. Anterior cingulate cortex in rodents: connections, visceral control functions, and implications for emotion. In: B. A. Vogt and M. Gabriel (eds.) *Neurobiology of Cingulate Cortex and Limbic Thalamus: A Comprehensive Handbook*. Boston, Mass.: Birkhauser, pp. 206–223.

Ovsiew, F., and Frim, D. M. 1997. Neurosurgery for psychiatric disorders. *J. Neurol. Neurosurg. Psychiatry* **63**:701–705. Editorial.

Panksepp, J., Herman, B., Conner, R., Bishop, P., and Scott, J. P. 1978. The biology of social attachments: opiates alleviate separation distress. *Biol. Psychiatry* **13**:607–618.

Pardo, J. V., Pardo, P. J., Janer, K. W., and Raichle, M. E. 1990. The anterior cingulate cortex mediates processing selection in the Stroop attentional conflict paradigm. *Proc. Natl. Acad. Sci. U. S. A.* **87**:256–259.

Pedersen, C. A., Caldwell, J. D., Walker, C., Ayers, G., and Mason, G. A. 1994. Oxytocin activates postpartum onset of rat maternal behavior in the ventral tegmental and medial preoptic areas. *Behav. Neurosci.* **108**:1163–1171.

Picard, N., and Strick, P. L. 1996. Motor areas of the medial wall: a review of their location and functional activation. *Cereb. Cortex* **6**:342–353.

Pool, K. D., Devous, M. D. Sr., Freman, F. J., Watson, B. C., and Finitzo, T. 1991. Regional cerebral blood flow in developmental stutters. *Arch Neurol.* **48**:509–512.

Posner, M. I., and Dehaene, S. 1994. Attentional networks. *Trends Neurosci.* **17**:75–79.

Poynton, A. M., Kartsounis, L. D., and Bridges, P. K. 1995. A prospective clinical study of stereotactic subcaudate tractotomy. *Psychol. Med.* **25**:763–770.

Raichle, M. E., Fiez, J. A., Videen, T. O., MacLeod, A.-M. K., Pardo, J. V., Fox, P. T., and Petersen, S. E. 1994. Practice-related changes in human brain functional anatomy during nonmotor learning. *Cereb. Cortex* **4**:8–26.

Rapoport, J. L., and Inoff-Germain, G. 1997. Medical and surgical treatment of obsessive-compulsive disorder. *Neurol. Clin. North Am.* **15**:421–428.

Rauch, S. L., Jenike, M. A., Alpert, N. M., Baer, L., Breiter, H. C. R., Savage, C. R., and Fischman, A. J. 1994. Regional cerebral blood flow measured during symptom provocation in obsessive-compulsive disorder using oxygen 15-labeled carbon dioxide and positron emission tomography. *Arch. Gen. Psychiatry* **51**:62–70.

Shah, N. J., Marshall, J. C., Zafiris, O., Schwab, A., Zilles, K., Markowitsch, H. J., and Fink, G. R. 2001. The neural correlates of person familiarity. A functional magnetic resonance imaging study with clinical implications. Brain **124**:804–815.

Silbersweig, D. A., Stern, E., Frith, C., Cahill, C., Holmes, A., Grootoonk, S., Seaward, J., McKenna, P., Chua, S. E., and Schnorr, L. 1995. A functional neuroanatomy of hallucinations in schizophrenia. *Nature* **378**:176–799.

Steinfels, G., Heym, J., Strecker, R., and Jacobs, B. 1983. Behavioral correlates of dopaminergic unit activity in freely moving cats. *Brain Res.* **158**:217–228.

Sutherland, R. J., and Hoesing, J. M. 1993. Posterior cingulate cortex and spatial memory: a microlimnology analysis. In: B. A. Vogt and M. Gabriel (eds.) *Neurobiology of Cingulate Cortex and Limbic Thalamus: A Comprehensive Handbook*. Boston, Mass.: Birkhauser, pp. 461–477.

Swedo, S. E., Schapiro, M. B., Grady, C. L., Cheslow, D. L., Leonard, H. L., Kumar, A., Friedland, R., Rapoport, S. I., and Rapoport, J. L. 1989. Cerebral glucose metabolism in childhood-onset obsessive-compulsive disorder. *Arch. Gen. Psychiatry* **146**:246–249.

Swedo, S. E., Pietrini, P., Leonard, H. L., Schapiro, M. B., Rettew, D. C., Goldberger, E. L., Rapoport, S. I., Rapoport, J. L., and Grady, C. L. 1992. Cerebral glucose metabolism in childhood-onset obsessive-compulsive disorder. Revisualization during pharmacotherapy. *Arch. Gen. Psychiatry* **49**:690–694.

Talbot, J. D., Marrett, S., Evans, A. C., Meyer, E., Bushnell, M. C., and Duncan, G. H. 1991. Multiple representations of pain in human cerebral cortex. *Science* **251**:1355–1358.

Tamminga, C. A., Thaker, G. K., Buchanan, R., Kirkpatric, B., Alphs, G. D., Chase, T. N., and Carpenter, W. T. 1992. Limbic system abnormalities identified in schizophrenia using positron emission tomography with fluorodeoxyglucose and neocortical alterations with deficit syndrome. *Arch. Gen. Psychiatry* **49**:522–530.

Van Hoesen, G. W., Morecraft, R. J., and Vogt, B. A. 1993. Connections of the monkey cingulate cortex. In: B. A. Vogt and M. Gabriel (eds.) *Neurobiology of Cingulate Cortex and Limbic Thalamus: A Comprehensive Handbook*. Boston, Mass.: Birkhauser, pp. 249–286.

Vogt, B. A. 1993. Structural organization of the cingulate cortex. In: B. A. Vogt and M. Gabriel (eds.) *Neurobiology of Cingulate Cortex and Limbic Thalamus: A Comprehensive Handbook*. Boston, Mass.: Birkhauser, pp. 19–70.

Vogt, B. A., Sikes, R. W., and Vogt, L. J. 1993. Anterior cingulate cortex and the medial pain system. In: B. A. Vogt and M. Gabriel (eds.) *Neurobiology of Cingulate Cortex and Limbic Thalamus: A Comprehensive Handbook*. Boston, Mass.: Birkhauser, pp. 313–344.

13 Limbic system: overview

The term *limbic lobe* was used by the French physician, Paul Broca, to designate the structures on the limbus or margin of the neocortex. These structures lie in a C-shaped arch on the medial and basilar surfaces of the cerebral hemispheres that surround the lateral ventricles (Figure 13.1). Broca defined the limbic lobe as the parahippocampal and cingulate gyri (*le grand lobe limbique*). In addition to the limbic cortex, a number of subcortical structures can be added to make up what is usually considered the limbic system. The subcortical structures include the hippocampus, the amygdala, and the septal nuclei. Depending on the author, the list of limbic structures can be expanded to include portions of the hypothalamus and thalamus, the habenula, the raphe nuclei, the ventral tegmental nucleus, the nucleus accumbens, the basal nucleus (of Meynert), the posterior frontal orbital cortex, and others (Trimble, 1991; Van Hoesen *et al.*, 1996).

The limbic system works in collaboration with other brain systems. Therefore, a more complete theory of the function of the limbic system can be developed only in tandem with a more complete understanding of the entire brain. The limbic system provides the animal with a means of coping with the environment and with other members of the species found in that environment. More basic parts of the system are concerned with primal activities (i.e., food and sex), while others are related to feelings and emotions. More sophisticated parts of the system combine the external and internal inputs into one whole reality. This chapter attempts to present an overview of the limbic system.

Imaging studies show that the localization of pathological functioning in schizophrenia is predominantly in the anterior cingulate and hippocampal/parahippocampal cortices (Tamminga, 1998). The limbic cortices are a major target of dopaminergic fibers, and dopamine has been implicated in schizophrenia (see Chapter 3). In addition, the highest concentration of NMDA-sensitive glutamate receptors is found in the hippocampus and anterior cingulate cortex. Glutamate also has been implicated in schizophrenia (Tamminga, 1998).

Anatomy

The basic anatomical components of the limbic system include:
Cortical structures
- Parahippocampal gyrus
- Cingulate gyrus.

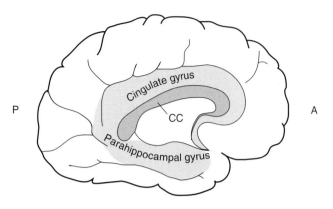

Figure 13.1.   The limbic lobe consists of the parahippocampal gyrus and cingulate gyrus, which form an arc around the corpus callosum (see Figure 12.1). A, anterior; P, posterior; CC, corpus callosum.

Subcortical structures
- Hippocampal formation
- Amygdaloid nuclear complex
- Septal nuclei.

Structures that are closely linked with the limbic system include:
- Olfactory system
- Sensory association cortices
- Hypothalamus
- Nucleus accumbens
- Orbital prefrontal cortex.

The limbic system is the anatomical substrate of behaviors including social behaviors that assure the survival of the individual and of the species. Social interaction in many species continues to rely on the importance of olfactory cues. Olfactory cues are of lesser importance to humans but the emotions and behaviors controlled by the limbic system remain critical for human survival. The complex interconnections that allow the limbic system to perform its many functions can be simplified into two subsystems. The hippocampus and septal nuclei make up one subsystem; the hippocampal formation is associated with memory. The second subsystem revolves around the amygdala and is involved with the assignment of anxiety to sensory stimuli. A brief discussion of the olfactory system is followed by an overall view of the interactions of limbic structures and their interactions.

Olfactory structures

The olfactory system plays an important role in limbic function in many animals. The olfactory stria are made up of fibers that arise from the olfactory bulb and terminate in limbic structures (Figure 13.2; nos. 1 and 2 in Figure 13.3). The targets of these olfactory

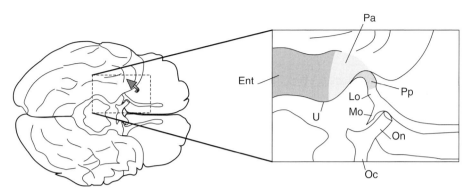

Figure 13.2.   The ventromedial temporal lobe is rolled back (arrow) and enlarged to show the components of the pyriform lobe (compare with Figure 5.2). These components include the prepyriform area (Pp), the periamygdaloid area (Pa) and the entorhinal area (Ent). Other structures include the lateral olfactory stria (Lo), medial olfactory stria (Mo), uncus (U), optic nerve (On), and optic chiasm (Oc).

fibers include prepyriform and pyriform areas, the entorhinal cortex, and the underlying amygdala (see Figures 11.6 and 13.2). For many years these connections led authors to assume that the limbic system processed olfactory cues.

Olfactory connections with the limbic structures account for the emotional aspects of olfaction. The olfactory cues are vital to many animals for appropriate social interaction and for affiliative behavior. Olfactory cues, however, are relatively unimportant to humans.

The hippocampal formation and related structures

The parahippocampal gyrus

The rostral parahippocampal gyrus includes portions of the pyriform lobe and receives primary olfactory information. The caudal part of the parahippocampal gyrus is represented by the entorhinal cortex (see Figures 11.2 and 13.2). The primary source of input into the entorhinal cortex is the multimodal association areas of the cortex. The entorhinal cortex represents the port of entry into the hippocampal formation (see Chapter 11).

The hippocampal formation

The hippocampal formation consists of the hippocampus proper along with the dentate gyrus and the subiculum (see Figure 11.2). Sensory signals are directed toward the hippocampus by way of relays in the entorhinal cortex and the dentate gyrus (see Figures 11.3 and 13.4). In addition to information arriving from the entorhinal cortex, there is input from the hypothalamus, the septal nuclei, and the amygdala.

Outgoing projections from the hippocampal formation are represented by the axons of the pyramidal neurons of the hippocampus as well as axons from the subiculum. These axons are distributed largely through the fornix (2, Figure 13.5). The fornix projects to the septal nuclei, to the ventromedial hypothalamus and to the mamillary bodies of the

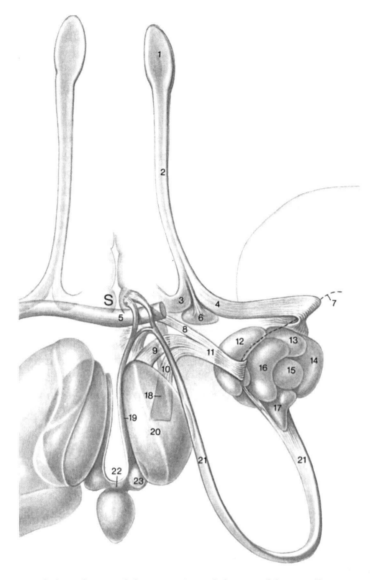

Figure 13.3.   Dorsal view of some of the connections of the amygdala. 1–4, olfactory structures; 5, anterior commissure; 6, olfactory tubercle; 7, limen insulae; 8, diagonal band (of Broca); 9, inferior thalamic peduncle; 10, medial telencephalic fasciculus; 11, ventral amygdalofugal pathway; 12–17, amygdala; 18, lateral hypothalamic area; 19–20, nucleus and stria medullaris; 21, stria terminalis; 22, habenular commissure; 23, habenular nuclei; S, septal nuclei. (Modified with permission from Nieuwenhuys, R., Voogd, J., and Van Huijzen, C. 1988. *The human nervous system*. New York: Springer-Verlag.)

hypothalamus (20, Figure 13.5). The fibers of the fornix that terminate in the septal nuclei make up the precommissural fornix (14, Figure 13.5). The fibers from the hippocampus to the septal nuclei contribute to the "septohippocampal axis," which is especially important to nonprimate mammals. Other fibers project directly to the amygdala (Canteras and Swanson, 1992).

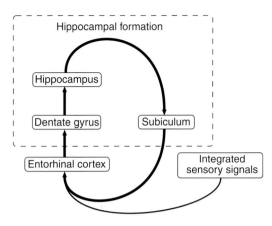

Figure 13.4.   The hippocampal formation consists of the dentate gyrus, the subiculum, and the hippocampus proper. Sensory signals enter the hippocampal formation by way of the entorhinal cortex. A feedback loop exists between the hippocampus and the entorhinal cortex. This circuit facilitates the memory function of the hippocampus.

Septal nuclei and nucleus accumbens

The septum pellucidum is a thin, membranous midline structure that separates the left and right lateral ventricles (see Figure 7.1). The space between the two leaflets of the septum pellucidum is called the cavum septum pellucidum. The cavum is seen during fetal development but normally disappears during infancy. The nuclei that make up the septal complex are situated below the corpus callosum and just in front of the anterior commissure. The lateral septal nucleus lies on the lateral aspect of the base of the septum pellucidum (see Figure 7.1). Just below and slightly medial to the lateral septal nucleus is the medial septal nucleus. Both of these nuclei are relatively small. The nucleus of the

Clinical vignettes

Case 1

A 35-year-old patient with a history of treatment-resistant schizophrenia since age 21 was readmitted for an acute exacerbation. The patient had a significant formal thought disorder with loosening of association and tangential speech. Neurological examination revealed subtle dysmetria and dysdiadochokinesia of the left arm. A computed tomographic (CT) scan revealed a large, cyst-like structure interposed between the bodies of the lateral ventricles (Wolf *et al.*, 1994). Agenesis of the septum pellucidum has been described in some cases of chronic psychosis but much less frequently than agenesis of the cavum septum pellucidum. Direct pathways from the cerebellum to the septum may be related to the dysmetria (Heath *et al.*, 1978).

Case 2

A 31-year-old male patient presented with a long history of chronic paranoid schizophrenia that was unresponsive to treatment. He had a history of enuresis and febrile seizures between the ages of 2 and 4 and was reported to be notably awkward at sports as a child. He also had developed polydipsia after the onset of psychosis. On examination he demonstrated difficulty with tandem walking. He had a total IQ score of 120 with 136 for verbal and 95 for performance. A magnetic resonance imaging (MRI) scan revealed the absence of the septum pellucidum and marked dilation of the lateral ventricles (Wolf *et al.*, 1994). Lesions of dysgenesis of the septal region may have cognitive or emotional manifestations, or both, given the region's key role in the limbic system.

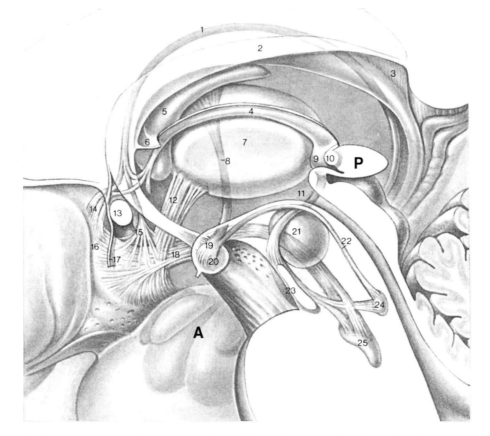

Figure 13.5.   Limbic system structures located close to the midline.1, stria terminalis; 2–3, fornix and commissure; 4, stria medullaris; 6, medial thalamic nuclei; 8, mammillothalamic tract; 9, habenular nuclei; 10, habenular commissure; 11, habenulointerpeduncular tract; 12, inferior thalamic peduncle; 13, anterior commissure; 14, precommissural fornix; 15, stria terminalis; 17, lamina terminalis; 18, medial forebrain bundle; 20, mammillary body; 21, red nucleus; 22, mammillotegmental tract; 23, interpeduncular nucleus; 24, dorsal tegmental nucleus; 25, central superior nucleus (raphe); A, amygdaloid nuclear complex; P, pineal. (Modified with permission from Nieuwenhuys, R., Voogd, J., and Van Huijzen, C. 1988. *The human nervous system.* New York: Springer-Verlag.)

diagonal band of Broca is included as part of the septal nuclear complex. All of these nuclei are important sources of acetylcholine (Gaykema *et al.*, 1990). The nucleus accumbens lies immediately lateral to the septal nuclei. It is generally considered to be part of the corpus striatum (see Chapter 7).

Amygdaloid nuclear complex

The many nuclei of the amygdaloid nuclear complex are summarized in Chapter 11 (see 12–17, Figure 13.3). Overall, the amygdala has access to integrated sensory information from higher-order cortical areas. The sensory information that reaches the amygdala provides details that help identify the object rather than determine its location (Amaral *et al.*, 1992). Auditory signals may arrive directly from the medial geniculate body (Norita and Kawamura, 1980). Dopaminergic fibers arrive from the ventral tegmental area

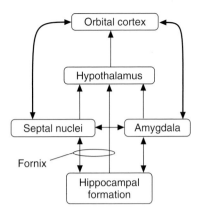

Figure 13.6.   The amygdala and septal nuclei both interact directly with the orbital cortex. Hippocampal input to the orbital cortex is by way of the hypothalamus.

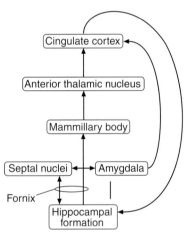

Figure 13.7.   The amygdala projects to the cingulate gyrus via the stria terminalis and the ventral amygdalofugal pathway. The septal nuclei and amygdala interact with the hippocampus and the circuit of Papez.

(see Figure 10.3). Other connections link the amygdala directly with the orbital cortex of the frontal lobe (Figure 13.6). The extended amygdala consists of a corridor of cells that extend forward from the amygdala to the nucleus accumbens (Alheid and Heimer, 1996). In addition, a special relationship exists between the amygdala and the hippocampal formation (Figure 13.7). There are direct fibers between these two limbic structures as well as an indirect link from the amygdala back to the hippocampal formation by way of the entorhinal cortex (see Figures 11.3, 13.6, and 13.7).

One group of fibers that leaves the amygdala makes up the stria terminalis, which arches dorsally and terminates in the hypothalamus, thalamus, and nucleus accumbens (21, Figure 13.3; 1, Figure 13.5). A second contingent of fibers projects ventrally from the amygdala to the septal nuclei, the nucleus accumbens, and the orbital cortex as well as to the hypothalamus and thalamus (8–11, Figure 13.3; Gloor, 1997).

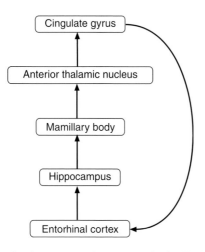

Figure 13.8.   The classic circuit of Papez provides feedback to the hippocampus by way of the cingulate gyrus (compare with Figure 12.3). The fornix connects the hippocampus with the mammillary body. The mammillothalamic tract ascends to the anterior thalamic nucleus. The cingulum contains the efferents from the cingulate gyrus to the entorhinal cortex.

Behavioral considerations

The limbic system has extensive connections within itself and with almost all other areas of the brain. Most of the data supporting such circuitry come from animal work. It should be noted that although much of the limbic circuitry has been identified, the specific contributions of each circuit to our emotional and cognitive behaviors are not yet fully known.

The loop formed by the hippocampus, fornix, mammillary bodies, mammillothalamic tract, anterior thalamic nuclei, cingulate gyrus, and projections back to the hippocampus form the circuit of Papez (see Figures 12.3 and 13.8). Papez (1937) described this circuit as the substrate of "a harmonious mechanism which may elaborate the functions of central emotions."

In a recent review article, strongly recommended for readers who wish to expand their understanding of limbic connectivity, two functional divisions of the limbic system were suggested (Mega *et al.*, 1997). An older paleocortical division has the amygdala and orbital prefrontal cortex at its center. The newer archicortical division has the hippocampus and cingulate cortex at its center. The older division functions in the integration of affect, drive, and object association, while the newer division functions in explicit sensory processing, encoding, and attentional control. The authors suggest that the distinction between the orbital prefrontal/amygdala division (emotional associations and appetitive drives) and the hippocampal/cingulate division (mnemonic and attentional processes) can further our interpretation of limbic system disorders. They further suggest that psychiatric disorders can be reinterpreted within a brain-based framework of limbic dysfunction and divided into three general groups: decreased (e.g., depression, Kluver–Bucy), increased (e.g., mania, obsessive-compulsive disorder), and dysfunctional (e.g., psychosis) limbic syndromes.

Hippocampal formation and related structures

The hippocampal formation is of primary importance in the storage and in the recall of new information in the form of declarative memory (see Chapter 11). Declarative memory is based on configural learning in both space and time. Nondeclarative memory (e.g., motor skills, habits, emotions) is independent of the hippocampus (Squire, 1992). The hippocampal formation retains new information for only a short time. The long-term storage of new information is dependent on neocortical areas and may be coincident with the same sensory association areas that first supplied the information to the hippocampal formation. Feedback signals from the hippocampus to sensory association areas may be important in the consolidation of new memory. The hippocampal–entorhinal circuit provides a feedback pathway and is hypothesized to be a reinforcement circuit that lowers the threshold of the neurons of the entorhinal cortex in order to more quickly recognize a pattern of sensory signals (See Figure 13.4.) (Buzsaki *et al.*, 1990).

Memory is believed to reflect a conceptual cognitive map that is inherent to the hippocampal formation and possibly to the hippocampus itself (Jarrard, 1993). Verbal and contextual memory may have developed from mechanisms already in place in the hippocampal formation. The mapping concept has been extended by some authors to include linguistic and semantic relationships (Gloor, 1997).

Bilateral damage to the hippocampal formation has a devastating effect on the ability to store and recall new information. Even minor damage to the hippocampus can produce a significant and lasting memory impairment (Zola-Morgan and Squire, 1993). Left temporal lobe damage affects verbal learning, whereas right temporal lobe damage affects nonverbal learning.

Projections from the hippocampal formation make up the fornix, and many of the fibers of the fornix terminate in the septal nuclei and in the mammillary bodies. (S in Figure 13.3; 20 in Figure 13.5. See also Figures 13.6 and 13.7.)

Lesions of the fornix are reported to produce amnesia (Von Cramon and Schuri, 1992). Lesions seen in the mammillary bodies in Korsakoff's syndrome also correlate with amnesia (Kopelman, 1995). Damage to other related structures including the medial thalamus (see Chapter 9) can also produce amnesia.

The theta rhythm is an electroencephalographic (EEG) pattern ranging from 4 to 12 Hz that has been recorded from the hippocampus of rodents and rabbits during certain behavioral conditions (Vanderwolf, 1988). It has been speculated that the theta rhythm is important in arousal and in the creation of a spatial map that is conducive to learning. Surprisingly the theta rhythm appears to be absent in primates and humans (Huh *et al.*, 1990).

Septal nuclei and nucleus accumbens

The septal nuclei have been implicated in memory (S, Figure 13.3).

They, along with the basal nucleus (of Meynert), are cholinergic nuclei and exhibit degeneration in Alzheimer's disease (Arendt *et al.*, 1983; Coyle *et al.*, 1983). Lesions in humans that include the septal area can produce memory loss along with hyperemotionality (Bondi *et al.*, 1993).

A cavity in the septum pellucidum (cavum septum pellucidum) of varying size has been reported to be found in up to 85% of the population (Figure 13.9; Nopoulos *et al.*, 1996, 1997). The presence or absence of a cavum septum pellucidum does not differentiate between control and psychiatric patients. However, a significant number of moderate to large (grade 3–4) cavum septi pellucidi were found only in schizophrenics (Shioiri *et al.*, 1996) and in patients with affective disorder and

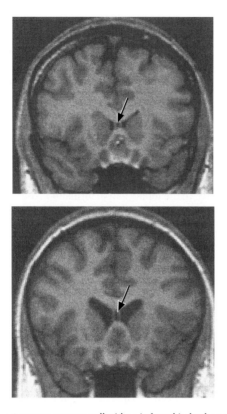

Figure 13.9.   A cavum septum pellucidum is found in both normal and schizophrenic populations; however, it is consistently
larger in schizophrenics. The cavum septum pellucidum in normals is rated "small" (top arrow) when seen on up
to two contiguous magnetic resonance (MR) 1.5-mm coronal slices. The cavum septum pellucidum is rated
"large" when seen on at least four contiguous MR 1.5-mm coronal slices (bottom arrow). (Modified with
permission from Nopoulos, P., Swaze, V., Flaum, M., Ehrhardt, J. C., Yuh, W. T., and Andreasen, N. C. 1997.
Cavum septi pellucidi in normals and patients with schizophrenia as detected by magnetic resonance imaging.
Biol. Psychiatry 41:1102–1108.)

schizotypal personality disorder (Kwon *et al.*, 1998). The closure of the cavum is influenced devel-
opmentally by enlargement of the corpus callosum and hippocampus. The large cavum may reflect
the relatively small size of the corpus callosum and hippocampus during the developmental period
when the cavum normally closes. This is consistent with the finding that the severity of cavum
septum pellucidum enlargement is believed to correlate with childhood-onset schizophrenia
(Nopoulos *et al.*, 1998).

The nucleus accumbens is well recognized as a reward center of the brain (see Figures 7.1 and 13.10).
The action of mood-elevating drugs is believed to coincide with dopamine release in the nucleus
accumbens (Self and Nestler, 1995). Accumbal neurons increased activity with the onset of cocaine
administration (Peoples *et al.*, 2004). In contrast, drugs that block the dopamine receptor sites result
in an increase in alcohol consumption in rats (Dyr *et al.*, 1993). Components of drug withdrawal
correlate with a decrease in dopamine release and an increase in acetylcholine release in the nucleus
accumbens (Rossetti *et al.*, 1992). Anxiety coincident with drug withdrawal may be due to an increase
in activity in the amygdala subsequent to a decrease in dopamine from the ventral tegmental area

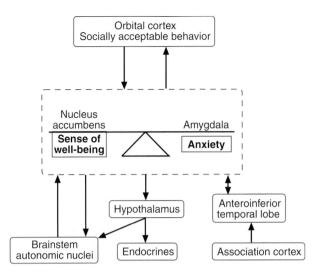

Figure 13.10. A speculative overall scheme of the elements of the limbic system suggests that a balance normally exists between the septal nuclei (contentment) and the amygdala (anxiety). Incoming sensations are identified by cortical association areas and are labeled with a degree of familiarity by the anterior inferior temporal lobe, including the hippocampus. The orbital cortex serves as a reservoir of past experience with social situations. The assignment of emotion by the septal–amygdala complex is influenced by the current autonomic state. The septal–amygdala complex effects emotional responses via the hypothalamus and brainstem autonomic centers.

(Pilotte and Sharpe, 1996). A decrease in dopamine in the amygdala and hippocampus is hypothesized to produce anxiety or cravings, or both, for substances that provide temporary relief by releasing dopamine (Blum *et al.*, 1996).

Women showed reduced activation of the μ-opoid system in the accumbens nucleus ipsilateral to a pain stimulus when compared with men (Zubieta *et al.*, 2002). Theoretically this reduction would allow more efficient pain transmission and is consistent with studies that found that women show higher perceptual responses to pain (Fillingim and Maixner, 1995; Coghill *et al.*, 1999). Women also are diagnosed more frequently with persistent pain conditions (Unruh, 1996).

Amygdala and related structures

New incoming sensory signals arriving at the sensory association cortices are made available simultaneously to the amygdala and the hippocampus. The hippocampus recalls specific facets of the sensory experience and links them with details of past events, especially with regard to visual signals. It has been suggested that sensory information reaches the amygdala by two routes. One route is direct via the thalamus and supports a quick, primitive emotional response. The second route is indirect via the cortex and results in a slower, more cognitive response (Kandel and Kupfermann, 1995).

Once the stimulus arrives in the amygdala it is recognized and an affective dimension is attached to the stimulus. Evidence suggests that the amygdala represents the central fear system and that it is critical in the acquisition and expression of conditioned fear as well as anxiety (Davis, 1992). The appropriate emotional significance is attached if the current event occurs in the context of a previously learned psychoaffective atmosphere related to social events and other forms of affiliative behavior. The amygdala responds by activating three sets of connections. First, the amygdala recruits appropriate autonomic and endocrine responses through its connections with the hypothalamus and brainstem. Second, the amygdala sends signals back to the hippocampus to reaffirm the emotional significance of the signals that have simultaneously entered the hippocampus. Finally both the hippocampus and the amygdala project signals back to the sensory association cortices, where, with time, the memory of the event is probably created. The next time the same constellation of sensory signals arrives at the sensory association cortex the learned emotional response will be elicited more efficiently. If, in the future, less than the entire set of sensory signals is experienced, the amygdala–hippocampus axis may be triggered to respond with the same emotions (Kesner, 1992).

Connections between the amygdala and the orbital prefrontal cortex are important in formulating reactions to socially significant stimuli and for controlling aggressive behavior (De Bruin, 1990). In some cases a minimal set of stimuli may be able to reactivate a vague recollection of a past experience without the specifics of that experience, producing the sense of déjà vu (Gloor, 1997). Connections with the posterior cingulate gyrus have been implicated to be important in the conscious appreciation of anxiety (McGuire et al., 1994); however, others believe that the prefrontal cortex is of particular importance in the appreciation of emotions generated in the amygdala (Kandel and Kupfermann, 1995).

A bilateral lesion of the anterior temporal lobe produced a marked change in the behavior of the normally aggressive rhesus monkey (Kluver and Bucy, 1939). Lesioned animals were remarkably tame. Fear and aggression were lost. When released in the wild the monkeys showed no aggressive response when attacked by strangers. They were aloof of the social group and lost all social status. Although in the laboratory they exhibited abnormal sexual behavior with greatly increased autoerotic homosexual or heterosexual activity, they engaged in no sexual behavior in the wild. Mothers lost interest in their infants. Oral behavior was exaggerated and they examined everything orally. They became indiscriminate in their dietary preferences. They ate previously rejected foods and ate nonfood items including feces. They exhibited hypermetamorphosis, which is a tendency to attend to and to react to every visual stimulus. At the same time they exhibited visual agnosia. These behaviors make up the Kluver–Bucy syndrome.

Further behavioral considerations

Kluver–Bucy syndrome

The complete Kluver–Bucy syndrome is seldom seen in humans. Humans with bilateral temporal lobe damage who are described as exhibiting the Kluver–Bucy syndrome are very placid and are indiscriminate in dietary preferences. Several have died from stuffing their mouths with inedible objects (e.g., Styrofoam cups, surgical gauze, toilet paper, etc.; Mendez and Foti, 1997).The patients examined all objects orally. Hypersexuality is rare; however, inappropriate sexual commentary is common (Trimble et al., 1997).

Temporal lobe epilepsy

A full-blown temporal lobe seizure is often preceded by an aura indicating limbic involvement. The aura may include olfactory hallucinations, visceral sensations, fear, déjà vu, and motor automatisms. Behavioral disorders may be seen in the interictal period (Trimble et al., 1997). These disorders include depression, schizophreniform psychosis, and an interictal behavior syndrome that consists of affective disturbances and long-term personality changes. Delusions may appear several years after the onset of seizures.

A subset of these patients present with the Gastaut–Geschwind syndrome, which consists of a constellation of behaviors that include hyperreligiosity, hypergraphia, exaggerated philosophical concerns, sexual dysfunction, and irritability. This syndrome has been subdivided into three subgroups of behavior (Bear, 1986). The first is an alteration of physiological drives including sexual behavior, aggression, and fear. The second is a preoccupation with religious, moral, and philosophical concepts. Finally, the patient is unable to terminate an idea, often during a conversation, and to move on to another topic.

Patients with temporal lobe epilepsy may exhibit hyperemotionality and increased aggression. Thirty percent of psychiatric patients with intermittent violent outbursts have temporal lobe epilepsy (Elliot, 1992). Projections from the temporolimbic area to the brainstem periaqueductal gray and raphe nuclei (see Figures 10.1–10.4 and 11.6) may account for the decreased levels of serotonin reported to be associated with violent behavior and suicide (Marazziti and Conti, 1991).

Hallucinations and delusions are associated with limbic dysfunction that involves both superficial and deep structures of the temporal lobe (Yudofsky and Hales, 1992). The delusions are often of the paranoid type and are seen in approximately 10% of patients who suffer from temporal lobe epilepsy. Delusions are more often seen if the left temporal lobe is involved, whereas the presence of auditory or visual hallucinations correlates with right temporal lobe epilepsy. Recruitment of the frontal lobe may be required together with temporal lobe activity in order to produce a delusion (Trimble *et al.*, 1997).

Other considerations

Episodes of transient sadness experienced by a group of healthy women activated bilateral limbic and paralimbic structures as measured by relative blood flow. In contrast, transient happiness corresponded with no regions of increased activity but did correspond with widespread reductions in blood flow, especially in the right prefrontal and bilateral temporoparietal regions (George *et al.*, 1995).

Intravenous procaine activates limbic structures in animals; in humans, it evokes emotional and psychosensory experiences, including dysphoria, euphoria, fear, and hallucinations. Procaine-induced auditory hallucinations correlate with superior temporal activation. Procaine-induced visual hallucinations correlated with left mesial occipital lobe and amygdala activation coupled with right anterior cingulate and lateral frontal lobe activation (Ketter *et al.*, 1996). Increases in brain activity bilaterally following procaine injection have been reported in limbic areas, including the parahippocampal gyri, insula, and anterior cingulate cortex (Servan-Schreiber and Perlstein, 1997). Videotape stimuli increase blood flow in the amygdala and anterior cingulate gyrus of recovering cocaine addicts when compared with life-long abstainers (Childress *et al.*, 1999).

SELECT BIBLIOGRAPHY

J. P. Aggleton ed. The Amygdala. *Neurobiological Aspects of Emotion, Memory, and Mental Dysfunction.* (New York: Wiley-Liss, 1992.)
— ed. *The Amygdala. A Functional Analysis*, 2nd edn. (Oxford UK: Oxford University Press, 2000.)

A. Bjorklund, T. Hokfelt, and L.W. Swanson eds. *Handbook of Chemical Neuroanatomy*, vol. **5**. *Integrated Systems of the CNS.* Part I. Hypothalamus, Hippocampus, Amygdala, Retina. (New York: Elsevier, 1987.)

B.K. Doane, and K.F. Livingston eds. *The Limbic System: Functional Organization and Clinical Disorders.* (New York: Raven Press, 1986.)

P. Gloor, *The Temporal Lobe and Limbic System.* (New York: Oxford University Press, 1997.)

P.W. Kalivas, and C.D. Baraes eds. *Limbic Motor Circuits and Neuropsychiatry.* (Ann Arbor, Mich.: CRC Press, 1993.)

J. LeDoux, *The Emotional Brain.* (New York: Simon and Schuster, 1996.)

E.T. Rolls, *The Brain and Emotion.* (New York: Oxford University Press, 1999.)

REFERENCES

Alheid, G. F., and Heimer, L. 1996. Theories of basal forebrain organization and the "emotional motor system." In: G. Holstege, R. Bandler, and C.B. Saper (eds.) *The Emotional Motor System.* Amsterdam: Elsevier pp. 461–484.

Amaral, D.G., Price, J.L., Pitkanen, A., and Carmichael, S.T. 1992. Anatomical organization of the primate amygdaloid complex. In: J.P. Aggleton (ed.) *The Amygdala: Neurobiological Aspects of Emotion, Memory, and Mental Dysfunction.* New York: Wiley-Liss, pp. 1–66.

Arendt, T., Bigl, V., Arendt, A., and Tennstedt, A. 1983. Loss of neurons in the nucleus basalis of Meynert in Alzheimer's disease, paralysis agitans and Korsakoff's disease. *Acta Neuropathol.* **61**:101–108.

Bear, D. 1986. Behavioural changes in temporal lobe epilepsy: conflict, confusion, challenge. In: M.R. Trimble and T.G. Bolwig (eds.) *Aspects of Epilepsy and Psychiatry.* Chichester, England: Wiley, pp. 19–30.

Blum, K., Cull, J.G., Braverman, E.R., and Comings, D.E. 1996. Reward deficiency syndrome. *Am. Sci.* **84**:132–145.

Bondi, M.W., Kaszniak, A.W., Rapcsak, S.Z., and Butters, M. 1993. Implicit and explicit memory following anterior communicating artery aneurysm rupture. *Brain Cogn.* **22**:213–229.

Buzsaki, G., Chen, L.S., and Gage, F.H. 1990. Spatial organization of physiological activity in the hippocampus regions: relevance to memory formation. In: J. Storm-Mathisen, R. Zimmer, and O. Ottersen (eds.) Understanding the brain through the hippocampus. *Prog. Brain Res.* **83**:257–268.

Canteras, N.S., and Swanson, L.W. 1992. Projections of the ventral subiculum to the amygdala, septum, and hypothalamus: an PHAL anterograde tract-tracing study in the rat. *J. Comp. Neurol.* **324**:180–194.

Childress, A.R., Mozley, P.D., McElgin, W., Fitzgerald, J., Reivich, M., and O'Brien, C.P. 1999. Limbic activation during cue-induced cocaine craving. *Am. J. Psychiatry* **156**:11–18.

Coghill, R., Sang, C., Maisog, J. and Iadarola, M. 1999. Pain intensity processing within the human brain: a bilateral, distributed mechanism. *J. Neurophysiol.* **82**:1934–1943.

Coyle, J.T., Price, D.L., and DeLong, M.R. 1983. Alzheimer's disease: a disorder of cortical cholinergic innervation. *Science* **219**:1184–1190.

Davis, M. 1992. The role of the amygdala in fear and anxiety. *Annu. Rev. Neurosci.* **15**:353–375.

De Bruin, J.P.C. 1990. Social behaviour and the prefrontal cortex. In: H.B.M. Uylings, C.G. Van Eden, J.P.C. De Gruin, M.A. Corner, and M.G.P. Feenstra (eds.) The Prefrontal Cortex: Its Structure, Function and Pathology. *Prog. Brain Res.* **85**:485–497.

Dyr, W., McBride, W. J., Lumeng, T. K., and Murphy, J. M. 1993. Effects of D1 and D2 dopamine receptor agents on ethanol consumption in the high-alcohol-drinking (HAD) line of rats. *Alcohol* **10**:207–212.

Elliot, F. A. 1992. Violence: the neurological contribution: an overview. *Arch. Neurol.* **49**:595–603.

Fillingham, R., and Maixner, W. 1995. Gender differences in the responses to noxious stimuli. *Pain Forum* **4**:209–221.

Gaykema, R. P. A., Luiten, P. G. M., Nyakas, C., and Traber, J. 1990. Cortical projection patterns of the medial septum-diagonal band complex. *J. Comp. Neurol.* **293**:103–124.

George, M. S., Ketter, T. A., Parekh, P. I., Horwitz, B., Herscovitch, P., and Post, R. M. 1995. Brain activity during transient sadness and happiness in healthy women. *Am. J. Psychiatry* **152**:341–351.

Gloor, P. 1997. *The Temporal Lobe and Limbic System.* New York: Oxford University Press.

Heath, R., Dempsy, C., Fontana, C., and Myers, W. 1978. Cerebellar stimulation: effects on septal region, hippocampus, and amygdala of cats and rats. *Biol. Psychiatry* **13**:501–529.

Huh, K., Meador, K. J., Lee, G. P., Loring, D. W., Murrow, A. M., King, D. W., Gallagher, B. B., Smith, J. R., and Flanigin, H. F. 1990. Human hippocampal EEG: effects of behavioral activation. *Neurology* **40**:1177–1181.

Jarrard, L. E. 1993. On the role of the hippocampus in learning and memory in the rat. *Behav. Neurol. Biol.* **60**:9–26.

Kandel, E., and Kupfermann, I. 1995. Emotional states. In: E. R. Kandel, J. H. Schwartz, and T. M. Jessell (eds.) *Essentials of Neural Science and Behavior.* Norwalk, Conn.: Appleton and Lange, pp. 595–612.

Kesner, R. P. 1992. Learning and memory in rats with an emphasis on the role of the amygdala. In: J. Aggleton (ed.) *The Amygdala.* New York: Wiley, pp. 379–400.

Ketter, T. A., Andreaseon, P. J., George, M. S., Lee, C., Gill, D. S., Parekh, P. I., Willis, M. W., Herscovitch, P., and Post, R. M. 1996. Anterior paralimbic mediation of procaine-induced emotional and psychosensory experiences. *Arch. Gen. Psychiatry* **53**:59–69.

Kluver, H., and Bucy, P. C. 1939. Preliminary analysis of functions of the temporal lobe in monkeys. *Arch. Neurol. Psychiatry* **42**:979–1000.

Kopelman, M. D. 1995. The Korsakoff syndrome. *Br. J. Psychiatry* **166**:154–173.

Kwon, J. S., Shenton, M. E., Hirayasu, Y., Salisbury, D. F., Fischer, I. A., Dickey, C. C., Yurgelun-Todd, D., Tohen, M., Kikinis, R., Jolesz, F. A., and McCarley, R. W. 1998. MRI study of cavum septi pellucidi in schizophrenia, affective disorder, and schizotypal personality disorder. *Am. J. Psychiatry* **155**:509–515.

Marazziti, D., and Conti, L. 1991. Aggression, hyperactivity, and platelet IMI-binding. *Acta Psychiatr. Scand.* **84**:209–211.

McGuire, P. K., Bench, C. J., Frith, C. D., Marks, I. M., Frackowiak, R. S. J., and Dolan, R. J. 1994. Functional anatomy of obsessive-compulsive phenomena. *Br. J. Psychol.* **164**:459–468.

Mega, M. S., Cummings, J. C., Salloway, S., and Malloy, P. 1997. The limbic system: an anatomic, phylogenetic, and clinical perspective. *J. Neuropsychiatry Clin. Neurosci.* **9**:315–330.

Mendez, M. F., and Foti, D. 1997. Lethal hyperoral behavior from the Kluver–Bucy syndrome. *J. Neurol. Neurosurg. Psychiatry* **62**:293–294.

Nieuwenhuys, R., Voogd, J., and Van Huijzen, C. 1988. *The Human Nervous System.* New York: Springer-Verlag.

Nopoulos, P., Swayze, V., and Andreasen, N. C. 1996. Pattern of brain morphology in patients with schizophrenia and large cavum septi pellucidi. *J. Neuropsychiatry. Clin. Neurosci.* **8**:147–152.

Nopoulos, P., Swayze, V., Flaum, M., Ehrhardt, J. C., Yuh, W. T., and Andreasen, N. C. 1997. Cavum septi pellucidi in normals and patients with schizophrenia as detected by magnetic resonance imaging. *Biol. Psychiatry* **41**:1102–1108.

Nopoulos, P. C., Giedd, J. N., Andreasen, N. C., and Rapoport, J. L. 1998. Frequency and severity of enlarged cavum septi pellucidi in childhood-onset schizophrenia. *Am. J. Psychiatry* **155**:1074–1079.

Norita, M., and Kawamura, K. 1980. Subcortical afferents to monkey amygdala: an HRP study. *Brain Res.* **190**:225–230.

Papez, J. W. 1937. A proposed mechanism of emotion. *Arch. Neurol. Psychiatry* **38**:725–743.

Peoples, L., Lynch, K. G., Lesnock, J., and Gangdhar, N. 2004. Accumbal neural response during the initiation and maintenance of intravenous cocaine self-administration. *J. Neurophysiol.* **91**(1):314–323.

Pilotte, N. S., and Sharpe, L. G. 1996. Cocaine withdrawal alters regulatory elements of dopamine neurons. In: M. D. Majewska (ed.) *Neurotoxicity and Neuropathology Associated with Cocaine Abuse.* Rockville, Md.: National Institutes of Health, pp. 193–202.

Rossetti, Z. L., Hmaidan, Y., and Gessa, G. L. 1992. Marked inhibition of mesolimbic dopamine release: a common feature of ethanol, morphine, cocaine and amphetamine abstinence in rats. *Eur. J. Pharmacol.* **221**:227–234.

Self, D. W., and Nestler, E. J. 1995. Molecular mechanisms of drug reinforcement and addiction. *Annu. Rev. Neurosci.* **18**:463–495.

Servan-Schreiber, D., and Perlstein, W. M. 1997. Pharmacologic activation of limbic structures and neuroimaging studies of emotions. *J. Clin. Psychiatry* **58** (Suppl. 16):13–15.

Shioiri, T., Oshitani, Y., Kato, T., Murashita, J., Hamakawa, H., Inubushi, T., Nagata, T., and Takahashi, S. 1996. Prevalence of cavum septum pellucidum detected by MRI in patients with bipolar disorder, major depression and schizophrenia. *Psychol. Med.* **26**:431–434.

Squire, L. R. 1992. Memory and the hippocampus: a synthesis from findings with rats, monkeys, and humans. *Psychol. Rev.* **99**:195–231.

Tamminga, C. A. 1998. Schizophrenia and glutamatergic transmission. *Crit. Rev. Neurobiol.* **12**:21–36.

Trimble, M. R. 1991. *The Psychoses of Epilepsy.* New York: Raven Press.

Trimble, M. R., Mendez, M. F., and Cummings, J. L. 1997. Neuropsychiatric symptoms from the temporolimbic lobes. *J. Neuropsychiatry Clin. Neurosci.* **9**:429–438.

Unruh, A. 1996. Gender variations in clinical pain experience. *Pain* **65**:123–167.

Van Hoesen, G. W., Morecraft, R. J., and Semendeferi, K. 1996. Functional neuroanatomy of the limbic system and prefrontal cortex. In: B. S. Fogel, R. B. Schiffer, and S. M. Rao (eds.) *Neuropsychiatry.* Baltimore, Md.: Williams and Wilkins, pp. 113–143.

Vanderwolf, C. H. 1988. Cerebral activity and behavior: control by central cholinergic and serotonergic systems. *Int. Rev. Neurobiol.* **30**:225–340.

Von Cramon, D. Y., and Schuri, U. 1992. The septo-hippocampal pathways and their relevance to human memory: a case report. *Cortex* **28**:411–422.

Wolf, S. S., Hyde, T. M., and Weinberger, D. R. 1994. Malformations of the septum pellucidum: two distinctive cases in association with schizophrenia. *J. Psychiatry Neurosci.* **19**:140–144.

Yudofsky, S. C, and Hales, R. E (eds.). 1992. *The American Psychiatric Press Textbook of Neuropsychiatry,* 2nd edn. Washington, D. C.: American Psychiatric Press.

Zola-Morgan, S. M., and Squire, L. R. 1993. Neuroanatomy of memory. *Annu. Rev. Neurosci.* **16**:547–563.

Zubieta, J. -K., Smith, Y. R., Bueller, J. A., Xu, Y., Kilbourn, M. R., Jewett, D. M., Meyer, C. R., Koeppe, R. A., and Stohler, C. S. 2002. μ-Opioid receptor-mediated antinociceptive responses differ in men and women. *J. Neurosci.* **22**(12):5100–5107.

14 Interhemispheric connections and laterality

A hallmark of human brain function is cerebral lateralization and specialization. This specialization necessitates an efficient interhemispheric communication system. No other mammal possesses the degree of localization of function seen in the human. Only the human brain has the intellectual and computational capabilities necessary to study how neural systems both generate and respond to the intense information demands of the environment.

At first glance the anatomical brain appears largely symmetrical. More careful analysis reveals "typical counterclockwise hemispheric torque," which is reflected in the fact that the left parieto-occipital region is wider and extends further posteriorly than the right. On the right side the frontal lobe is larger than the left and extends further anteriorly (Glicksohn and Myslobodsky, 1993). This difference is called *petalia* (Hadziselimovic and Cus, 1966). Fiber bundles interconnect the left and right sides. It must be assumed that these bundles play a role in the behavioral specializations that are reflected in the laterality of behavior.

Cerebral blood flow is greater on the right than on the left in infants. Left parietal dominance emerges at about 2½ years concordant with the onset of right-handedness and improved motor skills. Cerebral blood flow dominance shifts from right to left during the third year of life (Chiron *et al.*, 1997).

Speech has long been recognized to be localized in the left (dominant) hemisphere. The right hemisphere has been hypothesized to be specialized in emotional and visuospatial functions that are important in survival of the species (Geschwind and Galaburda, 1985). Norepinephrine and serotonergic pathways project more heavily to the right hemisphere (Robinson, 1985).

Interhemispheric communication

Corpus callosum

The corpus callosum is larger in the human than in any other mammal. It is a broad thick plate of fibers that reciprocally interconnects broad regions of the corresponding lobes of the cortex of the left and right side (Figures 14.1–14.3). The fibers of the corpus callosum make up the floor of the longitudinal cerebral fissure, form most of the roof of the lateral ventricle, and fan out in a massive callosal radiation as they distribute to various cortical regions.

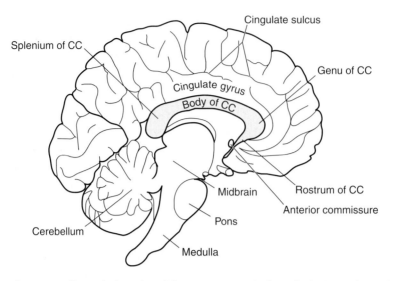

Figure 14.1.   The corpus callosum (CC) consists of the rostrum, genu, body, and splenium. It forms the floor of the longitudinal cerebral fissure and lies below the cingulate gyrus.

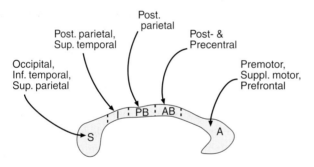

Figure 14.2.   Cortical areas whose fibers contribute to each subdivision are indicated. The corpus callosum can be divided approximately in half by the junction of the anterior midbody (AB) and the posterior midbody (PB). The anterior one-third includes the rostrum, genu, and anterior body (A). The splenium (S) accounts for about the posterior one-fifth of the corpus callosum. I, isthmus.

The corpus callosum can be divided into a series of function-specific channels (Zaidel *et al.*, 1990), which include the following.

- Rostrum, genu, and anterior body (Figures 14.1 and 14.2). These make up the anterior one-third of the corpus callosum. These anterior channels contain interconnecting fibers from the prefrontal, premotor, supplementary, and possibly anteroinferior parietal cortex. Anterior callosal channels are important for the interhemispheric transfer of control signals.

- Anterior midbody. The anterior midbody contains fibers that interconnect the precentral and postcentral gyri and possibly the midtemporal cortex. This channel is particularly important because it interconnects the primary motor cortex.

Frontal pole

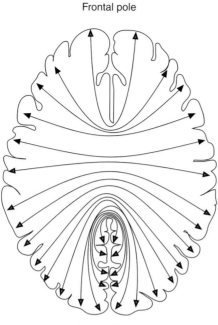

Occipital pole

Figure 14.3.   Diagrammatic horizontal section of the brain shows the corpus callosum interconnecting the cortex on each side.

- Posterior midbody. The posterior midbody interconnects the postcentral gyrus, the posterior parietal cortex, and possibly the midtemporal cortex. The two midbody channels coordinate motor activity across the midline.
- Isthmus. The isthmus interconnects the posterior parietal and superior temporal cortex, including the auditory cortex.
- Splenium. The splenium contains fibers that interconnect the inferior and ventral temporal cortices as well as the visual cortex of the occipital lobe. The more posterior channels interconnect sensory signals such as visual, auditory, and touch. The anterior corpus callosum is organized topographically but the splenium contains fibers that represent all sensory areas including olfaction.

A lesion sparing the splenium often results in minimal loss of function (Berlucchi, 2004).

The between-hemisphere corticocortical pathways and within-hemisphere corticocortical pathways have a common embryological origin (Trevarthen, 1990). Many of the fibers are unmyelinated, indicating that interhemisphere information transfer is relatively slow. In addition to providing communication between the left and right hemisphere, many of the same neurons that give rise to the callosal fibers also give rise to within-hemisphere collateral fibers. Wherever the callosal fibers terminate in the contralateral hemisphere, the collateral fibers end in the homologous region of the ipsilateral hemisphere. These are referred to as *symmetrical heterotopic connections* and are common in association regions of the cortex (Liederman, 1995).

The corpus callosum provides a channel for communication between the two hemispheres. It serves three categories of tasks. First, callosal relay tasks are those tasks that can be performed by only one hemisphere. The corpus callosum allows stimuli to be relayed from one hemisphere to the other where the task can be performed. Second, it provides for coordination of direct access tasks, which are tasks that can be performed by either hemisphere. Third, it provides for transfer of signals for tasks that require the interaction of both hemispheres (Zaidel, 1995).

Some investigators speculate that maturation of the corpus callosum is a prerequisite to the finalization of hemispheric specialization. In humans, completion of callosal myelination approximately coincides with puberty. The splenium tends to contain more fibers in females than males, although there is significant overlap in the number of fibers between sexes.

The midsagittal area of the corpus callosum is significantly larger in the female rat than in the male. Early postnatal exposure to cocaine abolishes this sexual dimorphism (Ojima *et al.*, 1996).

Disconnection of the hemispheres ("split brain") in an adult produces few disturbances of ordinary daily behavior, temperament, or intellect. Visual signals reach both sides of the cortex by way of fibers that cross in the optic chiasm and auditory signals that cross in the brainstem. Special tests that project sensory signals to either the left or right side have been performed. Results indicate that identical signals presented to the opposite cortex may sometimes produce conflicting emotional responses.

The presence of a number of small tracts interconnecting the left and right temporal lobes allows abnormal ongoing epileptic activity to be transmitted between the two lobes without necessarily involving the much larger corpus callosum. Since the corpus callosum is not involved, generalization of the epileptic activity may not occur. In such cases, the patient may be able to maintain some contact with the environment while at the same time experiencing a complex partial seizure. This should not be taken as evidence that the seizure is of psychogenic origin (pseudoseizure).

Signs and symptoms of complete callosal damage may include left ideomotor apraxia, right or bilateral construction apraxia, left agraphia, left tactile anomia, left alien hand sign, impaired bimanual coordination, alexia in the left visual field, anomia for objects felt with the left hand, and left visualanomia. Obvious symptoms usually appear only after large callosal lesions (Peru *et al.*, 2003). Certain lesions involving the corpus callosum, or association areas of the cortex that give rise to commissural fibers, produce disturbances of brain functions collectively known as disconnection syndromes. Split-brain patients may be slow to respond. Once one hemisphere is activated, it may be very difficult for the split-brain patient to activate the inactivated hemisphere. In such a situation, Sperry (1962) questioned whether consciousness may have been shifted entirely to the active hemisphere. A common sequela of callosectomy is neglect.

Clinical vignette

A 38-year-old right-handed woman developed a personality change over a two-month period. She became progressively apathetic and disengaged. On examination, she had prominent psychomotor slowing, pallor of the left optic disc, left central facial nerve weakness, gait instability, sensory loss on the left side of her body, and upper motor neuron signs. Magnetic resonance imaging disclosed multiple subcortical and periventricular lesions and pronounced atrophy of the corpus callosum (Figure 14.4). An eventual frontal brain biopsy confirmed the presence of advanced multiple sclerosis.

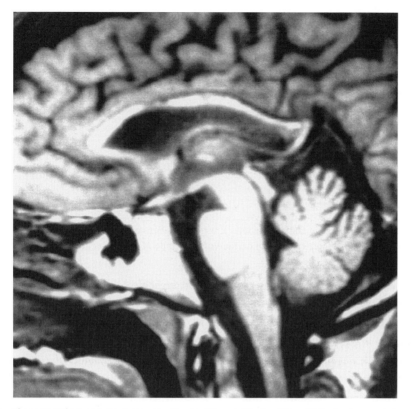

Figure 14.4. The patient's magnetic resonance image (T1-weighted, mid-sagittal view) revealed marked thinning of the corpus callosum as a result of demyelination. (Reprinted with permission from Mendez, 1995.)

Her neuropsychological evaluation disclosed an interhemispheric disconnection syndrome from demyelination of her corpus callosum. She could formulate and write sentences with her right hand but not with her left. She could draw and copy figures with her left hand but not with her right. The spatial elements of her constructions were worse with her right hand than with her left hand. She had greater trouble naming items placed out-of-sight in her left hand as compared to her right hand. With her left hand, the patient had difficulty saluting, miming the use of a toothbrush, flipping a coin, pretending to comb her hair, and other praxis tasks. Finally, on a tachistoscopic task, the patient could not read any of the items presented in her left hemifield.

There is a significant tendency to neglect left-sided targets, and it is argued that this is due to underactivation of the nondominant hemisphere (Liederman, 1995). Mutism following callosal section is an extreme example of such an imbalance. Mutism is more common if speech is centered in one hemisphere and control of the dominant hand in the opposite hemisphere. The role of the corpus callosum in conscious awareness and cognitively determined behavior continues to be the subject of much research.

A role for the corpus callosum in the pathogenesis of schizophrenia has been suggested (Crow, 1997). Nasrallah (1985) proposed a mechanism for schizophrenic signs and symptoms based on a body of evidence pointing to a disturbance of interhemispheric integration. Velek *et al.* (1988) reported a case of congenital agenesis of the corpus callosum that presented with strong features of first-rank

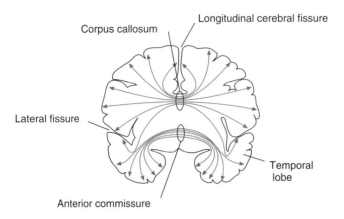

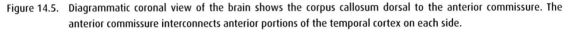

Figure 14.5.   Diagrammatic coronal view of the brain shows the corpus callosum dorsal to the anterior commissure. The anterior commissure interconnects anterior portions of the temporal cortex on each side.

Schneiderian symptoms. The posterior subregions and the body of the corpus callosum were found to be significantly smaller in individuals with autism (Piven *et al.*, 1997). The lack of normal asymmetry is also reported in schizophrenia (Crow, 1990, 1997).

A reduction in the total midsagittal corpus callosum area along with a reduction in the overall centerline length was seen in adults with Tourette's syndrome (Peterson *et al.*, 1994). In contrast, the anterior corpus callosum was significantly larger in children with Tourette's syndrome but significantly smaller in children with attention-deficit hyperactivity disorder (Baumgardner *et al.*, 1996). Alterations in the size of the corpus callosum may reflect alterations in the cortical areas served by the corpus callosum.

A rather intriguing disorder called *alien hand sign* can develop with a lesion that involves the region of the anterior corpus callosum (see Chapter 6). Reportedly there is a feeling of loss of voluntary control over the nondominant hand (Brion and Jednyak, 1972). A feeling of estrangement for the nondominant hand (*la main étrangère*) is reported. Other features include a tendency for the arm to drift off and assume odd postures, especially when the eyes are closed or when there is intermanual conflict or competition. Indeed, studies of patients in whom the corpus callosum has been sectioned have led to the notion that these individuals function with two independent minds, the left under the control of consciousness and the right largely functioning unconsciously and automatically (Bogen, 1993).

Anterior commissure

The anterior commissure is a small compact bundle that crosses the midline rostral to the fornix (Figures 14.1, 14.5, and 14.6). This commissure consists of two divisions that are not distinguishable on gross examination: a small anterior division that interconnects olfactory structures on either side, and a large posterior division that connects the anterior, middle, and inferotemporal regions.

The role of the anterior commissure remains unresolved (Zaidel, 1995). Prenatal stress in rats disrupts sexual differentiation and sexual behavior. The anterior division of the anterior commissure is

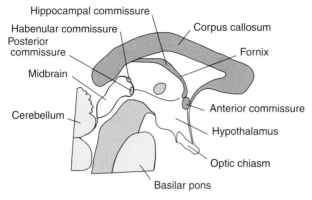

Figure 14.6.   Diagrammatic midline view of the brain shows five commissures: the corpus callosum, the anterior commissure, the posterior commissure, the hippocampal commissure, and the habenular commissure.

sexually dimorphic in rats, and prenatal stress eliminates the male–female difference (Jones *et al.*, 1997). The number of axons in the anterior commissure is 17% greater in mice with a hereditary absence of the corpus callosum. However, the regions of the brain served by the axons remain the same (Livy *et al.*, 1997). It is hypothesized that the larger anterior commissure seen in females provides for better intercommunication between the two amygdaloid nuclei and predisposes females to be more emotionally intelligent and socially sensitive (Joseph, 1993).

Hippocampal commissure

The hippocampal commissure (fornical commissure or psalterium) consists of fibers that originate in the hippocampus and cross the midline beneath the splenium of the corpus callosum (see Figure 14.6). This commissure interconnects the hippocampus of both sides and is poorly developed in the human.

Supraoptic commissure

The small supraoptic commissure lies dorsal to the optic chiasm (see Figure 14.6). It consists of several bundles of fine fibers that cross the midline. Included among these bundles is the hypothalamic commissure, which fans out into the lateral preoptic-hypothalamic area. A ventrally located bundle (ventral supraoptic decussation) is thought to arise from the reticular formation of the rostral pons and ascends in association with fibers of the medial longitudinal fasciculus. A dorsally located bundle (dorsal supraoptic decussation) may interconnect parts of the basal ganglia.

Papez (1937) believed that these decussations linked the thalamus with the hypothalamus and suggested that they played a role in emotions and in emotional expression.

Habenular commissure

The habenular commissure lies immediately beneath the pineal and is a small commissure whose fibers originate from the stria medullaris (see Figure 14.6). Some of these fibers link the habenula with the superior colliculus. Other fibers within the habenular commissure interconnect the amygdala and the hippocampus of the two sides. The function of this commissure is not known.

Posterior commissure

The posterior commissure lies at the junction of the midbrain and diencephalon (see Figure 14.6). It contains fibers that join the pretectal nuclei as well as fibers that interconnect oculomotor control nuclei located in the periaqueductal gray of the midbrain.

These fibers are important in the pupillary reflex and in lid and vertical eye movements (Yun *et al.*, 1995; Kokkoroyannis *et al.*, 1996).

Hemispheric specialization

The anatomical projection of fibers to primary regions of the cortex is generally equally distributed between the hemispheres. In contrast, control of many complex functions is markedly asymmetrical. It is possible that complex functions can be more efficiently executed in a restricted unilateral site, while relying on transcortical fibers to interconnect with the contralateral hemisphere.

Some asymmetry may be localized to specific lobes of the cerebral cortex and is discussed below. Asymmetries that involve the entire hemisphere are presented in this section.

Left hemisphere

Language is the first area of behavior for which hemispheric dominance was demonstrated. The left hemisphere is dominant for linguistic functions in approximately 98% of individuals. The left hemisphere is specialized for the manipulation of numbers in the process of calculation.

Roughly 90% of the population is right-handed. In these people the left hemisphere is specialized for fine motor control. Most left-handed people, however, have their speech centers located in the left hemisphere.

The supratemporal plane (planum temporale), a region generally included in Wernicke's area, is larger on the left side of the brain in 65% of individuals. The right planum is larger in only about 10% of brains (Geschwind and Levitsky, 1968). This asymmetry is speculated to play a role in the left hemispheric language superiority.

The left cerebral hemisphere of right-handers is believed to be specialized for tool use. The network responsible for this function favors the inferior parietal lobule and the middle frontal gyrus. A second network that controls hand-to-target interaction is located slightly superior in the intraparietal and dorsal premotor area becomes activated contralateral to the hand being used at the time (Johnson and Grafton, 2003).

Right hemisphere

Complex nonlinguistic perceptual skills, facial recognition, and spatial distribution of attention are centered in the right hemisphere. Patients with right hemisphere lesions, especially in the posterior areas, have a much greater impairment in complex visuospatial tasks than do those with equivalent left-sided lesions. The identification of faces is a most complex perceptual task that is also of great biological importance (see Chapter 5, Inferior temporal and fusiform gyrus, p. 63). Under certain circumstances either hemisphere can recognize faces. However, the right hemisphere is specialized in face recognition (Sergent, 1995; Mandal and Ambady, 2004). Recent works point to the fact that the right hemisphere is also specialized for determining the distribution of attention within the extrapersonal space. This leads to marked contralateral neglect after right hemispheric injury. Contralateral neglect is seldom seen after the occurrence of a left hemisphere lesion.

The right hemisphere is more important than the left both in experiencing and in expressing emotions. It contains records of prototypic facial emotional representations. These records are innate and appear to be localized to the temporal lobe (Heilman and Bowers, 1996). Limbic and temporal association areas were more activated on the right during sexual arousal in men (Stoléru *et al.*, 1999).

Lesions in the right temporoparietal area can produce receptive aprosodia, disrupting the patient's ability to understand, name, or discriminate emotional expressions. Patients with right hemisphere stroke can be impaired at recognizing facial displays. Right hemisphere lesions may impair the patient's ability to determine if two faces, previously unknown to the patient, are the same or different people. Patients with right hemisphere lesions are impaired at determining the emotional content of verbal descriptions (Blonder *et al.*, 1991a).

Clinical vignette

A 76-year-old right-handed man developed environmental disorientation after a stroke. He had difficulty finding his way in the hospital and in his neighborhood. He had special problems with corridors, public bathrooms, and theaters. At one point, he could not get out of a public bathroom because he could not find the exit. He was able to read a map, draw an accurate floor plan of his house, and give verbal directions of familiar routes, yet he quickly got lost when taken out on familiar routes.

This patient had a relatively isolated environmental disorientation, or topographagnosia, from a stroke involving the parahippocampal place area located in the right hemisphere. His neurological examination was otherwise remarkable only for a visual field deficit in his upper left quadrant. Magnetic resonance imaging confirmed the presence of an infarction involving the right posterior–inferior temporal and occipital lobes (see Figure 14.7).

Patients with left hemisphere lesions tend to be agitated, anxious, and depressed ("catastrophic reaction"), whereas those with right hemisphere lesions tend to be indifferent to their predicament or may even be mildly euphoric. The patient's inability to express emotion may contribute to the appearance of indifference. Deficits in the display of emotional expressions are associated with right frontal lesions similar to lesions in the left hemisphere that cause Broca's aphasia. A deficit in the expression of emotion is termed *expressive aprosodia*. Patients with right hemisphere lesions are less emotionally expressive (Blonder *et al.*, 1991b).

Frontal hemisphere activation is asymmetrical in patients with panic disorder. Right frontal activation appears to represent acute activation of avoidance-withdrawal and is associated with negative emotions (Wiedemann *et al.*, 1999).

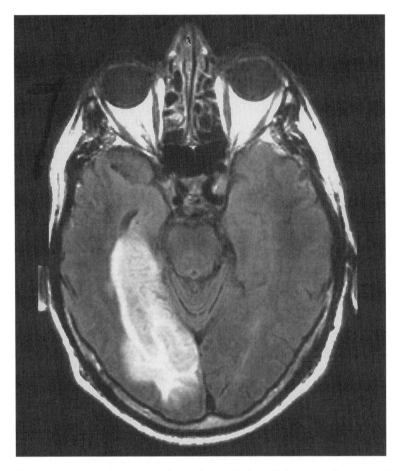

Figure 14.7.   The patient's magnetic resonance image (FLAIR, horizontal view) revealed a posterior circulation stroke in the right medial occipitotemporal region extending to the presumed parahippocampal place area. (Reprinted with permission from Mendez and Cherrier, 2003.)

Lobular specializations

Occipitoparietal lobe

A lesion of the inferiomesial aspect of the left occipitotemporal lobe below the splenium of the corpus callosum can produce color agnosia. The patient can sort colors according to hue but cannot name colors. These patients usually also have right homonymous hemianopia and alexia.

A lesion of the right occipitotemporal region can produce prosopagnosia, although this disorder is more frequently seen after the occurrence of a bilateral lesion. The patient with prosopagnosia is unable to recognize familiar faces, often including his or her own face.

A large lesion of the parietal lobe can produce sensory neglect in the contralateral hemifield. The right lobe plays a greater role in controlling attention and contains a map of both visual fields, and therefore sensory neglect is more often seen after the occurrence of a right-sided parietal lesion. A lesion in the right parietal lobe can produce confusion and disorientation for place. A patient with a large left-sided parietal lesion involving the supramarginal gyrus may react inappropriately to painful stimuli. Patients who demonstrate construction apraxia after a parietal lobe lesion may differ in their ability to draw based on the side of the lesion. With a right-sided parietal lesion, the drawing maintains its complexity, but the left side of the drawing is missing. With a left-sided lesion, the drawing is symmetrical, but details are missing and it is drawn slowly. Gerstmann's syndrome is seen following a left-sided parietal (angular gyrus) lesion (see Chapter 4, p. 48).

Temporal lobe

Both visual and auditory responses can result from stimulation of the temporal lobe; however, these responses are seen more often when the right temporal lobe is stimulated (Gloor, 1990). Cell densities in the left hippocampus were found to be greater than in the right hippocampus of men. The left planum temporale is larger in females than in males, but the asymmetry seen in the planum temporale in males is not present in females. No differences were seen between sexes or between hemispheres for the primary auditory area (Heschl's gyrus) (Kulynych *et al.*, 1994). Asymmetries in women are less apparent in both the planum temporale and the hippocampus (Zaidel *et al.*, 1994).

Patients with lesions of the temporal lobe that affect audition have difficulty distinguishing words if the lesion is on the left and difficulty distinguishing nonverbal sounds, including music, if the lesion is on the right. Left temporal lobe lesions that affect memory involve the loss of language-related information. Right temporal lesions affect the memory of musical melodies and of geometric shapes.

Lesions of the left posterior superior temporal gyrus including BA 22 produce receptive aphasia (Wernicke's). Comprehension of verbal language is primarily affected. If the lesion extends into the inferior parietal lobe, reading may also be affected. In some left-handed individuals, the left hemisphere may be dominant for comprehension whereas the right hemisphere is dominant for the production of speech.

Patients with epileptogenic foci localized to the left temporal lobe tend to be paranoid and to exhibit schizophrenia-like and antisocial behavior. Patients with right-sided temporal foci tend to show emotional extremes, manic-depressive symptoms, and denial (Sherwin *et al.*, 1982; Bear, 1986). Exceptions have been reported in which patients with right-sided foci present with thought disturbances (Sherwin, 1982).

A lesion of the right posterior temporoparietal area can produce aprosodia in which patients are unable to appreciate the emotional content of speech based on pitch and intonation, although they comprehend the semantic meaning. In contrast, a person with Wernicke's aphasia will not understand the meaning of the words but will react to the emotion (e.g., anger) expressed by the speaker.

Volume of the left temporal lobe is reduced in schizophrenics (Turetsky *et al.*, 1994), and the left lateral fissure is larger (Rubin *et al.*, 1993). Male schizophrenic patients demonstrated a smaller superior temporal gyrus than that of male control subjects. Female schizophrenics demonstrated less laterality than did female controls (Reite *et al.*, 1997). The left temporal lobe exhibits higher metabolic activity than the right. Whether there is a left hypometabolism or a right hypermetabolism when compared with normals remains an open question (Gur *et al.*, 1995).

Surgical removal of portions of the temporal lobe is sometimes effective in the treatment of epilepsy. It is essential to determine the hemisphere that is dominant for language and speech before surgery. The lateral portion of the temporal lobe, which contains the receptive speech area, is served by the middle cerebral artery (see Figure 2.5). The Wada test can be used in this situation to determine laterality. In this Wada test, short-acting barbiturates are injected into the internal carotid artery. Aphasia is induced when the barbiturate perfuses the dominant hemisphere. More recently, the use of transcranial magnetic stimulation (TMS) has been proposed as a less invasive procedure to determine language and speech dominance (Pascual-Leone *et al.*, 1991).

Frontal lobe

The pars opercularis (Broca's region) is larger in the left than in the right frontal lobe (Geshchwind and Galaburda, 1985). Folds surrounding the lateral fissure appear earlier on the right than on the left side (Simonds and Scheibel, 1989).

The left frontal region is proposed to be responsible for approach behavior, including planning, intention and self-regulation. The right frontal region is responsible for withdrawal (Davidson, 1995). Ten-month-old infants who cry frequently show more right frontal activation (Fox and Davidson, 1986). Children at 38 months of age who spent more time proximal to their mother in a novel situation were judged to be inhibited and showed greater right frontal activation than uninhibited children (Davidson, 1995).

A lesion of the opercular portion of the inferior frontal gyrus (BA 44 and 45) on the left side produces expressive aphasia (Broca's aphasia). Comprehension of speech is intact but speech production is reduced. The patient with expressive aphasia speaks slowly and with effort.

A lesion of the right premotor area (BA 6 and 8) of the frontal lobe can produce hemiakinesia in which the patient cannot look toward and has difficulty reaching into the opposite hemifield. Hemiakinesia produced by a left premotor area lesion is seen less frequently, and when it appears it is less pronounced. The right hemisphere mediates attention to both hemifields, whereas the left directs attention only to the right hemifield (Knight, 1984).

Patients with a lesion of the left hemisphere tend to be anxious, tearful, depressed, and abusive. Patients with right-sided lesions may be inappropriately cheerful. The degree of emotional involvement, irrespective of side of involvement, is greater if the lesion is closer to the frontal pole. Activation of the left frontal lobe in normal subjects correlates with heightened approach-related positive affect, whereas activation of the right frontal lobe correlates with withdrawal-related negative affect (Wheeler *et al.*, 1993). Patients with unipolar depression exhibit hypometabolism in the left anterolateral prefrontal cortex (George *et al.*, 1993). It is suggested that frontal lobe emotional asymmetry may reflect subcortical asymmetries such as catecholamine asymmetries in the amygdala and thalamus (Jacobs and Snyder, 1996). The normal frontal lobe asymmetry is reversed in autistic subjects (Nowell *et al.*, 1990).

Subcortical regions

The lenticular nucleus (globus pallidus and putamen) is normally larger on the left than on the right. This asymmetry in the lenticular nucleus is missing in children and adults with Tourette's syndrome (Yank *et al.,* 1995). Changes seen in caudate nucleus glucose metabolism following treatment for obsessive-compulsive disorder indicate greater dysfunction on the right side in this disorder (Baxter *et al.,* 1990). Patients with Parkinson's disease who have symptoms that primarily reflect a left-sided lesion are more depressed (Starkstein *et al.,* 1990). The depression may be the result of disruption of connections between the basal ganglia and the frontal cortex (Mayberg, 1992).

Activation of the right side was seen during the recall of painful memories in patients with posttraumatic stress disorder (see Figure 11.5). Right-sided activation was not seen during recall of neutral memories. It was suggested that the results reflected activation of the right amygdala. The patients also showed deactivation of Broca's area. The authors suggested that this may reflect the difficulty these patients have in cognitively reconstructing their traumatic experience (Rauch *et al.,* 1996).

SELECT BIBLIOGRAPHY

P. W. Brazis, J. C. Masdeu, and J. Biller, *Localization in Clinical Neurology.* (Boston, Mass.: Little, Brown, 1990.)

R. J. Davidson, and K. Hugdahl, *Brain Asymmetry.* (Cambridge, Mass.: MIT Press, 1995.)

R. D. Nass, and M. S. Gazzaniga, Cerebral lateralization and specialization in human central nervous system. In *Handbook of Physiology – The Nervous System,* ed. N. Plum, F. Plum and V. B. Mountcastle. (Bethesda, Md.: American Physiological Society, 1987.)

M. R. Trimble, *Biological Psychiatry.* (New York: Wiley, 1988.)

REFERENCES

Baumgardner, T. L., Singer, H. S., Denckla, M. B., Rubin, M. A., Abrams, M. T., Colli, M. J., and Reiss, A. L. 1996. Corpus callosum morphology in children with Tourette syndrome and attention deficit hyperactivity disorder. *Neurology* **47**:477–482.

Baxter, L. R., Schwartz, J. M., Guze, B. H., Bergman, K., and Szuba, M. P. 1990. Neuroimaging in obsessive-compulsive disorder: seeking the mediating neuroanatomy. In: M. A. Jenike, L. Baer, and W. E. Minichiello (eds.) *Obsessive-Compulsive Disorders: Theory and Management.* Littleton, Mass: Year Book Medical Publishers.

Bear, D. 1986. Hemispheric asymmetries in emotional function: a reflection of lateral specialization in cortical-limbic connections. In: B. K. Doane and K. E. Livingston (eds.) *The Limbic System: Functional Organization and Clinical Disorders.* New York: Raven Press, pp. 29–42.

Berlucchi, G. 2004. Some effects of cortical and callosal damage on conscious and unconscious processing of visual information and other sensory inputs. *Prog. Brain Res.* **144**:79–93.

Blonder, L. X., Bowers, D., and Heilman, K. M. 1991a. The role of the right hemisphere on emotional communication. *Brain* **114**:1115–1127.

Blonder, L., Burns, A., Bowers, D., Moore, R., and Heilman, K. 1991b. Right hemisphere expressivity during natural conversation (abstract). *J. Clin. Exp. Neuropsychol.* **13**:85.

Bogen, J. E. 1993. The callosal syndromes. In: K. M. Heilman, and E. Valenstein (eds.) *Clinical Neuropsychology*, 3rd edn. New York: Oxford University Press, pp. 337–407.

Brion, S., and Jednyak, C. P. 1972. Troubles du transfert interhemispherique. *Rev. Neurol.* **126**:257–266.

Chiron, C., Jambaque, I., Nabbout, R., Lounes, R., Syrota, A., and Dulac, O. 1997. The right brain hemisphere is dominant in human infants. *Brain* **120**:1057–1065.

Crow, T. J. 1990. Temporal lobe asymmetries as the key to the etiology of schizophrenia. *Schizophr. Bull.* **16**:433–443.

Crow, T. J. 1997. Temporolimbic or transcallosal connections: where is the primary lesion in schizophrenia and what is its nature? *Schizophr. Bull.* **23**:521–523.

Davidson, R. J. 1995. Cerebral asymmetry, emotion, and affective style. In: R. J. Davidson, and K. Hugdahl (eds.) *Brain Asymmetry*. Cambridge, Mass.: MIT Press, pp. 361–387.

Fox, N. A., and Davidson, R. J. 1986. Taste-elicited changes in facial signs of emotion and the asymmetry of brain electrical activity in human newborns. *Neuropsychologia* **24**:417–422.

George, M. S., Ketter, T. A., and Post, R. M. 1993. SPECT and PET imaging in mood disorders. *J. Clin. Psychiatry* **54** (Suppl. 11):6–13.

Geschwind, N., and Galaburda, A. M. 1985. Cerebral lateralization. *Arch. Neurol.* **42**:428–459.

Geschwind, N., and Levitsky, W. 1968. Human brain: left-right asymmetries in temporal speech region. *Science* **161**:186–187.

Glicksohn, J., and Myslobodsky, M. S. 1993. The presentation of patterns of structural brain asymmetry in normal individuals. *Neuropsychologia* **31**:145–159.

Gloor, P. 1990. Experimental phenomena of temporal lobe epilepsy: facts and hypotheses. *Brain* **113**:1673–1694.

Gur, R. E., Mozley, P. D., Resnick, S. M., Mozley, L. H., Shtasel, D. L., Gallacher, F., Arnold, S. E., Karp, J. S., Alavi, A., Reivich, M., and Gur, R. C. 1995. Resting cerebral glucose metabolism in first-episode and previously treated patients with schizophrenia relates to clinical features. *Arch. Gen. Psychiatry* **52**:657–667.

Hadziselimovic, H., and Cus, M. 1966. The appearance of internal structures of the brain in relation to configuration of the human skull. *Acta Anat. (Basel)* **63**:289–299.

Heilman, K. M., and Bowers, D. 1996. Emotional disorders associated with hemispheric dysfunction. In: B. S. Fogel, R. B. Schiffer, and S. M. Rao (eds.) *Neuropsychology*. Baltimore, Md.: Williams and Wilkins, pp. 401–406.

Jacobs, G. D., and Snyder, D. 1996. Frontal brain asymmetry predicts affective style in men. *Behav. Neurosci.* **110**:3–6.

Johnson, S. H., and Grafton, S. T. 2003. From "acting on" to "acting with": the functional anatomy of object-oriented action schemata. *Prog. Brain Res.* **142**:127–139.

Jones, H. E., Ruscio, M. A., Keyser, L. A., Gonzalez, C., Billack, B., Rowe, R., Hancock, C., Lambert, K. G., and Kinsley, C. H. 1997. Prenatal stress alters the size of the rostral anterior commissure in rats. *Brain Res. Bull.* **42**:341–346.

Joseph, R. 1993. *The Naked Neuron: Evolution and the Languages of the Body and Brain*. New York: Plenum Press.

Knight, R. T. 1984. Decreased response to novel stimuli after prefrontal lesions in man. *Electroencephalogr. Clin. Neurophysiol.* **59**:9.

Kokkoroyannis, T., Scudder, C. A., Balaban, C. D., Highstein, S. M., and Moschovakis, A. K. 1996. Anatomy and physiology of the primate interstitial nucleus of Cajal. I. *Efferent projections. J. Neurophysiol.* **75**:725–739.

Kulynych, J. J., Vladar, K., Jones, D. W., and Weinberger, D. R. 1994. Gender differences in the normal lateralization of the supratemporal cortex: MRI surface-rendering morphometry of Heschl's gyrus and the planum temporale. *Cerebr. Cortex* **4**:107–118.

Liederman, J. 1995. A reinterpretation of the split-brain syndrome: implications for the function of corticocortical fibers. In: R. J. Davidson, and K. Hugdahl (eds.) *Brain Asymmetry*. Cambridge, Mass.: MIT Press, pp. 451–490.

Livy, D. J., Schalomon, P. M., Roy, M., Zacharias, M. C., Pimenta, J., Lent, R., and Wahlsten, D. 1997. Increased axon number in the anterior commissure of mice lacking a corpus callosum. *Exp. Neurol.* **146**:491–501.

Mandal, M. K., and Ambady, N. 2004. Laterality of facial expressions of emotion: universal and culture-specific influences. *Behav. Neurol.* **15**:23–34.

Mayberg, H. S. 1992 Neuroimaging studies of depression in neurological disease. In: S. E. Starkstein, and R. G. Robinson (eds.) *Depression in Neurologic Disease*. Baltimore, Md.: Johns Hopkins University Press.

Mendez, M. F., 1995. The neuropsychiatry of multiple sclerosis. *Int. J. Psychiatry Med.* **25**:123–135.

Mendez, M. F., and Cherrier, M. M. 2003. Agnosia for scenes in topogragnosia. *Neuropsychologia* **10**:1387–1395.

Nasrallah, H. A. 1985. The unintegrated right cerebral hemispheric consciousness as alien intruder: a possible mechanism for Schneiderian delusions in schizophrenia. *Compr. Psychiatry* **26**:273–282.

Nowell, M. A., Hacknery, D. B., Muraki, A. S., and Coleman, M. 1990. Varied MR appearance of autism: fifty three pediatric patients having full autistic syndrome. *Magn. Reson. Imaging* **8**:811–816.

Ojima, E., Abiru, H., and Fukui, Y. 1996. Effects of cocaine on the rat cerebral commissure. *Int. J. Dev. Neurosci.* **14**:649–654.

Papez, J. W. 1937. A proposed mechanism of emotion. *Arch. Neurol. Psychiatry* **38**:725–743.

Pascual-Leone, A., Gates, J. R., and Dhuna, A. 1991. Induction of speech arrest and counting errors with rapid-rate transcranial magnetic stimulation. *Neurology* **41**:697–702.

Peru, A., Beltramello, A., Moro, V., Sattibaldi, L., and Berlucchi, G. 2003. Temporal and permanent signs of interhemispheric disconnection after traumatic brain injury. *Neuropsychologia* **41**:634–643.

Peterson, B. S., Leckman, J. F., and Duncan, J. 1994. Corpus callosum morphology from MR images in Tourette's syndrome. *Psychiatry Res.* **55**:85–99.

Piven, J., Bailey, J., Ranson, B. J., and Arndt, S. 1997. An MRI study of the corpus callosum in autism. *Am. J. Psychiatry* **154**:1051–1056.

Rauch, S. L., van der Kolk, B. A., Fisler, R. E., Alpert, N. M., Orr, S. P., Savage, C. R., Fischman, A. J., Jenike, M. A., and Pitman, R. K. 1996. A symptom provocation study of posttraumatic stress disorder using positron emission tomography and script-driven imagery. *Arch. Gen. Psychiatry* **53**:380–387.

Reite, M., Sheeder, J., Teale, P., Adams, M., Richardson, D., Simon, J., Jones, R. H., and Rojas, D. C. 1997. Magnetic source imaging evidence of sex differences in cerebral lateralization in schizophrenia. *Arch. Gen. Psychiatry* **54**:433–440.

Robinson, R. G. 1985. Lateralized behavioral and neurochemical consequences of unilateral brain injury in rats. In: S. D. Glick (ed.) *Cerebral Lateralization in Nonhuman Species*. New York: Academic Press, pp. 135–156.

Rubin, P., Karle, A., Moller-Madsen, S., Hertel, C., Povlsen, U. J., Noring, U., and Hemingsen, R. 1993. Computerised tomography in newly diagnosed schizophrenia and schizophreniform disorder: a controlled blind study. *Br. J. Psychiatry* **163**:604–612.

Sergent, J. 1995. Hemispheric contribution to face processing: patterns of convergence and divergence. In: R. J. Davidson, and K. Hugdahl (eds.) *Brain Asymmetry*. Cambridge, Mass.: MIT Press, pp. 157–181.

Sherwin, I. 1982. The effect of the location of an epileptogenic lesion on the occurrence of psychosis in epilepsy. In: W. Koella, and M. R. Trimble (eds.) *Temporal Lobe Epilepsy, Mania, and Schizophrenia and the Limbic System*. Basel: Karger, pp. 81–97.

Sherwin, I., Peron-Magnan, P., Bancaud, J., Bonis, A., and Talairach, J. 1982. Prevalence of psychosis in epilepsy as a function of the laterality of the epileptogenic lesion. *Arch. Neurol.* **39**:621–625.

Simonds, R. J., and Scheibel, A. B. 1989. The postnatal development of the motor speech area: a preliminary study. *Brain Lang.* **37**:42–58.

Sperry, R. 1962. Some general aspects of interhemispheric integration. In: V. B. Mountcastle (ed.) *Interhemispheric Relations and Cerebral Dominance*. Baltimore, Md.: Johns Hopkins Press, pp. 43–49.

Starkstein, S. E., Cohen, B. S., Fedoroff, P., Parikh, R. M., Price, T. R., and Robinson, R. G. 1990. Relationship between anxiety disorders and depressive disorders in patients with cerebrovascular injury. *Arch. Gen. Psychiatry* **47**:246–251.

Stoléru, S., Grégoire, M.-C., Gérard, D., Decety, J., Lafarge, E., Cinotti, L., Lavenne, F., LeBars, D., Vernet-Maury, E., Rada, H., Collet, C., Mazoyer, B., Forest, M. G., Magnin, F., Spira, A., and Comar, D. 1999. Neuroanatomical correlates of visually evoked sexual arousal in human males. *Arch. Sex. Behav.* **28**(1):1–21.

Trevarthen, C. 1990. Growth and eduction in the hemispheres. In: C. Trevarthen (ed.) *Brain Circuits and Functions of the Mind*. Cambridge, England: Cambridge University Press, pp. 334–363.

Turetsky, B. I., Cowell, P. E., Gur, R. C., Grossman, R. I., and Gur, R. E. 1994. Frontal and temporal lobe brain volumes in schizophrenia: relationship to symptomatology and clinical subtype. Presented at the 49th Annual Meeting for the Society for Biological Psychiatry, 21 May, 1994, Philadelphia, Pa.

Velek, M., White, L. E., Williams, J. P., Stafford, R. L., and Marco, L. A. 1988. Psychosis in a case of corpus callosum agenesis. *Alabama Med.* **58**:27–29.

Wheeler, R. E., Davidson, R. J., and Tomarken, A. J. 1993. Frontal brain asymmetry and emotional reactivity: a biological substrate of affective style. *Psychophysiology* **30**:82–89.

Wiedemann, G., Pauli, P., Dengler, W., Lutzenberger, W., Birbaumer, N., and Buchkremer, G. 1999. Frontal brain asymmetry as a biological substrate of emotions in patients with panic disorders. *Arch. Gen. Psychiatry* **56**:78–84.

Yank, M., Yazgan, B. P., Wexler, B. E., and Leckman, J. F. 1995. Behavioral laterality in individuals with Gilles de la Tourette Syndrome and basal ganglia alterations: a preliminary report. *Biol. Psychiatry* **38**:386–390.

Yun, S., Shoumura, K., Ichinohe, N., Hirama, H., and Amayasu, H. 1995. Functional and anatomical fiber analysis of the posterior commissure (PC) in the cat: evidence for PC fibers of which stimulation elicits non-oculosympathetic pupillary dilation. *J. Hirnforsch* **36**:29–50.

Zaidel, E. 1995. Interhemispheric transfer in the split brain: long-term status following complete cerebral commissurotomy. In: R. J. Davidson and K. Hugdahl (eds.) *Brain Asymmetry*. Cambridge, Mass.: MIT Press, pp. 491–532.

Zaidel, E., Clarke, J. and Suyenobu, B., 1990. Hemispheric independence: a paradigm case for cognitive neuroscience. In: A. B. Scheibel, and A. F. Wechsler (eds.) *Neurobiology of Higher Cognitive Function*. New York: Guilford Press, pp. 297–362.

Zaidel, D. W., Esiri, M. M., and Oxbury, J. M. 1994. Sex-related asymmetries in the morphology of the left and right hippocampi? *J. Neurol.* **241**:620–623.

Index